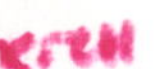

LIVESTOCK HOUSING

Livestock Housing

Edited by

C.M. Wathes

Animal Science and Engineering Division
Silsoe Research Institute
Wrest Park
Silsoe
Bedford MK45 4HS
UK

and

D.R. Charles

ADAS
Chalfont Drive
Nottingham NG8 3SN
UK

CAB INTERNATIONAL

CAB INTERNATIONAL
Wallingford
Oxon OX10 8DE
UK

Tel: Wallingford (0491) 832111
Telex: 847964 (COMAGG G)
Telecom Gold/Dialcom: 84: CAU001
Fax: (0491) 833508

A catalogue entry for this book is available from the British Library.

ISBN 0 85198 774 5

Disclaimer

While every effort has been made to ensure that the information and advice in this book is complete and correct at the time of going to press, neither the publishers, editors nor contributing authors accept liability for any error or omission in the content, or for any loss, damage or accident arising from the use of this book.

Typeset by Solidus (Bristol) Limited
Printed and bound in the UK at the University Press, Cambridge

Contents

Contributors

R.W. Blowey *Wood Veterinary Group, 124 Stroud Road, Gloucester GL1 5JN, UK*

C.R. Boon *Animal Science and Engineering Division, Silsoe Research Institute, Wrest Park, Silsoe, Bedford MK45 4HS, UK*

Dr D.R. Charles *ADAS Nottingham, Chalfont Drive, Nottingham NG8 3SN, UK*

Dr J.A. Clark *Department of Physiology and Environmental Science, University of Nottingham, Sutton Bonington Campus, Loughborough, Leicestershire LE12 5RD, UK*

Dr A.F. Clarke *Equine Research Centre, University of Guelph, Guelph, Ontario, Canada N1G 2W1*

H.A. Elson *ADAS Nottingham, Chalfont Drive, Nottingham NG8 3SN, UK*

Professor J. Hartung *Tierärtzliche Hochschule Hannover, Institut für Tierhygiene und Tierschutz, 30559 Hannover, Bünteweg 17p, Germany*

M.P.S. Haywood *ADAS Nottingham, Chalfont Drive, Nottingham NG8 3SN, UK*

N.G. Lawrence (deceased) *ADAS, Woodthorne, Wergs Road, Wolverhampton WV6 8TQ, UK*

DR A.J. MCARTHUR *Department of Physiology and Environmental Science, University of Nottingham, Sutton Bonington Campus, Loughborough, Leicestershire LE12 5RD, UK*

DR D.R. MERCER *ADAS Nottingham, Chalfont Drive, Nottingham NG8 3SN, UK*

DR C.J. NICOL *Department of Clinical Veterinary Science, University of Bristol, Langford House, Langford, Bristol BS18 7DU, UK*

J.E. OWEN *Farm Buildings Research Team, ADAS Bridgets, Coley Park, Reading RG1 6DE, UK*

DR J.M. RANDALL *Animal Science and Engineering Division, Silsoe Research Institute, Wrest Park, Silsoe, Bedford MK45 4HS, UK*

C.F.R. SLADE *ADAS, Woodthorne, Wergs Road, Wolverhampton WV6 8TQ, UK*

A.T. SMITH *ADAS, Woodthorne, Wergs Road, Wolverhampton WV6 8TQ, UK*

MISS L. STUBBINGS *ADAS, 4 Brewery Yard, Sudborough, Kettering, Northants NN14 3BT, UK*

PROFESSOR C.M. WATHES *Animal Science and Engineering Division, Silsoe Research Institute, Wrest Park, Silsoe, Bedford MK45 4HS, UK*

PROFESSOR A.J.F. WEBSTER *Department of Clinical Veterinary Science, University of Bristol, Langford House, Langford, Bristol BS18 7DU, UK*

Preface

This book addresses all those who are concerned with the needs of *housed* livestock, set in the context of best commercial practice. It is relevant to both animal scientists and engineers, as well as those who work in the livestock industry. It describes – and in some cases attempts to reconcile – the interests of consumers, farmers and farm animals in the provision of livestock accommodation suitable to their various needs. It presents the important principles and processes by which livestock housing affects animal health, welfare and productivity, and shows how an understanding of these can be translated into practical specifications for housing designs.

The emphasis throughout this book is on the building as a means to an environmental end. For much of their lives animals occupy their man-made environments, yet few housing systems are centred entirely about the animal. This book redresses this limitation of current housing by focusing on the biological responses and welfare needs of the animal, but also accepts the need for commercial and economic criteria in agricultural production.

Animals have been kept in stables or byres since at least Roman times. The earliest housing not only provided shelter against the extremes of winter or summer weather but also gave protection against predators. In many cases housing was shared with the peasant. Over the centuries, agricultural wisdom revealed a strong link between the environment and animal well-being and productivity, although the underlying physiological mechanisms were not elucidated until the 19th and 20th centuries. Building designs and construction methods also evolved slowly, often with much success in meeting both the farmer's and his animals' needs. A notable example is the stable, the design of which has changed little over the past two centuries. Sadly, these early lessons are sometimes forgotten and key features of successful stable designs can be omitted, even in new constructions.

The 20th century saw the introduction of many diverse forms of livestock housing that are often associated with intensification. When introduced, these innovations represented the forefront of animal husbandry and their widespread adoption indicated their commercial success. With hindsight and changes in public acceptability, some of these forms of housing can be criticized today on grounds of welfare or rural pollution. However, good progress has been made by agricultural scientists, engineers and farmers in the design and operation of livestock housing. This progress results from advances in our understanding of environmental physiology and technological developments such as systems of mechanical ventilation. Similar advances can be expected from current research in animal behaviour.

It is now possible to make more detailed assessments than hitherto of the biological requirements and responses of the animals, before designers consider structural and engineering aspects of the building. Much of the financial guesswork has been removed by current design techniques. Investment decisions for some farm species can be made given the financial penalties of deviations from the optimum environment. An important example is environmental temperature, which affects considerably the type of structure and control chosen. Many years ago the effects of another key variable – namely light – on poultry were discovered to be so crucial that radical building designs were required for the purposes of light control. Our understanding of ventilation requirements is, perhaps, less complete, though the early pioneers of the subject would probably be astonished by the complexity and detail now discussed in several chapters of this book.

Few authors could do justice to all the nuances and subtleties of livestock housing. Consequently, contributions to this book have been solicited from specialists in a range of topics. The book does not offer a complete prescription since this is not always available and, in any case, animals often adapt well enough to their buildings. Nor does it contain detailed accounts of construction techniques: there are many practical texts available on this subject, (e.g. Barnes, M. and Mander, C. (1992) *Farm Building Construction,* 2nd edn. Farming Press, Ipswich). The early chapters consider the environmental needs and responses of farm animals and are followed by a detailed account of the engineering systems by which these needs can be met. Finally, there are descriptions of housing for each of the major farm animals, as well as the horse.

C.M. Wathes
D.R. Charles

Acknowledgements

The editors gratefully acknowledge the patience shown by the authors and publishers in the preparation of this book. Not only have they responded well to our coercion and critical review but they have at all times retained a sense of humour and proportion during the protracted revisions. Special thanks must go to Miss Loraine Clark of Silsoe Research Institute; on her capable shoulders fell many administrative and secretarial tasks which she undertook with her customary enthusiasm and goodwill.

Animal Requirements

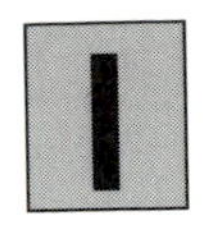

1 Comparative Climatic Requirements

D.R. CHARLES
ADAS Nottingham, UK

Introduction – Climatic Factors to be Considered

Dry bulb air temperature is the climatic variable most commonly measured and described in the theory and practice of livestock housing. It is far from the whole story, and it does not even fully describe the demand of the environment for heat from the animal. It is, however, often the most influential single variable, and usually the easiest to measure in routine daily monitoring.

The demand for heat which the environment makes of the animal is influenced by temperature, air speed, humidity, the radiative environment, the conductive properties of the surfaces in contact with the animal, as well as some non-climatic factors such as stocking density and group size. Several authors have proposed and precisely defined indices for the combined effect of temperature and other variables on the demand for heat from the animal. A recent rather comprehensive example is that of McArthur (1990). Strictly, these indices can only be used in accordance with their specific definitions, and when all the relevant variables are quantified. In this chapter an approximation referred to as the effective temperature is used in certain circumstances, but only as defined in context.

The thermoneutral zone

Chapter 5 deals in detail with the thermal relations of animals, but for the purposes of this chapter it is necessary to offer brief definitions of a few terms. Within the thermoneutral zone metabolic heat production and energy expenditure are minimal, most productive processes are at their most efficient, and the animal is probably thermally comfortable. The zone is

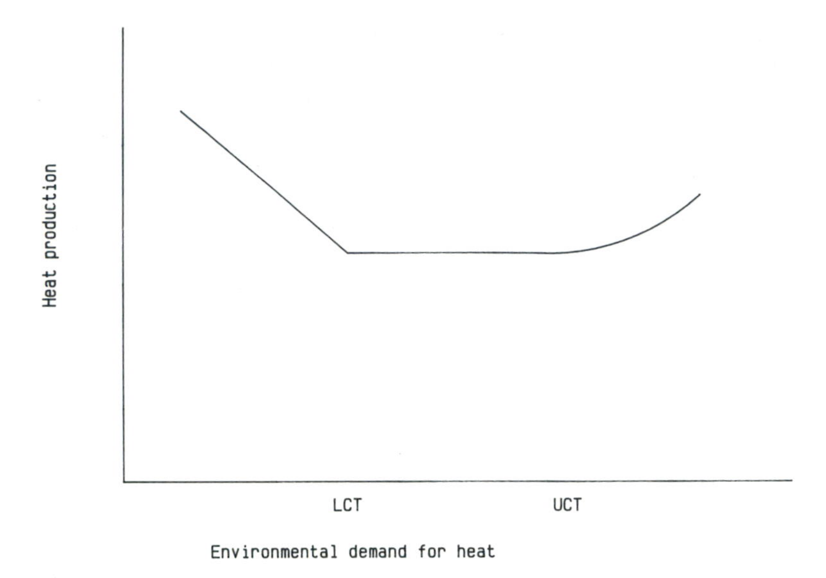

Fig. 1.1. The thermoneutral zone.

bounded by the lower critical temperature (LCT) and the upper critical temperature (UCT). Within the zone the regulation of body temperature is physical (e.g. by the adjustment of insulation) but below LCT and above UCT there are energy costs of thermoregulation (Fig. 1.1).

The climatic environment also includes light, several aspects of which sometimes have their separate effects, namely photoperiod, light intensity and light colour.

Finally, the composition of the air surrounding the animal is important, and in housing practice this means ventilation. Consideration needs to be given to levels of gases (oxygen, carbon dioxide, water vapour, and a wide range of gaseous pollutants of animal, excretal, bedding or microbiological origin). These pollutants are usually only present at low concentration, but some of them, such as ammonia, are potentially influential on performance and animal welfare.

The building and its ventilation equipment are capable of modifying all these factors, and there are both production and welfare reasons to concern ourselves with the modifications. In this chapter the emphasis is on production, mainly for reasons of the historical development of the objective information, but also because other chapters place the emphasis on welfare.

Historical Background

The idea that a building can be used to modify the climatic environment of farm animals in order to affect performance is not new. The Roman agricultural author Lucius Junius Moderatus Columella, writing '... of the fattening and cramming of hens ...' suggested: '... an exceeding warm place of very little light is required for this purpose, wherein the fowls may be shut up one by one in very narrow coops ...'.

Modern objective investigation of the effects of the indoor environment developed in the 19th century, after the chemists of the 18th century had discovered that life involved the combustion of oxygen.

Liebig (1803–1873) realized that there is a connection between food and warmth, and his influence had substantial effects on 19th-century agricultural writers. Playfair (1844) wrote that warmth is the equivalent of food. Childer (1840) measured and compared the consumption of turnips, and the growth rate, of Leicester wether sheep indoors and outside, and found that the indoor sheep ate less and grew faster. In a textbook of about the same period Mechi (1857), quoted by Scott Watson and Hobbs (1937), advised, 'Let us keep our cattle warm and dry and well fed and we shall seldom feel the cramp in our pockets.' From the late 19th century onwards several authors built animal calorimeters to measure heat production and metabolism, usually with a view to improving the precision of feeding. By the mid-20th century the science of bioenergetics was thoroughly and elegantly capable of generating quantitative practical suggestions on the thermal and gaseous requirements of animals (e.g. Mitchell and Kelley, 1933; Brody, 1945; Kleiber, 1961, 1975; Blaxter, 1962, 1975). For some species, particularly poultry, the responses to the light environment were also becoming well defined (Parkhurst, 1928; Morris, 1968).

Principles and Applied Climatic Physiology

Despite the illustrious history of bioenergetics, attempts are often made to design systems starting from engineering and building constraints. It is better to start from the needs of the animals. A four-stage approach has been found to be useful:

1. The quantitative responses of the animals to climatic factors are analysed.
2. These responses are evaluated in cash terms if possible.
3. Designs of housing and ventilation systems to provide the best environment are developed if appropriate, though some classes of stock neither need nor justify housing.

Attention should be paid at this stage to aspects of the design relevant to animal health (see Chapter 2) and animal welfare (Chapters 3 and 4).

4. Finally, the results are monitored, these days usually by data logging, to check the physical performance of the system.

An alternative strategy to stages 1 and 2, particularly relevant to animal welfare, is operant conditioning. The animal is permitted to demonstrate its preferences for environmental factors, usually by choosing within gradients of a factor, or choosing to work for an environmental reward (see Chapter 4).

Thermal environment

Stages 1 and 2 have been, for good reasons, applied differently to two groups of farm species. Using a classification based on Webster (1981), and on the classical description of thermoneutrality (e.g. Kleiber, 1961; see this volume, Chapters 3 and 5), the groups are defined below:

- *Group I* Animals thermoregulating mainly by varying heat production within normal operating temperatures, and often kept below their theomoneutral zone under normal farm conditions. This group contains most classes of poultry and pigs.

  The characteristics are: small animals of low individual value, which are managed and researched as populations rather than as individuals, normally fed to appetite, with a very narrow thermoneutral zone, and for which production response curves are available.
- *Group II* Animals thermoregulating mainly by adjusting evaporation rate and tissue insulation at normal operating temperatures. This group includes ruminants and horses. The characteristics are: large animals of high individual value, which are managed and researched as individuals, for which production response curves are scarce and climatic physiology well understood, but which are not always fed to appetite.

The production response curves available for Group I are generally empirical, and as such are not always robust over time as genetic changes take place, but they lend themselves well to cost–benefit evaluation within well-defined limits. To generate experimental data capable of proper exploitation often requires complex statistical design (Dillon, 1977; Fisher and Boorman, 1986). Because of *ad libitum* feeding there are often important interactions between environment and nutrition, which must be taken into account both in experimental work and in practical application. Thus the response curves available, and quoted below, have generally been produced in population-size climate rooms capable of including nutritional treatments within rooms.

For Group II animals, large population experiments would be prohibitively expensive, but the calorimetry which has been done provides fairly thorough information on the thermoneutral zone and on factors affecting it.

For Group I the effect of environment on nutrition is through its effect on voluntary feed intake, since the animals use adjustment of feed intake as the means of balancing energy intake against heat loss, thus stabilizing body temperature. Since feed intake is adjusted to affect energy intake it may be necessary to reformulate the feed as the environment changes, so as to maintain the intake of protein, vitamins and minerals, the requirements for which are independent of environment.

For Group II animals, often fed a predetermined allowance of feed, or attempting to eat to requirements but limited by constraints such as feed quality or availability (Forbes, 1986), the energy available for production is that which is left after heat losses have been met.

Utilization of energy and protein

As the early writers realized, animal life includes a combustion process, and the conversion of feed energy to product energy is most efficient, by definition, when the amount of energy used by the animal for the maintenance of its body is minimal. This is the most efficient state, both from the point of view of survival of a wild animal or agricultural efficiency of a domestic one.

The energy released on complete combustion of a feed is called the gross energy of that feed (GE) (Fig. 1.2). The digestible energy (DE) is that fraction of the gross energy remaining after substraction of the energy content of the faeces. The energy ultimately useful to the animal's metabolic

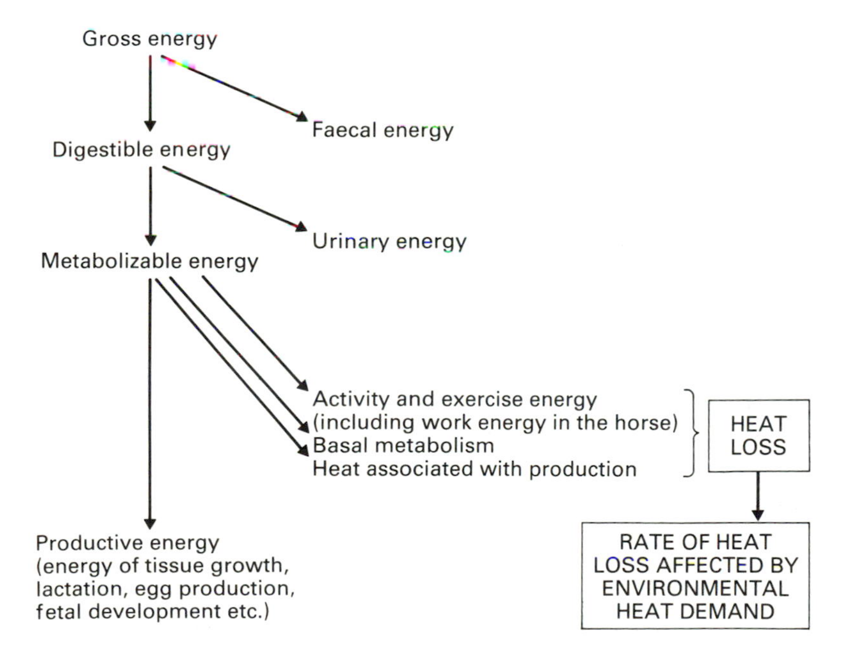

Fig. 1.2. Fate of food energy.

processes, called the metabolizable energy (ME) is the digestible energy *less* the urinary energy. In pigs, ruminants and horses faecal and urinary energy are measured separately, after the collection of the separate excreta, but in poultry droppings energy accounts for both. In ruminant and poultry nutrition it is conventional to describe diets in terms of ME, but in pig and horse nutrition DE is usually used. Highly productive farm animals convert ME to product energy (PE) with an efficiency of about 0.2 to 0.4 in the thermoneutral zone. Outside the zone efficiencies are lower due to the use of ME for cold thermogenesis (keeping warm) or for heat dissipation. Within the zone the exact efficiencies depend on the level of production, since the conversion of ME to eggs, milk, growth, or wool growth all take place with their own specific utilization efficiencies (see ARC, 1980).

The conversion of feed-digestible protein to product protein is *per se* independent of temperature, but is apparently temperature dependent because energy balance affects potential production, through energy availability after the demands of the environment, and sometimes also via effects on voluntary feed intake.

Light

Several production processes exploit ovulation, and in some species photoperiod is the trigger for seasonal breeding. Artificial lighting can be used to regulate or to reinforce the stimuli. The mediation is via the hypothalamus and pituitary gonadotrophins. Some species ovulate in response to long days and some to short days. Examples of long-day species are chickens, turkeys, geese and ducks. Short-day species include sheep and goats. There are some indications of weak photoperiodic seasonal breeding responses in cattle, horses and rabbits. Photoperiod may affect coat growth in cattle, wool growth in sheep, and milk yield and feed intake in dairy cattle, but it is usually only in egg production of hens that artificial daylength control is sometimes taken to the point of the deliberate exclusion of natural light.

There have been successful experimental applications of photoperiod in other species, however. Seasonality of breeding in ewes can be manipulated photoperiodically, though the technique has not been much exploited in practice because its commercial benefits are usually considered outweighed by the cost and practical disadvantages of the need to house. More recently it has been shown that long days have been associated with increased growth rate in sheep, cattle and deer, and with increased milk yield (e.g. Forbes, 1982; Tucker, 1985). The use of photoperiod to influence ovulation in mares is practised.

Hitherto, light intensity and light colour recommendations for species other than poultry have generally been for the benefit of the working conditions of the staff rather than for any animal response or requirement.

About 200 lux is often suggested, and this should be suitable for the needs of the stock.

Important features of the photoperiodic response have been most thoroughly examined in poultry, but may be generally applicable, as follows:

1. Change in daylength is more important than absolute daylength.
2. The operative wavelength is probably about 600–750 nm (according to work on the duck).
3. There may be a threshold intensity below which the animals treat the intensity as darkness (0.4 lux in the chicken, and perhaps as high as 200 lux in applications such as the use of reducing photoperiods for the induction of ovulation in sheep, and increasing photoperiods for the same purpose in mares).

Air supply

There are two ventilation requirements, not one. The maximum requirement is the amount of air necessary to prevent the building overheating due to metabolic heat. This dictates the capacity of a ventilation system. The minimum ventilation requirement is the amount of air required to provide oxygen and to remove carbon dioxide, ammonia, dust, and other excretory and microbiological by-products. Typical standards are carbon dioxide kept below 0.3%, and ammonia kept below 25 ppm. (See Chapters 6 and 7 and Table 1.1 for details.) Table 1.2. compares the housing requirements for the main groups of farm animals, and for the horse.

Table 1.1. Typical ventilation rate requirements.

Animal	Minimum	Maximum
Poultry	$1.6 \times 10^{-4} m^3 s^{-1} kg^{0.75}$	$1.5 \times 10^{-3} m^3 s^{-1} kg^{0.75}$
Pigs	$2.1 \times 10^{-4} m^3 s^{-1} kg^{0.67}$	$2.1 \times 10^{-3} m^3 s^{-1} kg^{0.67}$
Ruminants	$0.35 m^3 h^{-1} kg^{-1}$	At least 10 × minimum
Horses	$0.4–0.7 m^3 h^{-1} kg^{-1}$	At least 10 × minimum

Source: Based on Charles (1981); Bruce (1981); Wathes *et al.* (1983); and Webster *et al.* (1987) and reproduced with permission.

Highly productive animals, such as high yielding dairy cows, need more generous allowances of air, due to their high metabolic rate. Another increment may be needed to allow for floor water in dairy cubicles.

Table 1.2. Comparative housing requirements.

Factor	Poultry	Pigs	Ruminants	Horses
Shelter	Yes	Yes	Yes	Yes
Controlled temperature	Yes	Yes	No	No
Controlled light	Yes	No	No	No
Wind proof	Yes	Yes	Yes	Yes
Draught proof	Yes	Yes	Yes	Yes
Light proof	Yes	No	No	No
Rain proof	Yes	Yes	Yes	Yes
Free from condensation	Yes	Yes	Yes	Yes

Specific Requirements

Temperature for poultry

At several centres, large replicated climate rooms have been used to measure the responses of populations of poultry to environment, in a way which permits statistical curve fitting and, from that, response modelling. For adult poultry dry bulb air temperature is normally an adequate descriptor of the thermal environment in draught-free houses. For young chicks and poults, before feathering is complete, air speed should be below 0.15 m s^{-1}.

In hot climates low relative humidity is required because the response of the birds to heat stress is panting, during which their rate of respiratory evaporation increases dramatically. Therefore, evaporative cooling of houses can only be used in hot dry climates.

Layers

As temperature is increased feed intake falls and so does egg weight. Up to about 20°C rate of lay can be partially maintained provided that nutrient intake is maintained by reformulation (Payne, 1967; Emmans and Charles, 1977; Marsden *et al.*, 1987) (Figs 1.3 and 1.4). The economic best temperature depends on the relative prices of feed and of eggs and can be calculated for any local market circumstances using models of the data (e.g. Charles, 1984). Often the economic optimum is about 21°C as measured in the gangways between the cages, which corresponds to about 24°C for non-cage systems.

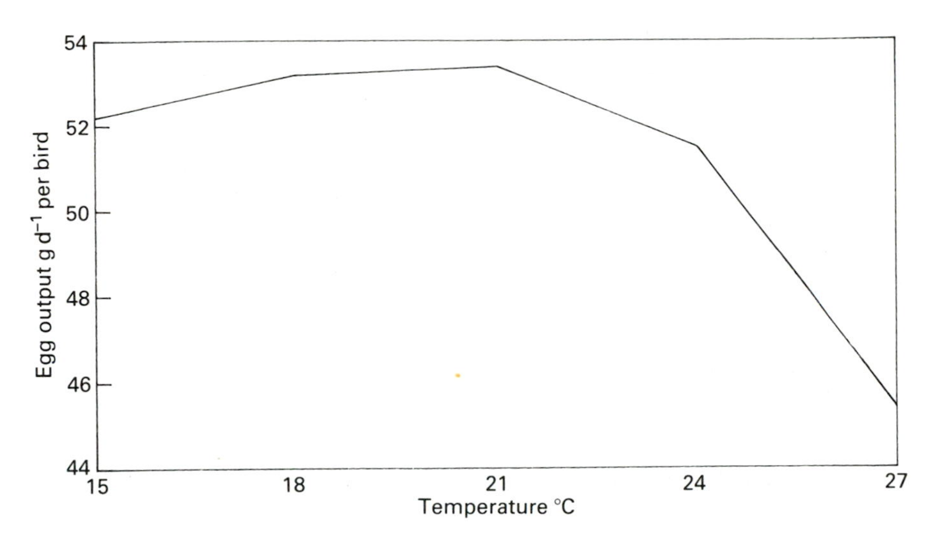

Fig. 1.3. Effect of temperature on egg output of brown egg layers (based on Charles, 1984).

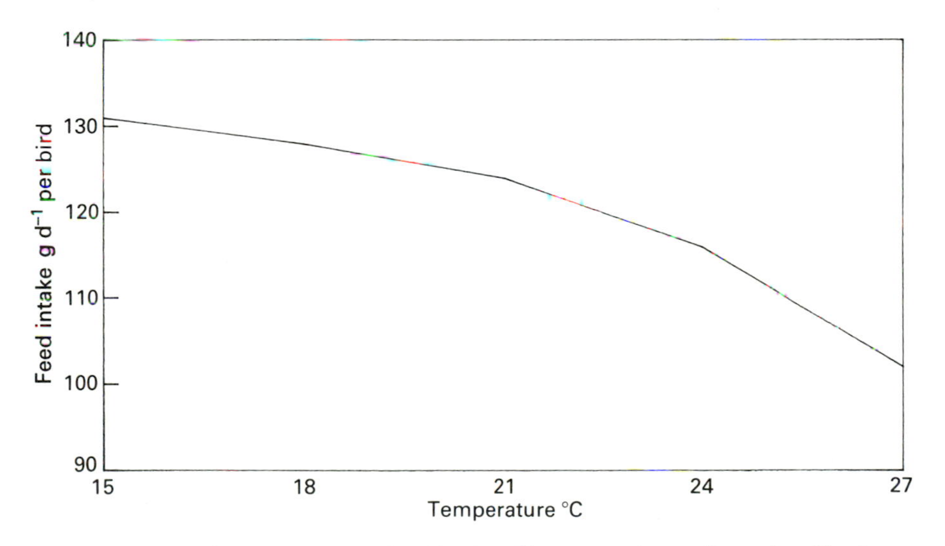

Fig. 1.4. Effect of temperature on feed intake of brown egg layers (based on Charles, 1984).

Broilers

At day-old, 31°C is probably suitable in draught-proof houses, reduced to 21°C at 17 to 21 days. In brooding systems using a high proportion of radiant heat lower background temperatures may be suitable, outside the brooder canopy. Chicks in such regimes are able to choose their own environment, though they need an attraction light in the radiant heated area (Alsam and Wathes, 1991a, b). During brooding the behaviour of the chicks gives a very good indication of the suitability of the thermal environment. After the brooding period growth rate and feed intake both decline as temperature is increased, and taking the money value of both into account the economic optimum depends upon the ratio between liveweight value and feed cost. At a ratio of 3:1 the optimum temperature is 21°C, and lower at higher ratios. The temperature requirements of broilers were reviewed by Charles (1986).

Turkeys

Growth rate and feed intake of growing turkeys are both depressed as temperature rises. The effect can only partially be prevented by dietary reformulation. Models of response are available, based on data reviewed by Charles (1989). The margin of liveweight value *less* feeding cost varies widely according to the market for which the birds are intended. It may be as low as 12–15°C for the high priced fresh trade, and as high as 20°C for the frozen trade.

Example prices date very quickly, so the values given in Table 1.3 are given merely to illustrate a principle.

To calculate specific example cost penalties, gross margin of product sale *less* feed cost is a good measure of the effect of thermal environmental variables. This is because it is generally safe to assume that changing the temperature will not affect such factors as labour or capital cost, and, as will be seen in Chapter 7, since most temperature changes are made merely by changing ventilation rate, there is no change in fuel cost. There may be trivial changes in electricity cost in the case of powered ventilation systems.

By definition the economic optimum temperature is that associated with the highest margin, and the cost penalty is the difference between the margin at the test temperature and the highest margin. The margins for poultry and pigs will be found to be very sensitive to price changes.

Air change rates for poultry

Table 1.1 gives some recommended rates for various classes and weights of poultry, based on maximum rates associated with limiting temperature lift above outside temperature to 3°C, and the air quality limits given above.

Lighting for poultry

Layers

Commercial exploitation of the photoperiodic response requires a short day

Table 1.3. Some effects of temperature on poultry calculated by models of the published data.

Temperature (°C)	Egg output (g day^{-1} per bird)	Eggs/hen housed, 52 weeks	Egg weight (g egg^{-1})	Feed intake (g day^{-1} per bird)	Cost* penalty of wrong temperature (p per bird year^{-1})
Layers – brown breeds					
15	52.2	284	65.5	131	61
18	53.2	290	65.5	128	22
21	53.4	293	65.0	124	0
24	51.5	289	63.5	116	5
27	45.4	267	60.7	102	64
(on a fixed diet, not reformulated for temperature)					
Laying hens – white breeds					
15	48.0	269	63.5	116	
18	50.8	285	63.5	112	†
21	51.7	293	63.0	108	N/A
24	49.9	288	61.7	102	
27	44.0	265	59.3	95	
(diet not reformulated at high temperature)					

Temperature (°C)	Liveweight (kg per bird)		Feed intake (kg per bird)		Cost penalty (p per bird)
	Males	Females	Males	Females	
Broilers, to 49 days of age					
10	2.93	2.42	6.15	5.40	10.5
15	2.99	2.48	5.95	5.20	3.6
20	2.96	2.45	5.65	4.92	0.3
25	2.83	2.32	5.26	4.52	0.6
30	2.60	2.09	4.78	4.03	4.6

Source: Data calculated from the model of Charles (1984).
See also Figs 1.3 and 1.4.

* At sample UK prices at the time of writing.
† White eggs were rare on the UK market at the time of writing.

(usually 8 hours) during rearing, followed by a step up from 18 weeks to 17 hours (e.g. Morris, 1968). The rate of step up suggested has usually been 15 to 20 minutes per week, though currently in some market circumstances faster rates are used for the first few weeks. The optimum depends on the relative monetary values of eggs and of egg size.

There has been interest in many countries in recent years in intermittent light regimes, and Rowland (1983) reviewed 75 papers, since when there have been several more. Some studies indicate a slight reduction in feed intake without reducing egg output, provided that nutrient intake is maintained.

Broilers

In the UK industry long days at low intensity (typically 1–2 lux) have traditionally been used, but there is some evidence that patterns involving intermittent lighting may be marginally beneficial.

Turkeys

In turkey breeder hens maximum egg production requires 14 to 16 hours of light per day at an intensity of at least 54 lux (Noll, 1989).

Temperature for pigs

In general, pigs should be kept at a temperature about 3°C above their lower critical temperature (LCT). By definition, energetic efficiency is maximized under such conditions, and pig comfort is probably also maximized.

However, even for a given age and weight of pig there is no single temperature which may be specified as the lower critical temperature, since the rate of heat loss from the pig is affected by several factors. The most important include group size (because of huddling effects), feeding level, air movement, the type, temperature and wetness of the floor, and the radiative environment. The physical mechanisms through which these factors have their influence are discussed in Chapter 5, but for the purposes of recommending house environments it is necessary to summarize in this chapter some of the consequences of the interactions between them.

Close (1981) and Bruce (1981) have reviewed and calculated the effects of several variables on LCT. Biological models have been developed by ADAS for the calculation of the combined effects of variables such as air speed, group size, floor type, body weight and feeding level on the growth of rationed pigs. For *ad libitum* fed pigs feed digestible energy is taken into account rather than feeding level. The models are quantitative literature reviews, in which published, and some unpublished, responses have been amalgamated in a biologically reasonable sequence, and then prices appended where appropriate. The literature reviewed includes the relevant references mentioned in this chapter, but many others besides.

Evidently, in order to minimize the detrimental effects of interacting factors on feed efficiency in cool conditions, housing should be draught free (air speed less than $0.15\,m\,s^{-1}$) and have dry floors, preferably made of non-conducting materials. Under hot conditions the pig can benefit from air movement and conductive floors.

Below LCT liveweight gain is likely to be depressed in the case of rationed pigs (i.e. those offered less than their *ad libitum* voluntary intake), and for *ad libitum* fed pigs feed intake will increase (Fig. 1.5). Close (1981) published a function relating the growth and feed intake to temperature for rationed pigs of 20–105 kg liveweight as follows:

$$DW = 26.26 + 1.48T - 0.015T^2 + 0.45I - 0.0002IT^2$$

where DW=body weight gain, $g\,kg^{-0.75}\,day^{-1}$; T=temperature, °C; I=feed intake, $g\,kg^{-0.75}\,day^{-1}$.

For *ad libitum* fed pigs from 18 to 90 kg body weight feed intake falls as temperature is increased (Close, 1989).

$$FI = 9.6 + 0.075T + 0.52W - 0.012TW$$

where T=temperature, °C; W=liveweight, kg; FI=metabolizable energy intake, $MJ\,day^{-1}$.

In the lactating sow temperature has pronounced effects on intake, for example $1.5\,MJ\,day^{-1}$ ME $°C^{-1}$, though at very high temperatures the effect may be greater, resulting in weight loss and reduced weaning weights of the piglets (Close, 1989).

The biological models described above can be used to calculate the cost

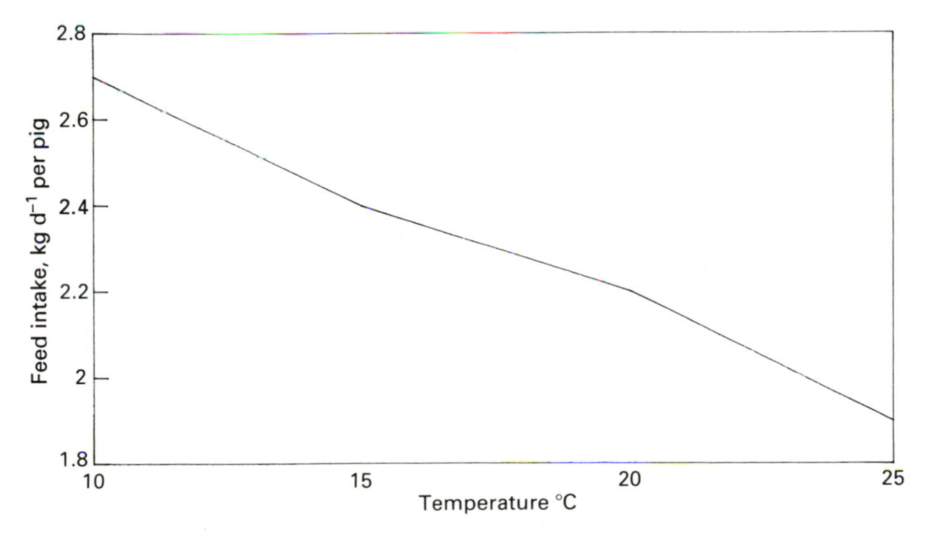

Fig. 1.5. Effect of temperature on *ad libitum* feed intake of 60 kg pigs (data from Table 1.5).

Table 1.4. Calculated effect of air speed and floor type on effective temperature and on cost penalty of temperature below LCT (rationed pigs).*

	Air temperature (°C)	Effective temperature (°C)		Depression in liveweight gain (g day^{-1})		Cost penalty (p kg^{-1} liveweight gain)	
Air speed (m s^{-1})		0.15	0.30	0.15	0.30	0.15	0.30
Fed 2.2 kg day^{-1}							
Insulated floor	9	10	8	0	6	0	1
	12	13	11	0	0	0	0
	15	16	14	0	0	0	0
	18	19	17	0	0	0	0
Fed 2 kg day^{-1}							
Concrete floor	9	7	5	19	36	1	3
	12	10	8	3	12	0	1
	15	13	11	0	1	0	0
	18	16	14	0	0	0	0
Fed 2 kg day^{-1}							
Wet concrete floor	9	6	4	27	47	2	3
	12	9	7	7	19	1	1
	15	12	10	0	3	0	1
	18	15	13	0	0	0	0

Source: The model used to calculate the data in this table is based mainly on Close (1981) and reproduced with permission.

*60 kg pigs in pens of 15, feed 13 MJ kg^{-1} DE @ £135 t^{-1}, liveweight value 90 p kg^{-1}.

consequences of temperatures below LCT in the case of rationed pigs, and to predict the feed intake of *ad libitum* fed pigs, taking into account the interacting environmental factors such as air speed.

Some example calculations from the models are given in Tables 1.4 and 1.5 (see also Fig. 1.5). Obviously the answers depend on the prices prevailing for pigs and for feed, but Table 1.4 gives some examples at sample UK prices at the time of writing. In the case of *ad libitum* fed pigs, feed intake is adjusted by the pig in order to maintain energy balance, but protein requirement is independent of temperature. Therefore, a diet adequate at low temperature to meet the potential protein deposition rate may be inadequate at high temperature. Likewise a diet adequate at high temperature may be wasteful of protein at low temperature, so that a prediction of feed intake is important in feed formulation work, and the nutritionist needs to know the environment for which his feeds are intended.

Table 1.5. Calculated effect of temperature on *ad libitum* feed intake of pigs.*

Liveweight (kg)	(°C)	Feed intake (kg day^{-1})
45	10	2.2
	15	2.0
	20	1.9
	25	1.7
60	10	2.7
	15	2.4
	20	2.2
	25	1.9
80	10	3.3
	15	3.0
	20	2.6
	25	2.2
100	10	3.9
	15	3.5
	20	3.0
	25	2.6

Source: The model used to calculate the data in this table is based partly on Close (1989) and is reproduced with permission. See also Fig. 1.5.

Note that breed, stock, air speed, floor type and management may cause large differences in these effects, but the trends are of interest.

*Feed 13 MJ kg^{-1}, draught free, insulated floor, 15 pigs per pen, gilts.

Air change rates for pigs

The values for air change rate given in Table 1.1 may be used to calculate the ventilation rates needed for any building, whether they are to be achieved by electric fans or by natural convection. The important design detail to bear in mind is that the metabolic weights in Table 1.1 must be calculated per pig and then multiplied by the number of pigs. It is not the total liveweight in the building which is raised to the power 0.67.

Temperature for ruminants

The larger farm animal species are much more temperature tolerant than pigs and poultry. But even large animals possess a band of temperature within which they are most energetically efficient, probably most comfortable, and probably at their most resistant to other stresses. However, this thermoneutral zone is generally wide, and often extends to much lower

Table 1.6. Calculated lower critical temperature for pre-ruminant calves.

	Air speed ($m s^{-1}$)	
	<0.2	0.45
Healthy		
Coat thickness (mm) 10	19°C	21°C
20	13°C	15°C
Scouring (coat 5% wetted)		
Coat thickness (mm) 10	26°C	26°C
20	21°C	22°C

Source: Data calculated using the model of Charles *et al.* (unpublished).

temperatures than those of pigs and poultry. Exceptions to this rule, among the larger species, are neonate and young animals, those which are sick, and under some circumstances those which are underfed or exposed to high air speeds – indoors or out – or which have wet coats, or some combination of all these.

Particular attention should be paid to the wide range of values of LCT for unweaned calves, which are particularly susceptible to draughts, and whose growth rate and health status may greatly influence their temperature requirement, through metabolic rate (Table 1.6).

Thus the aim is to provide an environment between the lower critical temperature and the upper critical temperature. The practical problem for stockmen and house designers is that the zone, while conveniently wide, moves about. This is because it is dependent on so many factors.

Factors affecting the lower critical temperature

The primary factors are the rate of heat production and the rate of heat loss. For any body weight the former is affected by metabolizable energy (ME) intake, the nature and digestibility of the feed, the level of production and the efficiency of utilization of ME for both maintenance and production, k (since a proportion $1 - k$ appears as heat), and by the amount of activity and locomotion. Heat loss is affected by coat thickness and coat thermal insulation, tissue insulation, the minimal rate of evaporative heat loss and the radiative environment.

Coat insulation is importantly affected by wetness and air speed. ARC (1980) and Charles, McArthur, Gregson and Crawshaw (unpublished) have reviewed the literature on these factors and the latter have developed a computer model for calculation of both LCT and the energy costs of cold.

Translation of these energy costs into equivalent cash costs is not quite so straightforward as it is for pigs and poultry, because large animals can often substantially buffer short-term energy deficit by losing weight, only to gain it again later. This is often acceptable husbandry, but it should be remembered that it is not free, since there are two inefficiencies of conversion involved if an animal calls upon reserves as an energy source, which happens with an efficiency of less than 1, and then replaces those reserves, also with an efficiency of less than 1. (Typical efficiencies are approximately 0.5 to 0.6.) In Tables 1.7, 1.8 and 1.9 apparent equivalent cash costs per animal per °C below LCT per day are given, but should be interpreted cautiously.

Factors affecting upper critical temperature

These include the level of feeding, the nature of the feed, and the level of production, as for LCT. Rate of heat loss is affected by the tissue and coat insulation, by the maximum rate of evaporation, and by the radiative environment. McArthur (1987) developed a model for the estimation of upper critical temperature (UCT), but it is much less easy to calculate than LCT, partly because evaporative heat loss regulation increases in phases as temperature rises. Skin temperature is the best simple indicator of evaporative events, but that will seldom be to hand, and certainly not at the design stage of an analysis or building project. McArthur (1990) modelled the effect of humidity and radiation on what he termed the standard environmental temperature, and found some potentially very large effects, so that high producing animals may sometimes be mildly heat stressed at surprisingly low temperatures.

However, despite these complications, some kind of design guidelines can be offered, in the form of tables of LCT, so that users can aim to keep the animals in environments just above LCT. Tables 1.6–1.9 provide values for LCT, and for the energy cost of temperatures below it, for a variety of

Table 1.7. Effects of weather on the energy requirements of beef cattle.*

Conditions	LCT (°C)	MJ day^{-1} °C^{-1} below LCT	p day^{-1} °C^{-1} below LCT
Dry, draught free	−9	–	–
4 m s^{-1} draught, coat 50% wet	+17	2	2

Source: Data calculated using the model of Charles *et al.* (unpublished).

*Gaining 0.75 kg day^{-1}, 400 kg liveweight, barley fed.
† Barley at £100 per tonne.

Table 1.8. Calculated effects of weather on the energy balance of dairy cows.*

Condition	LCT (°C)	MJ day^{-1} °C^{-1} below LCT	p day^{-1} °C^{-1} below LCT
Mild weather, draught-free holding area, yarded	−22	–	–
4 m s^{-1} wind, draughty holding area, raining, coat 30% wetted	−1	3	3

Source: Data calculated using the model of Charles *et al.* (unpublished).

*600 kg cow, 25 l day^{-1} yield, losing 0.5 kg day^{-1} body weight, fed silage and concentrates.
†At typical 1991 UK feed prices.

circumstances, as calculated by the model of Charles *et al.* (unpublished) In practical application of these values it must be remembered that the larger farm animals require fairly generous ventilation rates (see Table 1.1 and later chapters), and this requirement must not be compromised in the interests of temperature. Later chapters deal with the provision of air in practice.

Humidity is of little relevance to the response to cold unless the coat is wetted, but through evaporation rate it is relevant to upper critical temperature (UCT). High humidity depresses UCT, and is therefore a key determinant of the minimum ventilation rate requirements in Table 1.1. For example, fully fleeced ewes in poorly ventilated winter housing in temperate climates may be mildly heat stressed at temperatures as low as 10°C, according to both calculations of energy balance, and practical experience of appetite depression. Likewise high yielding dairy cows or fast growing beef cattle may experience slight depressions of performance due to mild heat stress if housed in inadequately ventilated accommodation at high humidity. Fertility of dairy cattle is depressed by mild heat stress.

Air change for ruminants

As seen above the minimum quantities of air in Table 1.1 are largely dictated by the need to control humidity, and also condensation. Buildings ventilated to provide for humidity control will normally also be adequately ventilated for the provision of oxygen, and the removal of carbon dioxide, ammonia, and other pollutants, though when calculating the size of the vents to supply air by buoyancy forces during winter occupancy it is advisable to allow at least double the vent sizes needed for humidity control in order to be sure of removing metabolic heat adequately on warm winter days. For summer occupancy much larger vents are needed so that the air change rate

Table 1.9. Effect of weather and management system on the energy requirements of ewes.*

Management system	Lower critical temperature (°C)	Effect on ME requirement per °C below LCT ($MJ\,day^{-1}$)	p day^{-1} $°C^{-1}$ below LCT†
1. Indoors, full fleece, dry, draught free	−8	0.2	0.2
2. Indoors, shorn, dry, draught free	17	0.4	0.5
3. Indoors, shorn, dry, draughty ($0.4\,m\,s^{-1}$)	18	0.4	0.5
4. Outdoors, dry, $4\,m\,s^{-1}$ wind speed	8	0.3	0.4
5. Outdoors, coat 30% wet, $4\,m\,s^{-1}$ wind	12	0.3	0.4
6. Outdoors, dry, $2.5\,m\,s^{-1}$ wind	2	0.2	0.2
7. Outdoors, coat 30% wet $2\,m\,s^{-1}$ wind	6	0.3	0.4
8. Outdoors, coat 20% wet, $4\,m\,s^{-1}$ wind, hill sheep climbing and ranging extensively	11	0.4	0.5

Source: Data calculated using the model of Charles *et al.* (unpublished).

* Pregnant 70 kg ewes, 75 days after conception, expecting twins. Assumptions include fleece thickness 50 mm, down cross type fleece (except No. 8).

† At sample UK prices at the time of writing.

Summary of conclusions from Table 1.9

Indoors, full fleece – No practical effect.
Indoors, shorn – Add 0.4 $MJ\,day^{-1}\,°C^{-1}$ below 17°C.
Outdoors, calm and dry – Add 0.2 $MJ\,day^{-1}\,°C^{-1}$ below 2°C.
Outdoors, windy and wet – Add 0.3 $MJ\,day^{-1}\,°C^{-1}$ below 12°C.

Notes: The above calculations are specific to the example assumptions. The results are very sensitive to fleece thickness and as pregnancy progresses the LCT will fall, *provided* that the ewes are offered and can eat enough dry matter to satisfy ME requirement. LCT rises at feeding levels below requirement. Note the substantial effects of shearing.

The LCT of newborn lambs is much higher, and may be as high as 25–33°C, depending on wind speed and coat wetness.

may be as generous as possible in order to cool the building as much as possible.

Temperature for horses

Adult horses are probably thermoneutral from about −10°C to +10°C according to work by McBride *et al.* (1983), although this work was on unacclimated animals over the short term. An unpublished version of the model of Charles *et al.* (unpublished) estimates the LCT of a 500 kg horse at rest to be within the range given by McBride *et al.* (1983), but very dependent on coat depth and air speed. Like all animals horses are intolerant of draughts, particularly after exercise or when clipped but not rugged, and therefore the air supply should not be associated with air speeds over $0.15\,m\,s^{-1}$.

Newborn foals are less tolerant of low temperature, and this can give difficulties when mare and foal share accommodation.

Air change for horses

Horses appear to be particularly susceptible to air quality, including high levels of ammonia, humidity, dusts and mould spores. These agents can cause respiratory stresses, which are particularly serious to the welfare and usefulness of an animal expected to perform exercise over a long life. The stressors operate as irritants or allergens (e.g. Webster *et al.*, 1987; Wathes, 1989), and some have been specifically associated with named disorders. An important example is the association between *Aspergillus fumigatus* and *Micropolyspora faeni* and chronic obstructive pulmonary disease (COPD) (McPherson *et al.*, 1979). Rye grass pollen also causes allergies, and ventilation is even more critical if the bedding or fodder is other than first class. Thus the values given in Table 1.1 for air change rates should be applied with a great deal of judgement, and of course without draughts. Grouped horses need more air per animal than individually housed horses.

References

Agricultural Research Council (1980) *The Nutrient Requirements of Ruminant Livestock.* Commonwealth Agricultural Bureaux, Farnham Royal.

Alsam, H. and Wathes, C.M. (1991a) Thermal preferences of chicks brooded at different air temperatures. *British Poultry Science* 32, 31–46.

Alsam, H. and Wathes, C.M. (1991b) Conjoint preferences of chicks for heat and light intensity. *British Poultry Science* 32, 899–916.

Blaxter, K.L. (1962) *The Energy Metabolism of Ruminants.* Hutchinson, London.

Blaxter, K.L. (1975) *The Energy Metabolism of Ruminants,* 2nd edn. Hutchinson, London.

Brody, S. (1945) *Bioenergetics and Growth.* Reinhold, New York.

Bruce, J.M. (1981) Ventilation and temperature control criteria for pigs. In: Clark, J.A. (ed.), *Environmental Aspects of Housing for Animal Production.* Butterworths, London, pp. 197–216.

Charles, D.R. (1981) Practical ventilation and temperature control. In: Clark, J.A. (ed.), *Environmental Aspects of Housing for Animal Production.* Butterworths, London, pp. 183–196.

Charles, D.R. (1984) A model of egg production. *British Poultry Science* 25, 309–321.

Charles, D.R. (1986) Temperature for broilers. *World's Poultry Science Journal* 43, 249–258.

Charles, D.R. (1989) Environmental responses of growing turkeys. In: Nixey, C. and Grey, T.C. (eds), *Turkey Science.* Butterworths, London, pp. 201–216.

Charles, D.R., McArthur, A.J., Gregson, K. and Crawshaw, R. (unpublished) A model of the winter energy balance of ruminants.

Childer, J.W. (1840) On shed feeding. *Journal of the Royal Agricultural Society of England* 1, 169–170.

Close, W.H. (1981) The climatic requirements of the pig. In: Clark, J.A. (ed.), *Environmental Aspects of Housing for Animal Production.* Butterworths, London, pp. 149–166.

Close, W.H. (1989) The influence of the thermal environment on the voluntary food intake of the pig. In: Forbes, J.M., Varley, M.A. and Lawrence, T.L.J. (eds), *The Voluntary Food Intake of Pigs.* British Society of Animal Production Occasional Publication No. 13, Edinburgh, pp. 87–96.

Dillon, J.L. (1977) *The Analysis of Response in Crop and Animal Production.* Pergamon, Oxford.

Emmans, G.C. and Charles, D.R. (1977) Climatic environment and poultry feeding in practice. In: Haresign, W., Swan H. and Lewis, D. (eds), *Nutrition and the Climatic Environment.* Butterworths, London, pp. 31–50.

Fisher, C. and Boorman, K.N. (1986) *Nutrient Requirements of Poultry and Nutritional Research.* Butterworths, London.

Forbes, J.M. (1982) Effects of lighting pattern on growth, lactation and food intake of sheep, cattle and deer. *Livestock Production Science* 9, 361–364.

Forbes, J.M. (1986) *The Voluntary Food Intake of Farm Animals.* Butterworths, London.

Kleiber, M. (1961) *The Fire of Life.* Wiley, New York.

Kleiber, M. (1975) *The Fire of Life,* 2nd edn. Krieger, New York.

McArthur, A.J. (1987) Thermal interaction between animal and microclimate: a comprehensive model. *Journal of Theoretical Biology* 126, 203–218.

McArthur, A.J. (1990) Thermal interaction between animal and environment: Specification of a 'Standard Environmental Temperature' for animals outdoors. *Journal of Theoretical Biology* 148, 331–343.

McBride, G.E., Christopherson, R.J. and Sauer, W.C. (1983) Metabolic responses of horses to cold stress. *Journal of Animal Science* 57 (Supplement), 175.

McPherson, E.A., Lawson, G.H.K., Murphy, J.R., Nicholson, J.M., Breeze, R.G. and Pirie, H.M. (1979) Chronic obstructive pulmonary disease in horses: Aetiological studies: Responses in intradermal and inhalation antigenic challenge. *Equine Veterinary Journal* 11, 159–166.

Marsden, A., Morris, T.R. and Cromarty, A. (1987) Effects of constant environmental temperatures on the performance of laying hens. *British Poultry Science* 28, 361–380.

Mechi, J.J. (1857) *How to Farm Profitably.*

Mitchell, H.H. and Kelley, M.A.R. (1933) Estimated data on the energy, gaseous, and water metabolism of poultry for use in planning the ventilation of poultry houses. *Journal of Agricultural Research* 47, 735–748.

Morris, T.R. (1968) Light requirements of the fowl. In: Carter, T.C. (ed.),

Environmental Control in Poultry Production. Oliver and Boyd, Edinburgh, pp. 15–39.

Noll, S. (1989) Management of breeding stock. In: Nixey, C. and Grey, T.C. (eds), *Turkey Science.* Butterworths, London, pp. 119–134.

Parkhurst, R.T. (1928) Artificial light for late hatched pullets. Eggs. *Scientific Poultry Breeders Association* Dec 1928, 270–271.

Payne, C.G. (1967) Environmental temperature and egg production. In: Carter, T.C. (ed.), *Environmental Control in Poultry Production.* Oliver and Boyd, Edinburgh, pp. 40–54.

Playfair, L. (1844) On the general principles of nutrition and on the food intake of cattle. *Journal of the Royal Agricultural Society of England* 4, 215–237.

Rowland, K.W. (1983) Interrupted lighting patterns for laying chickens: a review and evaluation. *World's Poultry Science Journal* 41, 5–9.

Scott Watson, J.A. and Hobbs, M.E. (1937) *Great Farmers.* Selwyn and Blount, London.

Tucker, H.A. (1985) Photoperiodic influences on milk production in dairy cows. In: Haresign, W. and Cole, D.J.A. (eds), *Recent Advances in Animal Nutrition.* Butterworths, London.

Wathes, C.M. (1989) Ventilation of stables. *Farm Buildings and Engineering* 6, 21–25.

Wathes, C.M., Jones, C.D.R. and Webster, A.J.F. (1983) Ventilation, air hygiene and animal health. *Veterinary Record* 113, 554–559.

Webster, A.J.F. (1981) Optimal housing criteria for ruminants. In: Clark, J.A. (ed.), *Environmental Aspects of Housing for Animal Production.* Butterworths, London, pp. 217–232.

Webster, A.J.F., Clarke, A.F., Madelin, T.M. and Wathes, C.M. (1987) Air hygiene in stables. 1. Effects of stable design, ventilation and management on the concentration of respirable dust. *Equine Veterinary Journal* 19, 448–453.

Environment and Animal Health

2

J. HARTUNG
Tierärtzliche Hochschule Hannover, Germany

Introduction

> It is essential to recognize and avoid those environmental factors which play a role in the development of diseases and may influence conditions and processes within the body.
>
> (Hippocrates, 400 BC)

The environment of modern housing systems has a major influence on animal welfare, health and performance. Although many classical diseases are controlled today, there remain a variety of environmental disorders which can cause considerable losses in performance and lives. Most of these problems occur in pig, poultry and calf production and include disorders of the digestive and respiratory tracts, cardiovascular system as well as the skin and skeleton. In milking cows, mastitis and lameness are typical disorders influenced by the environment. One German survey over nine years of mortality in pig production showed that 20% of all suckling pigs and 48% of all weaners died of viral gastroenteritis or coli enterotoxaemia, 21% of the store pigs suffered from pneumonia and 34% of fattening pig losses were due to cardiovascular failure (Hellmers, 1986). Total losses in fattening pig production are estimated to vary from 1 to 5% in Germany (Sommer, 1991). However, not all diseased pigs show clinical signs that can be detected in the confined conditions of some livestock systems. Often subclinical disease is apparent only at slaughter. An extensive epidemiological study on the relationship between pathological lesions at slaughter and growth performance of finishing pigs showed distinct differences in the daily gain (g day^{-1}) of pigs with pathological symptoms in comparison to the pigs of the same herds without lesions (Elbers, 1991). Table 2.1 indicates the

Table 2.1. Relationship between pathological lesions in finishing pigs at slaughter and growth performance in 155 herds.

Lesions	Number of pigs	Average daily weight gain	
		g day^{-1}	s.d.
Atrophic rhinitis	274	670	125
Pneumonia	32,260	687	104
Pleuritis	18,848	685	98
Abscess(es) in the lungs	1,128	682	113
Lungs impossible to mark	7,954	692	108
Arthritis	1,453	658	119
Inflammation of the leg	4,001	682	110
Inflammation of the tail	2,003	685	108
Skin lesions	1,691	676	107
Liver – partially affected	424	698	106
Liver – condemned	1,403	702	107
Bacterial examination	894	666	123
Disease free	28,973	729	104
Total number of pigs	101,306		

Source: Elbers, 1991.

Growth rates in pigs with lesions were significantly slower than disease free pigs ($P < 0.001$).

wide range of disorders which occur unseen in current production systems and the slower rates of growth.

Similarly, over the last 20 years there has been a change in the causes of rejection of broilers at meat inspection after slaughter. Respiratory diseases are still important while the disorders with the highest increase over the 20 years are skin diseases, in particular deep dermatitis (Table 2.2). Losses can reach 2 to 3% in individual broiler flocks (Frohne-Brinkmann, unpublished). The table also shows that even with modern husbandry systems, diseases causing heavy losses cannot be eliminated or avoided. The aetiology of most of the diseases quoted above is complex because a variety of external and internal factors are involved. For example, deep dermatitis is caused by common strains of *Escherichia coli* which are found in high numbers in broiler houses. The condition is more common in well fed, heavy birds, especially when stocking density is high and air quality is poor (Frohne-Brinkmann, unpublished).

This chapter considers the role of some of the most important environmental factors and conditions causing or contributing to the development of multifactorial disease in farm animals. Reference is also made to some internal factors and to stress.

Table 2.2. Rejection of broilers at meat inspection and affected organs. Percentage of total rejections.

Affected organs	A 1969	B 1979	C 1980	D 1988
Respiratory tract	45.2%	15.8%	–	29.5%
Skeleton	15.0%	48.1%	57.3%	18.1%
Digestive tract	6.6%	–	–	10.3%
Nervous system	3.8%	–	–	–
Urinary tract	2.4%	–	–	–
Reproductive system	1.8%	–	–	–
Skin/subcutis	1.4%	9.8%	16.7%	34.5%
Others	23.8%	26.3%	26.0%	7.6%

A = Papasolomontos *et al.*, 1969. C = Guarda *et al.*, 1980.
B = Bergmann and Scheer, 1979. D = Valentin *et al.*, 1988.

Recent Developments in Animal Farming

The development of modern, intensive animal production in developed countries started about 30–40 years ago: the overall trend is towards a significant increase in herd size kept on a diminishing number of farms. Undoubtedly, intensive systems considerably raised productivity aided by progress in animal breeding and nutrition. The most impressive example is egg production. In 1960, a laying hen produced 150 eggs; today annual outputs of over 300 eggs per hen are commonplace. At the same time, other structural changes in animal agriculture also occurred in the form of increased specialization and integration of production systems and marketing. To maximize the benefit of intensification, farms specialized in one species and increased the number of animals. In the 1970s and 1980s some East German dairy units comprised 2000 cows under one roof and piggeries with up to 200,000 sows, and fattening pigs in one closed system were built.

Similar developments on a smaller scale took place in other European countries. In the UK, the number of holdings with dairy cows dropped progressively from 188,000 in 1960 to 52,000 in 1986 (Fig. 2.1) while the herd size increased from 16 to 60 animals (Fig. 2.2). The number of farms with breeding pigs has fallen by a factor of 5 from 78,400 with an average herd size of 10 in 1967, to 15,700 with an average herd size of 52 by 1987. Since 1950 in one northern German district with a total area of only about 800 km^2, the animal population rose to more than 750,000 pigs (Fig. 2.3) and almost 13 million hens and broilers, thereby creating considerable problems of

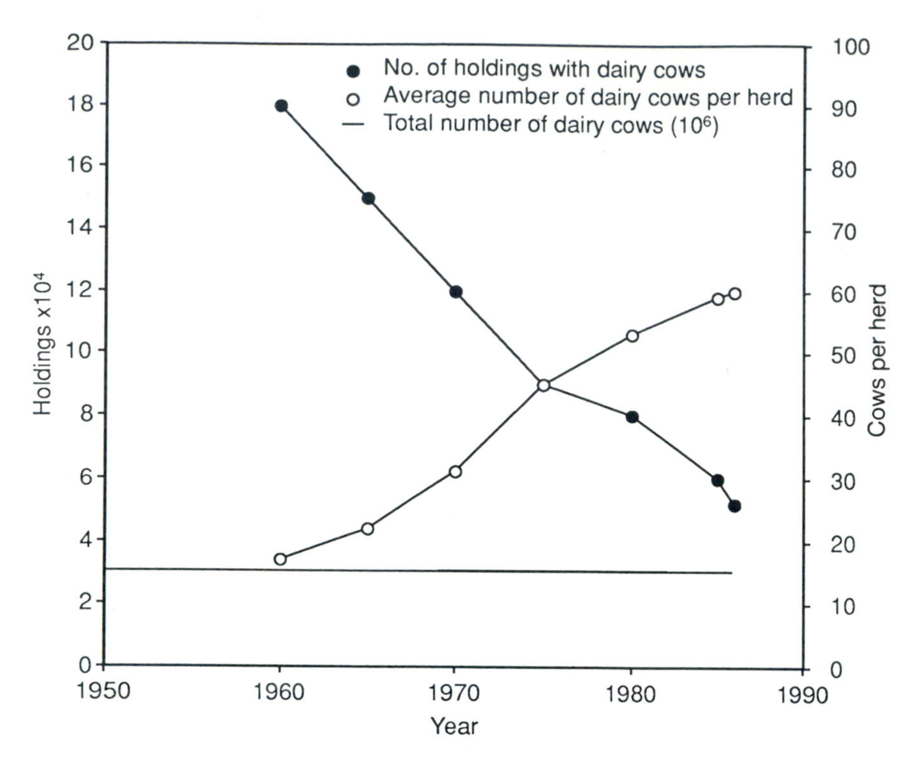

Fig. 2.1. Number of holdings with dairy cows, herd size and total number of cows in UK (after Marks, 1989).

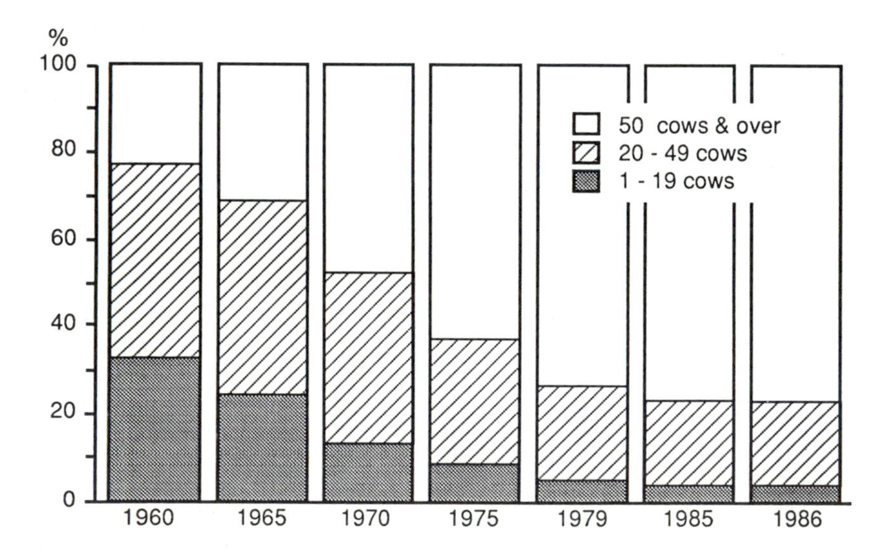

Fig. 2.2. Dairy herd size structure in UK (Marks, 1989).

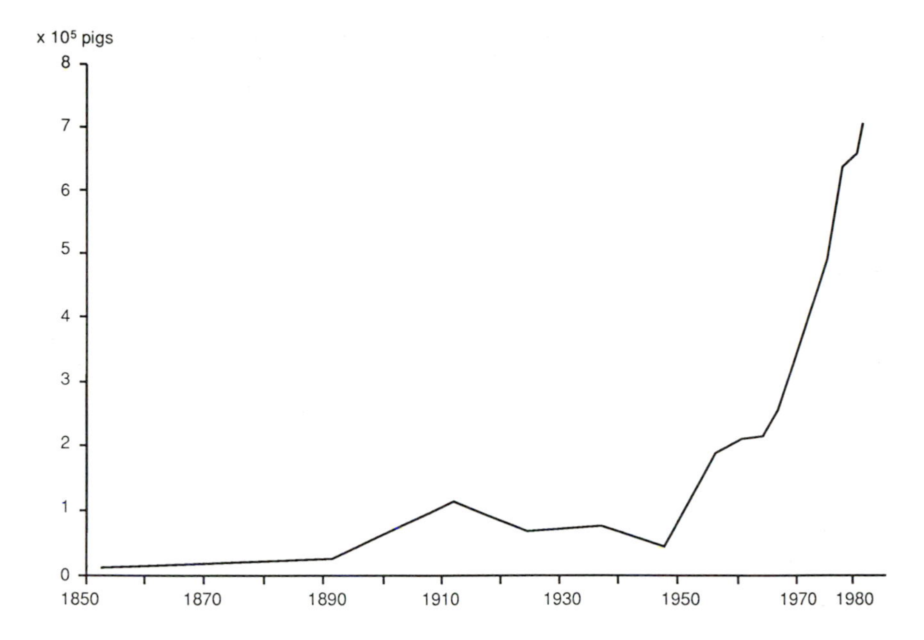

Fig. 2.3. Development of pig production in the district Vechta, North Germany since 1852 (Windhorst, 1984).

manure disposal and spread of diseases between farms (Strauch, 1987). More than 56% of all broilers in the UK are kept today in flocks of 100,000 and over. Under such conditions, the individual animal becomes less important and the treatment of an individual diseased animal is uneconomic. Interest focuses on the whole herd and its average gain or output, not on the fate of the individual animal. Thus, stocking densities of broilers can be raised to 35 $kg\,m^{-2}$ with good economic rewards. Pig units are often run with an airspace of less than 3 m^3 per animal to save investment in insulation and costs of heating. In many units, most classical diseases are well controlled by vaccination programmes and the prophylactic or therapeutic use of drugs via feedstuffs or water.

However, with the change to intensive systems with high animal densities on specialized farms, a change in the character of animal diseases took place. Diseases no longer followed the traditional pattern whereby one specific pathogen provoked clear clinical symptoms with a specific pathology. Intensification also meant that the animal became increasingly dependent on mechanical equipment for mechanical ventilation, feeding and manure removal. The considerable increase in herd size and the close contact between animals favours a quick passage of pathogens, which can lead to an increase in virulence and an increased infection pressure. Some animal breeds are productive but may lack sufficient disease resistance and

Table 2.3. Change of disease in poultry production after intensification.

Before 1960	After 1960
Monocausal infectious epidemics and enzootic infections, e.g. Newcastle disease	Multifactorial, multicausal infectious diseases and mixed infections, e.g. chronic infectious bronchitis
High morbidity and mortality	Morbidity less apparent, lower mortality
Economic losses because of low productivity not so important	High economic losses by drop in productivity

Source: Monreal, 1989.

are sensitive to relatively small perturbation in their artificial environment, such as in temperature or air supply. In contrast to the classical diseases of specific aetiology these new disorders are called multifactorial. Multifactorial diseases changed the pattern of diseases, morbidity, mortality and productivity considerably. Monreal (1989) sees three important differences between poultry production before and after intensification (Table 2.3).

Environmental Health and Multifactorial Diseases

One definition of health (Lapedes, 1978) is 'a state of dynamic equilibrium between an organism and its environment in which all functions of mind and body are normal'. Animal health is the state of an animal which is in dynamic equilibrium with the external conditions and his individual internal status. The animal is free of symptoms of disease or injury, its physiological and biochemical parameters lie in the normal ranges and it shows species-typical behavioural patterns. When health is in some sort of balance between internal and external factors, environmental conditions can decisively tip the balance out of level. Many diseases in modern animal farming are thought to have a direct link to the environment.

One definition of the environment for farm animals is the totality of external physical, chemical and biological factors that affect animal health, welfare and performance. Under natural conditions, this environment is complex, variable and can be hostile at times. Diurnal and geographical variations in temperature, rain and sunlight, may be combined with seasonal shortages of food and water. Animals employ their innate abilities – honed by experience to adapt and cope with these hazards. Furthermore, they are threatened by predators and a range of various parasitic and infectious diseases from which many may suffer or die.

The environment of modern livestock housing is completely different. It is devised and maintained by man and dominated by his needs. Animals have little opportunity to control their environment, e.g. to alter herd or group size or change floor and bedding facilities. However, they are protected against cold, rain and predators, sufficient food and water are supplied regularly and some diseases are immediately treated or prevented by vaccination. Consequently, when disease does occur under these man-made conditions, it may be accounted to man's error or lack of understanding.

The characteristic of a multifactorial disease is that there is a variety of internal and external factors involved and none of the factors alone can produce the disease itself. For this type of disease, the Henle–Koch postulates of causation cannot be applied because disease arises through a combination of infection and environmental stress (Webster, 1982). There are various formulations of the laws of causation, which are applicable to multifactorial infectious and non-infectious diseases. The unified concept of causation by Evans marshals formal epidemiological and other evidence to accumulate a case where a causal hypothesis can be sufficiently probable to

Table 2.4. External factors related to multifactorial diseases.

Housing	**Management**
Type of housing system	Stocking density
Floor	Care and treatment
Bedding	Management system (e.g. all in, all out)
Tethering	Milking system
Manure removal	Medication
Ventilation system	Vaccination
Feed and water supply	Disinfection
	Prophylactic hygiene
Environment	
Physical	**Feed and Water**
Temperature	Quantity
Relative humidity	Quality
Air velocity	Contaminants, e.g. toxins, mycotoxins
Ventilation rate	
Light	
Noise	
Chemical	
Gases	
Biological	
Microorganisms (pathogens)	
Dust	

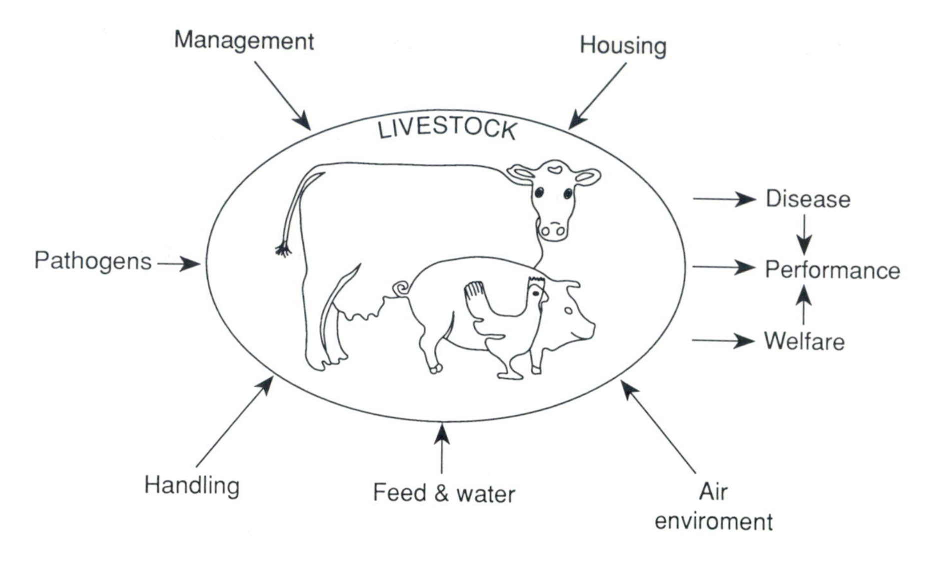

Fig. 2.4. Scheme of the external factors and pathogens acting on performance, health and welfare of livestock.

provide the rational basis for prophylactic and therapeutic measures (see Webster, 1982). Mayr (1984) explains the causation of modern infectious diseases by the relationships between pathogen, host, route of transmission and environment which makes the transition of an infection into a disease possible. The external factors representing the environment include the physical, chemical and biological environment, housing, management, feed and water; the most important factors are listed in Table 2.4. Together with pathogens or facultative pathogens these factors influence well-being, health and performance as shown in Fig. 2.4. A disease, however, will develop only if the 'internal factors' of the animal are unable to respond properly. The most important internal factors are genetic disposition (e.g. lack of resistance or adaptation, hormonal dysfunction) and immunity (e.g. maternal antibodies, immunosuppression) (Mayr, 1984; Monreal, 1989).

The environment also includes the building's structure and fittings. Use of incorrect materials or failure of components can lead to physical trauma and injury (see Chapter 3). Litterless systems with abrasive surfaces may lead to injuries of knees, joints and foot areas (Nilsson, 1992), causing suffering and local infections which may depress growth or milk yield. Poor air quality may enhance the growth of mycoplasma and other facultative pathogens and lead to pneumonia. Multifactorial diseases can be separated into infectious and non-infectious diseases and disorders such as atrophic rhinitis and lameness respectively (Webster, 1982). Both can lead to significant losses in productivity and even death; the most important are summarized in Table 2.5.

Table 2.5. Common multifactorial infectious diseases of farm animals attributed in major part to the housing environment.

		Factors implicated in causation	
Host	Disease	Pathogens	Environment
Cattle	Pneumonia 'Shipping Fever'	*Mycoplasma bovis, dispar* RSV, PI3 *P. haemolytica*, etc.	Crowding, poor feeding, changes, high relative humidity, 'stress'
	Environmental mastitis	*E. coli, Strep.uberis*	Contaminated bedding, stage of lactation
Pigs	Atrophic rhinitis Enzootic pneumonia	*Bordetella bronchiseptica* *Pasteurella multocida* *Mycoplasma suipneumoniae*	Crowding, poor ventilation, poor drainage, high relative humidity
	Diarrhoea	Rotavirus, *E. coli*, etc.	Weaning, hygiene, cold
Poultry	Infectious bronchitis Mycoplasmosis	IB virus *Mycoplasma* spp.	High temperatures, poor ventilation, high gas and dust levels, low humidity, lack of vitamin A, high stocking density
Horses	Obstructive pulmonary disease	*Micropolyspora faeni* *Aspergillus fumigatus*	Dusty feed and bedding, poor ventilation

Sources: Webster, 1985; Monreal, 1989.

There are numerous other diseases in farm animals which can be attributed to the environment, such as reticuloperitonitis traumatica and tail tip necrosis in cattle. Reticuloperitonitis occurs when a ruminant ingests a sharp edged foreign body, often a piece of metal, which is indigestible and does not pass through the rumen system. The foreign body remains in the reticulum and damages the stomach integument or can even penetrate the stomach wall and irritate the nearby pericardium. Usually the only way to remove the foreign body is by rumenotomy which is hazardous and reduces yield. The likely ingestion of foreign bodies is influenced by a variety of factors, including the type and frequency of feeding, feeding behaviour, age, yield and even the season (Table 2.6). Reticuloperitonitis can be avoided in part by careful preparation of feed and feeding several times per day to

Table 2.6. Environmental factors lowering or increasing the risk of reticuloperitonitis traumatica in cattle.

	Influence	
Factors	Protective	Harmful
Type of feed	Fresh green feed	Long fibre roughage
Frequency of feeding	High	Low
Husbandry	Grazing	All year indoors
Intake	Slow, small bites	Hasty
State of production	Dry cow Alternative rearing	High-yielding cow Intensive rearing
Age	< 2 years	> 2 years
Season	Summer, autumn	Winter, spring

Source: Stöber, 1989.

reduce hasty feed intake. Animals, which are older than two years, and high milking cows, which are kept all year indoors are most at risk (Stöber, 1989). Careful harvesting and processing of fodder is essential.

Tail tip necrosis occurs mainly in fattening bulls, which are loose housed on damaged, dirty concrete. Traumatic injuries of the tail lead to infection by various opportunistic bacteria. The critical animal density for fattening bulls of about 250kg liveweight lies between 160 and 210 $kg\,m^{-2}$ (Madsen and Nielsen, 1985). The most important environmental factors which increase or decrease the risk of disease are given in Table 2.7. Behavioural factors play a role too. At high animal densities the lower ranked animals are forced to move more often and can find laying space in the busiest and uncomfortable areas only. These animals are in particular prone to trauma at their resting place and they are also more likely to traumatize other animals because they are walking around more often. Animals which keep their tail close to their body when lying down show a lower incidence of injuries. This behaviour is likely to change when the air temperatures increase above comfortable levels. The simplest means of prevention is to reduce animal density which avoids unrest, unfavourably high temperatures and extensive soiling of the floor surfaces (Stöber, 1989). Productivity is not necessarily reduced because the daily weight gain and net return per animal are higher in moderately stocked pens (Blom, 1992).

In pig fattening production it is estimated that more than half of the overall losses (18%) are attributed to multifactorial infectious diseases

Table 2.7. Environmental factors lowering or increasing the risk of tip of tail necrosis in beef cattle.

	Influence	
Factors	Protective	Harmful
Animal density	$< 185\ kg\,m^{-2}$	$> 185\ kg\,m^{-2}$
Mean monthly indoor temperature	< 18°C	> 18°C
Floor surface	Slats with dry, clean, smooth edges	Slats with old, slippery, wet, soiled, sharp, broken edges
Feed	Rich in roughage	Succulent feed, silage
Rumination	High	Reduced
Faeces	Thick, pulpy	Soft, liquid

Source: Stöber, 1989.

(Bollwahn, 1989). However, disease and death will happen only if defence mechanisms are compromised. Because of the complexity of external and internal factors, which can vary significantly for the different species and husbandry conditions, it is useful to concentrate on the most important factors associated with multifactorial disease. These are: (i) air quality and indoor climate; (ii) housing and bedding; (iii) management and handling; (iv) environmental stress.

Air quality, indoor climate and disease

For housed animals the quality of the air is of considerable importance because the animal's respiratory and integumentary systems are in continuous contact with the air, which often contains numerous pollutants in various combinations and concentrations.

There are many examples indicating a direct relationship between incidence of respiratory disease and the air environment. In an early epidemiological study, Tielen (1977) showed that the incidence of pneumonia in 25,000 Dutch slaughtered pigs is distinctly higher in winter and spring than in summer and early autumn (Fig. 2.5). Ventilation rates in the cooler months are inevitably slow to conserve heat: the net result is poor air quality, especially high concentrations of ammonia and airborne dust, to which young pigs are particularly sensitive. Further evidence for the role of air quality in respiratory disease comes from the work of Dührsen (1982). A

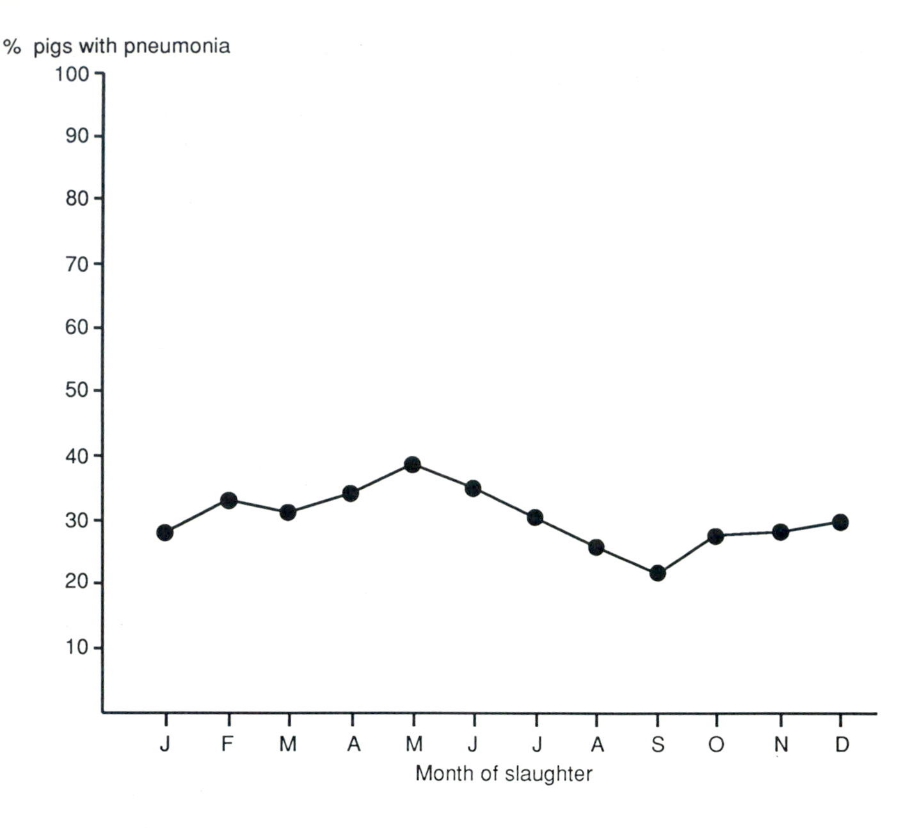

Fig. 2.5. Pneumonia in 25,000 slaughtered pigs (%) (Tielen, 1977).

high incidence of coughing on pig fattening farms was associated with high airborne bacteria concentrations, measured by sedimentation plates in colony-forming units (12 $cfu\,cm^{-2}min^{-1}$) and airborne dust levels (43 particles per cm^3) compared with controls in farms where hygiene was better (9 $cfu\,cm^{-2}min^{-1}$, and 13 particles per cm^3 respectively).

Gases and dust are the most important components of the aerial environment. In piggeries which were vacuum cleaned regularly once a week, the prevalence of pneumonia and other respiratory diseases dropped considerably (Table 2.8; Nilsson, 1984). A recent review of the effect of airborne particulates on livestock health and performance (Hartung, 1994) showed that dust and microorganisms in animal house air can lead to a mechanical irritation of the respiratory tract, specific infections, reduced resistance to infection and allergic disease and even toxic effects by bacterial and fungal toxins are possible (Table 2.9; Zeitler, 1988). More detailed information on air hygiene is given in Chapter 6.

Draught is often cited as one of the climatic stressors in pig housing. Under controlled conditions weaner pigs, aged 5 to 10 weeks were exposed

Table 2.8. Influence of dust vacuum cleaning on respiratory diseases in pigs at slaughter. Percentage of pigs showing disease.

Disease	No cleaning (770 pigs)	Vacuum cleaning (776 pigs)
Pneumonia	25.2%	9.4%
Pleuritis	6.9%	1.4%
Pericarditis	1.3%	1.0%
Perihepatitis	3.4%	1.7%

Source: Nilsson, 1984.

for 5 h each day to a draught of 0.99 ± $0.2 m s^{-1}$; in the control group the air velocity was $0.2 m s^{-1}$. Air temperature during the first 3 days was set at 24°C, 21°C for the next 17 days and 20°C thereafter. The relative humidity was 70%, ammonia concentration was below 10 ppm and carbon dioxide was below 0.2 vol %. Figure 2.6 shows that coughing in the experimental group increased significantly ($P \leq 0.05$) at about 20 days after start of draught. The frequency of coughing and sneezing was recorded during the first ten minutes after entering each room. It may be suggested that coughing and sneezing receptors in the upper respiratory tract were more frequently activated by the intermittent exposure to cold, dry air, acting as a stimulus, than in the control group. Table 2.10 shows that under random, intermittent draughts the incidence of sneezing, the number of pigs suffering from diarrhoea and the occurrence of ear lesions increased and the daily gain was lower compared with the control (Scheepens, 1991). Similar

Table 2.9. Possible influences of dust, microorganisms and gases on animal health.

Factor	Effect on the animal
High dust levels	Mechanical irritation and overloading of lung clearance; lesions of the mucous membranes
Specific microorganisms	Infectious disease
Dust, microorganisms + gases	Non-specific effects: defence mechanisms stressed and reduced resistance
Microorganisms + dust	Allergies: hypersensitivity reaction
Microorganisms + dust	Toxic effects: intoxication by bacterial/fungal toxins

Source: After Zeitler, 1988.

Table 2.10. Number of animals with clinical symptoms and decrease in daily gain of weaner pigs exposed to random, intermittent draught when compared to optimal housed weaners as a control. Both groups with $n = 45$ pigs.

	Sneezing	Diarrhoea	Ear lesions	Daily gain
Control	21	3	8	–
Intermittent draught	40	11	24	41 g/d
	($P < 0.001$)	($P < 0.005$)	($P < 0.005$)	($P < 0.05$)

Source: Scheepens, 1991.

results were reported by Mount and Start (1980). In contrast, Jacobsen *et al.* (1988) found no difference in growth performance when subjecting four-week-old weaned piglets to continuous (0.5 $m\,s^{-1}$; 25°C) or intermittent draught for four weeks. Verhagen (1987) assumes that the piglets acclimate within the first six days of such exposure to, for example, fluctuating temperatures (15–25°C) and no significant decrease in growth occurs.

It seems crucial for experiments like this that identical conditions of temperature and relative humidity can be established both in the control group and in the experimental group. The thermal demand of the animals is changing not only with decreasing temperatures but also with increasing relative humidity enhancing the cooling effect under draughts. It seems that animals which had not adapted to intermittent draughts are more prone to diseases, respiratory infections in particular, which may give rise to loss of appetite, decreased feed intake and, consequently, loss of performance and growth.

Under practical conditions, draught can often be caused by an insufficient air volume per animal at fast ventilation rates. There is clear evidence that small air volumes are associated with a high prevalence of lung disease (Table 2.11, Christiaens, 1987). Hilliger (1990) gives recommendations for minimum air volumes for various farm animals (Table 2.12). The smaller the air volume per animal the higher the requirements for the ventilation system and the more likely management failures increase risk of disease outbreaks.

The role of microbial pathogens acting with other factors, such as thermal and physical stress, has been demonstrated by Neumann (1988). Piglets were infected intranasally with *Pasteurella multocida* and then subjected to swimming exercise in cold water at 15°C for 5 to 70 minutes per day from 6 to 20 days of age. The daily liveweight gain was lowest in the infected experimentally cold-stressed group (Fig. 2.7). Fourteen days after nasal inoculation 39 of 42 thermo-physical stressed piglets developed a pneumonia compared with 7 of 38 in the infected unstressed controls.

Enzootic pneumonia in cattle is associated with a variety of factors

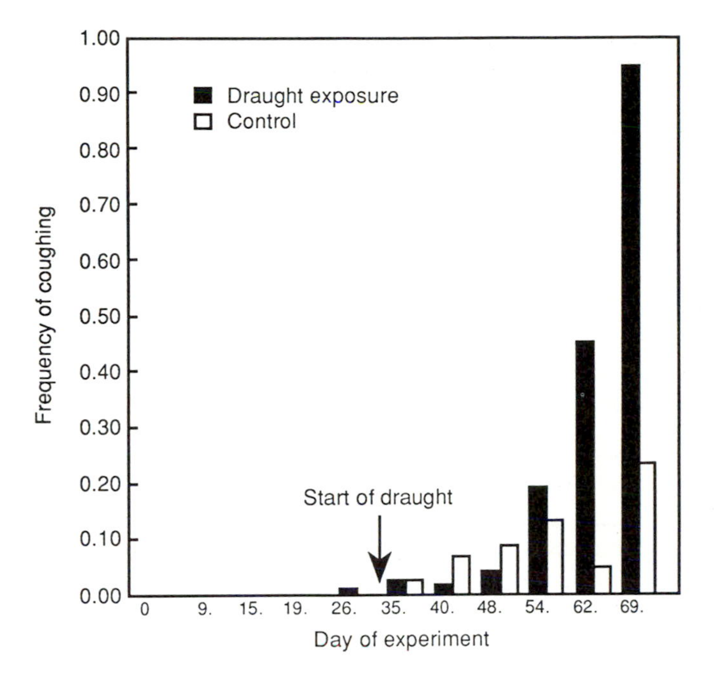

Fig. 2.6. Frequency of coughing in pigs exposed to daily draughts (Scheepens, 1991).

which can increase disease susceptibility (Stöber, 1989). These include high body weight in fast growing beef cattle or transport shipping fever, crowding and transit through several markets, aggressive encounters to establish social ranking in the group, change of animal house and group, high stocking densities, change of feed, variation in climatic conditions and air quality, immunosuppression by other infectious microorganisms, vaccination by live vaccines (e.g. BVD virus) and treatment with corticosteroids. An infection will happen only if the defence mechanisms of the

Table 2.11. Prevalence of affected lungs in 66 piggeries in relation to the air volume of the animal house.

Number of pig houses	Average volume (m^3 per pig)	Affected lungs (%)
30	3.6	< 25
20	3.3	25–35
16	3.1	> 35

Source: Christiaens, 1987.

Table 2.12. Minimum requirements for air volume per animal.

Animal type	Air volume (m^3 per animal)
Milking and dry cows	18
Heifers and beef	16
Calf (< 12 weeks)	5–8
Sow with litter	20
Sow without litter	7
Weaner (20 kg)	1
Fattening pig (100 kg)	3.5
Laying hen (floor keeping)	0.35
Laying hen (battery cages)	0.15
Horse	30

Source: Hilliger, 1990.

animal's respiratory tract such as surfactant factor, the clearance mechanism of bronchi and trachea, the cellular defence (macrophages, neutrophil granulocytes, lymphocytes, etc.) and the secretion of immunoglobulins (IgA, IgG) are impaired.

Housing and bedding

Mastitis is caused by microorganisms which penetrate the teat canal into the udder. Their origins are the housing environment, such as bedding or floor, or the milking machine. Floor type and the quality of bedding material have been shown to be important (Ekesbo, 1970). Loose housing and tie-stall barns with straw bedding have a lower incidence of teat injuries (1.4 and 3.9% respectively) and mastitis (6.8 and 8.6% respectively) than buildings without bedding material (10 and 17% respectively). Sawdust can be contaminated heavily with opportunistic bacterial pathogens (Schmidt *et al.*, 1985).

In tie-stall barns, mastitis and teat injuries seem to increase in particular when short stalls are used and stall partitions are inadequate, so that the teats of lying cows can be injured by the claws of their neighbours. However, only 20–25% of the variability in udder health between housing types may be attributed to environmental factors and other factors such as management, milking and genetic breed and improvement may play a considerable role. Hamann (1989) proposes a direct link between milk yield and resistance to mastitis (Fig. 2.8). With increasing milk yield, a reduction of local and systematic defence mechanisms can be observed. This may help to explain the higher incidence of mastitis in the early stage of lactation. The risk of mastitis also increases with age and udder forms which are less suitable for machine milking (Konermann, 1992).

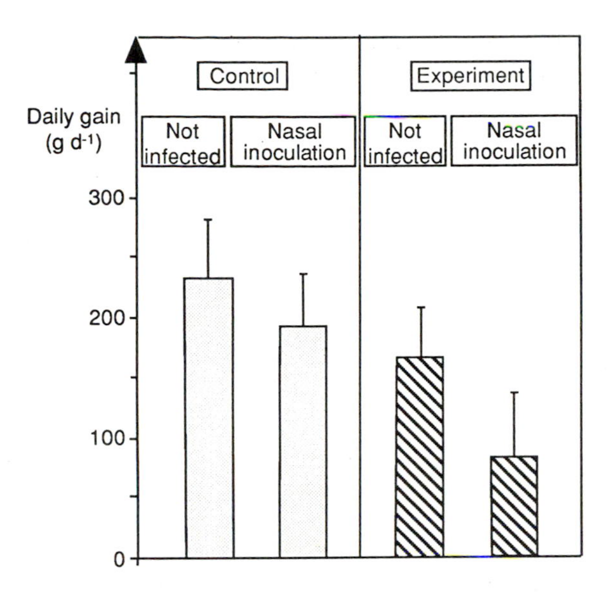

Fig. 2.7. Daily gain ($g\,d^{-1}$) of weaner pigs subjected to thermo-physical stress by swimming with and without intranasal infection by *Pasteurella multocida* (Carter type A) (Neumann, 1988).

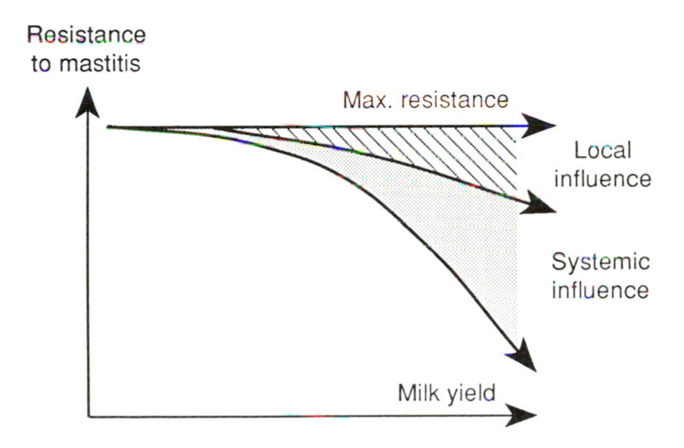

Fig. 2.8. Model of milk yield and resistance to mastitis (Hamann, 1989).

The teat is regularly contaminated by microorganisms but an infection of the udder takes place less than once per cow and lactation period. Biological, chemical and physical mechanisms act together and form a 'barrier' which prevents most infections. This barrier consists predominantly of five components which may vary according to the breed and genetics, the number and stage of lactations, and anatomical and physiological factors, e.g. the morphology of the teat, the teat canal diameter, the keratin layer of the teat canal, and muscle tension and the blood supply.

The morphology of the teat, together with the position of the blood vessels in the teat and its blood supply, are the fundamental defences of the teat canal. The tonus of the smooth muscle, the width of the test canal and the keratin cell layer contribute to this mechanism; tight closure of the teat canal by the teat muscles lowers the risk of microbial invasion. If an oedema of the udder occurs, for example at the beginning of the lactation period, then the blood supply can be insufficient and the barrier mechanisms impaired. Keratinization of the teat canal may also be incomplete after calving (Hamann, 1989).

Management and handling

The regime of stock supply and the use of quarantine facilities may also increase the risk of disease (Table 2.13). When animals are reared from a farmer's own stock then the risk of infectious disease is low because the animals have experience of the farm's microbial populations and a general herd immunity develops. When animals are supplied from off-farm sources, then the risk increases with the number of suppliers. All-in, all-out systems decrease the spread of disease because proper cleaning and disinfection procedures can be applied before the new animals arrive on the farm. Continuous systems should only be operated with quarantine facilities so that new animals may be observed and treated if necessary (Lotthammer, 1989).

Handling of animals, by farmers and stockmen – often referred to as the human factor – can affect performance and health. Aversive handling of pigs can reduce growth rate and reproduction and increase piglet mortality (Table 2.14). However, it seemed that the consistency of handling may be as crucial as its exact nature (Seabrook and Bartle, 1992).

Table 2.13. Risk of disease under different regimes of stock management.

Management	Risk of disease
Closed system (own stock)	–
Stock from one source	+
Stock supplied via dealers/markets	++
All-in, all-out system	–
Continuous system with quarantine	+
Continuous system without quarantine	+++

+ risk increased.

Table 2.14. The effects of handling treatments on the performance of pigs in experimental conditions.

	Handling treatments	
Performance criteria	Pleasant	Aversive
Growth rate 0–4 weeks (kg day^{-1})		
Study 1	0.205	0.192
Study 2	0.533	0.509
Study 3	0.656	0.641
Study 4	0.779	0.733
Study 5	0.455	0.404
Study 6	0.897	0.837
Study 7	0.709	0.669
Age of first detected oestrus (days)	169.0	171.8
Pregnancy rate (%)	88	33
Age for fully coordinated male mating response (days)	161	193
Piglets born alive per farrowing	10.1	9.3
Piglet mortality at 3 weeks (%)	11.1	15.2

Source: Seabrook and Bartle, 1992.

Environmental stress and disease

The term stress has attracted much attention since Selye described his general adaptation syndrome in the 1930s. However, a generally accepted definition is not yet available (Youssef, 1988). To some, stress is all factors of the environment which can damage or disturb an animal; to others, stress is the response to a challenge or it is the inability to cope with environmental demands (Ewbank, 1992). Selye (1974) proposed that stress is the non-specific response of the organism to any demand made upon it. Archer (1979) sees stress as the prolonged inability to remove sources of potential danger, leading to activation of systems beyond their range of maximum efficiency. In a similar way, Ewbank (1992) restricts stress to substantial responses to a noxious or potentially noxious stimulus. All relatively high levels of stressors which damage the animal and which cause suffering are termed distress or overstress (Ewbank, 1992), creating three classes of stress, e.g. stress that is low level and fully adaptive, overstress that is moderate level and probably adaptive, and distress that is high level with suffering.

In general terms, the concept of stress comprises the non-specific bodily response to a variety of environmental stimuli starting with the initial alarm reaction including the fight and flight response, followed by the state of resistance and possibly ending in the state of exhaustion. A stimulus is recognized by the organs of sense and stimulates the hypothalamus in the central nervous system where the adrenal medulla (sympathetic nervous system) will be activated and will immediately secrete adrenaline or noradrenaline into the blood. As a consequence, heart rate increases, blood sugar levels rise and the blood is redistributed from skin and viscera to muscles and brain in order to enable emergency reactions (flight or fight). At the same time corticotrophin releasing factor is produced, which stimulates the pituitary gland to form ACTH (corticotrophin) to initiate the formation and release of corticosteroids, e.g. such as cortisol from the adrenal cortex, which are seen as the adaptation hormones and have anti-inflammatory properties (resistance phase).

However, it seems possible that a chronic stressor may induce a corticosteroid response without an obvious flight or fight reaction. Prolonged stress response can lead to exhaustion of the adrenal cortex and impairment of the adaptative processes; if insufficient corticosteroids are produced the resistance of the organisms against the stressor is diminished. This can also have a negative effect on the infectious–defence mechanisms of animals. Long-term effects of this depletion can be as follows (Ewbank, 1992): structural damage, e.g. gastric ulceration, interference with immune function, decrease of growth, impairment of reproduction and changes in behaviour or even signs of suffering.

The quantification of stress remains difficult. The response of an animal to a stressor always takes place within species-related and individual limits. Biochemical, physiological and behavioural measurements and observations have to be evaluated within these limits (Dantzer and Mormede, 1983; Jasmin and Cantim, 1991). The biochemical investigations of stress hormones, such as catecholamines and corticosteroids (De Roth *et al.*, 1989; Shaw and Tume, 1992), reveal large individual variations. Therefore, it is necessary to combine endocrinological investigations with physiological and ethological measurements (Ladewig and von Borell, 1988). In addition, knowledge about the genetically-determined stress resistance of the animals under investigation is necessary (De Roth *et al.*, 1989).

Even with the above-mentioned combination of measurements it will be difficult to prove an exhaustion of the adaptative capacity of an animal in practice if clinical pathological symptoms are absent. But it is this pre-pathological phase (Moberg, 1987) which we must understand better. Today, measuring techniques are available which are able to monitor continuously body temperature and heart rate and which can take automatically multiple blood samples at various times without imposing a sampling stress. This may help to characterize the importance of single stresses in complex environments.

In agreement with Ewbank (1992), it seems useful to restrict the usage of the term stress and to specify in all investigations the distresses clearly with respect to type, intensity and duration and to try to indicate the severity of the stress response. This understanding may help us to create housing systems for farm animals, which are both suitable for the animals and acceptable for the farmer's economic needs. However, there will always exist some conflict between the various needs of animals and their keepers.

Conclusions

As a consequence of intensification of farm animal production, multifactorial diseases may occur which can cause suffering and economic losses. Housing conditions, management and handling of animals are the most important environmental factors which contribute to the development of these modern diseases. In order to improve these factors, it is necessary to define and quantify their separate contributions to environmental diseases. This may enable us to avoid those factors which cause the greatest harm. For example, there are no threshold levels for air pollutants. With regard to housing – but also in relation to other environmental factors – more attention should be paid to the animal's preferences in establishing housing environments and husbandry systems which are animal centred rather than man orientated. Although this concept may have some drawbacks because animals may not always choose in their long-term interests, it is a logical way to create new animal husbandry systems. Initial trends in this direction can be seen in the introduction of loose barns, outdoor pig and poultry units and the Louisiana-type broiler house, which give animals more freedom to move and make choices in a richer environment. A better understanding of the mechanisms of stress response in farm animals will also contribute to the development of animal-centred environments. New technical developments in animal farming, such as fully automated milking systems for cows (Frost *et al.*, 1993) and stress-free weighing facilities for pigs by image analysis techniques (Schofield, 1990), may give way to animal friendly, and at the same time, economic developments.

References

Archer, J. (1979) *Animals under Stress.* Edward Arnold, London.

Bergmann, V. and Scheer, J. (1979) Ökonomisch bedeutungsvolle Verlustursachen beim Schlachtgeflügel (Economically important losses in broiler production). *Mh. Vet.-Med.* 34, 543–547.

Blom, J.Y. (1992) Environment-dependent disease. In: Phillips, C. and Piggins, D. (eds), *Farm Animals and the Environment.* CAB International, Wallingford, UK, pp. 263–287.

Bollwahn, W. (1989) Infektiöse Faktorenkrankheiten beim Schwein (Infectious factorial diseases in pigs – pathogenesis and control). In: *Pathogenesis and Control of Factorial Diseases.* Proceedings 18th Congress, Deutsche Veterinärmedizinische Gesellschaft, Giessen, Bad Nauheim, pp. 59–67.

Christiaens, J.P.A. (1987) Gas concentrations and thermal features of the animal environment with respect to respiratory diseases in pig and poultry. In: Bruce, J.M. and Sommer, M. (eds), *Agriculture: Environmental Aspects of Respiratory Disease in Intensive Pig and Poultry Houses, Including the Implications for Human Health.* Proceedings of a meeting in Aberdeen 29–30 October 1986, Commission of the European Communities EUR 10820 EN, 29–43.

Dantzer, R. and Mormede, P. (1983) Stress in farm animals: a need for reevaluation. *Journal of Animal Science* 57, 6–18.

De Roth L., Vermette, L., Blouin, A. and Lariviere, N. (1989) Blood catecholamines in response to handling in normal and stress-susceptible swine. *Applied Animal Behaviour Science* 22, 11–16.

Dührsen, H.H. (1982) Vergleichende Prüfung mehrerer Stalluft- und Stallbaumerkmale von 20 Schweinemastställen im Landkreis Dithmarschen in je drei Jahreszeiten unter Berücksichtigung der Hustenhäufigkeit. (Comparison of some air quality parameters in 20 pig fattening units in the district Dithmarschen at three seasons in relation to the frequency of coughing). Diss. Vet. Med. (Thesis) Hannover.

Ekesbo, I. (1970) Traditional and modern barn environments related to animal health and welfare. Proceedings 11th Nordiske Veterinarkongres, Bergen, pp. 56–63.

Elbers, A.R.W. (1991) The use of slaughterhouse information in monitoring systems for herd health control in pigs. Thesis University of Utrecht, Netherlands.

Ewbank, R. (1992) Stress: a general overview. In: Phillips, C. and Piggins, D. (eds), *Farm Animals and the Environment.* CAB International, Wallingford, UK, pp. 255–262.

Frost, A.R., Street, M.J. and Hall, R.C. (1993) The development of a pneumatic robot for attaching a milking machine to a cow. *Mechatronics* 3, 409–418.

Guarda, F., Tezzo, G. and Bianchi, C. (1980) Sulla frequenza e natura delle lesioni osservate in broilers al macello (On frequency and kind of lesions observed in broilers at slaughter). *Clinica Veterinaria* 103, 437–439.

Hamann, J. (1989) Faktoren der Genese boviner subklinischer Mastitiden (Factors of the genesis of bovine sub-clinical mastitis). In: *Pathogenesis and Control of Factorial Diseases.* Proceedings 18th Congress, Deutsche Veterinärmedizinsche Gesellschaft, Giessen, Bad Nauheim, pp. 45–53.

Hartung, J. (1994) The effect of airborne particulates on livestock health and production. In: Ap Dewi, I., Axford, R.F.E., Fayez M. Marai, I. and Omed, H. (eds), *Pollution in Livestock Production Systems.* CAB International, Wallingford, UK, pp. 55–69.

Hellmers, B. (1986) Todesursachen bei Schweinen (Causes of deaths in pigs). Diss. Vet. Med. (Thesis), Hannover.

Hilliger, H.G. (1990) *Stallgebäude, Stalluft und Lüftung (Housing, air and ventilation).* Ferdinand Enke Verlag, Stuttgart.

Jacobson, L.D., Boedicker, J.J., Janni, K.A. and Noyes, E. (1988) *Performance and Immune Response of Nursery Piglets to Fluctuating Air Temperatures and Drafts.* Proceedings of the third international livestock environmental symposium, Toronto, Ontario, Canada, pp. 109–116.

Jasmin, G. and Cantim, M. (1991) Stress revisited: Neuroendocrinology of stress. In:

Jasmin, G. (ed.), *Methods and Achievements in Experimental Pathology*, Vol 14. Verlag Karger, Basel, pp. 1–174.

Konermann, H. (1992) Eutererkrankungen des Rindes – Ursachen und Bekämpfungsmöglichkeiten (Mastitis in cattle – aetiology and control). In: *Milchviehhaltung* (*Dairy Production*). Landwirtschaftsverlag Münster. Baubriefe Landwirtschaft 33, 12–20.

Ladewig, J. and von Borell, E. (1988) Ethological methods alone are not sufficient to measure the impact of environment on animal health and animal wellbeing. In: Unshelm, J., van Putten, G., Zeeb, K. and Ekesbo, I. (eds), *Proceedings of the International Congress on Applied Ethology in Farm Animals*. Skara 1988, KTBL, Darmstadt, pp. 95–102.

Lapedes, D.N. (ed.) (1978) *McGraw-Hill Dictionary of Scientific and Technical Terms*. McGraw-Hill Book Company, New York, London.

Lotthammer, K.H. (1989) Tierärztliche Aspekte der Kälberaufzucht and Rindermast (Veterinary aspects of calf rearing and beef production). In: *Kälberaufzucht, Jungviehhaltung, Rindermast* (*Calf and Heifer Rearing, Beef Production*). Landwirtschaftsverlag Münster. Baubriefe Landwirtschaft 31, 12–17.

Madsen, E.B. and Nielsen, K. (1985) A study of tail tip necrosis in young fattening bulls on slatted floors. *Nordisk Veterinaermedicin* 37, 349–357.

Marks, H.F. (1989) In: Britton, D.K. (ed.) *A Hundred Years of British Food and Farming*. Taylor and Francis, London, New York, Philadelphia.

Mayr, A. (1984) Allgemeine Infektions- und Seuchenlehre (Principles of infection and epidemics). In: Mayr, M. (ed.) *Medizinische Mikrobiologie, Infektions- und Seuchenlehre* (*Medical Microbiology, Infection and Epidemics*). Ferdinand Enke Verlag, Stuttgart, pp. 1–42.

Moberg, G.P, (1987) Problems in defining stress and distress in animals. *Journal of the American Veterinary Association* 191, 1207–1211.

Monreal, G. (1989) Infektöse Faktorenkrankheiten beim Geflügel (Infectious factorial diseases in poultry) In: *Pathogenesis and Control of Factorial Diseases*. Proceedings 18th Congress, Deutsche Veterinärmedizinische Gesellschaft, Giessen, Bad Nauheim, pp. 180–192.

Mount, L.E. and Start, I.B. (1980) A note on the effect of forced air movement and environmental temperature on weight gain in the pig after weaning. *Animal Production*. 30, 295–298.

Neumann, R. (1988) Der Schwimmtest für Saugferkel als Grundbelastungsmodell zur Untersuchung der Wirkung der Umwelt auf die Infektionsabwehr unter besonderer Berücksichtigung der experimentellen Infektion des Atmungstraktes. (The swim test for suckling pigs as model to investigate the effect of the environment on infect defense with particular respect to the artificial infection of the respiratory tract.) Thesis Vet. Med. University Leipzig.

Nilsson, C. (1984) Experiences with different methods of dust reduction in pig houses. In: Hilliger, H.G. (ed.), *Dust in Animal Houses*. Proceedings of German Vet. Association, 13–14 March, Hannover, pp. 90–91.

Nilsson, C. (1992) Walking and lying surfaces in livestock houses. In: Phillips, C. and Piggins, D. (eds), *Farm Animals and the Environment*. CAB International, Wallingford, UK, pp. 93–110.

Papasolomontos, P.A., Appleby, E.C. and Mayor, O.Y. (1969) Pathological findings in condemned chickens: A survey of 1000 carcases. *Veterinary Record* 85, 459–464.

Scheepens, C.J.M. (1991) Effects of draught as climatic stressor on the health status of weaned pigs. Thesis University of Utrecht, Netherlands.

Schmidt, M., Jørgensen, M., Møller-Madsen, A.A., Jensen, H., Horvath, Z., Keller, P. and Konggaard, S.P. (1985) Straw bedding for dairy cows. Report 593 from the National Institute of Animal Science, Copenhagen.

Schofield, C.P. (1990) Evaluation of image analysis as a means of estimating the weight of pigs. *Journal of Agricultural Engineering Research*, 47, 287–296.

Seabrook, M.F. and Bartle, N.C. (1992) Human factors. In: Phillips, C. and Piggins, D. (eds), *Farm Animals and the Environment*. CAB International, Wallingford, UK, pp. 111–125.

Selye, H. (1974) *Stress without Distress*. Lippincott, Philadelphia.

Shaw, F.D. and Tume, R.K. (1992) The assessment of pre-slaughter and slaughter treatments of livestock by measurement of plasma constitutents – a review of recent work. *Meat Science* 32, 311–329.

Sommer, H. (1991) Spezielle Hygiene Schwein (Special hygiene of pigs). In: Sommer, H., Greul, E. and Muller, W. *Hygiene der Rinder- und Schweineproduktion* (*Hygiene in Cattle and Pig Production*). Verlag Eugen Ulmer, Stuttgart, pp. 289–392.

Stöber, M. (1989) Zur Pathogenese multifaktoriell bedingter Krankheiten aus buiatrisch-klinischer Sicht (Pathogenesis of multifactorial diseases from the point of view of bovine medicine). In: *Pathogenesis and Control of Factorial Diseases*. Proceedings 18th Congress, Deutsche. Veterinärmedizinische Gesellschaft, Giessen, Bad Nauheim, pp. 19–35.

Strauch, D. (1987) Hygiene of animal waste management. In: Strauch, D. (ed.), *Animal Production and Animal Health*. Elsevier Science Publisher BV, Amsterdam, pp. 155–202.

Tielen, M.J.M. (1977) Stallklima und Tiergesundheit in Schweinemastbetrieben (Indoor climate and animal health in fattening piggeries). Publication of the Animal Health Office in Nord-Brabant, Boxtel, Netherlands.

Valentin, A., Bergmann, V., Scheer, J., Tschirch, I. and Leps, H. (1988) Tierverluste und Qualitätsminderungen durch Hauterkrankungen bei Schlachtgeflügel (Dead losses and losses of meat quality by skin disease in broilers). *Mh. Vet. -Med.* 43, 686–690.

Verhagen, J.M.F. (1987) Acclimation of growing pigs to climatic environment. PhD Thesis Agricultural University of Wageningen, The Netherlands, 128pp.

Webster, A.J.F. (1982) Improvements of environment, husbandry and feeding. In: Smith, H. and Payne, J.M. (eds), *The Control of Infectious Diseases in Farm Animals*. British Veterinary Association Trust, London, pp. 28–36.

Webster, A.J.F. (1985) Animal health and the housing environment. In: *Animal Health and Productivity*. Royal Agricultural Society of England, pp. 227–242.

Windhorst (1984) Ein neues Bild der Landwirtschaft (A new view of agriculture). In: Windhorst, H.W. (ed.), *Der Agrarwirtschaftsraum Oldenburg im Wandel* (*Agricultural Economy of Oldenburg in Changing Times*). Die Violette Reihe, No. 3, Vechtaer Druckerei und Verlag GmbH, Vechta, pp. 9–18.

Youssef, M.K. (1988) Animal stress and strain: definition and measurements. *Applied Animal Behaviour Science* 20, 119–126.

Zeitler, M. (1988) Hygienifische Bedeutung des Staubes- und Keimgehaltes der Stalluft (Hygienic significance of dust and bacteria in animal house air). *Bayerisches Landwirtschaftliches Jahrbuch* 65, 151–165.

3 Comfort and Injury

A.J.F. WEBSTER
Department of Clinical Veterinary Science,
University of Bristol, UK

All houses for livestock represent a compromise between cost, operating convenience and animal performance, itself defined by productivity, health and welfare. It is often assumed that these latter three objectives always go together – 'if the animals weren't happy/healthy they wouldn't grow so well'. There are, however, too many exceptions to this rule for our own comfort, many of which relate to the problem of chronic discomfort or the pain of chronic injury. There is good evidence, for example, that breeding females can sustain economic levels of production when suffering from bone fractures (laying hens: Gregory *et al.*, 1990), pressure sores (breeding sows: Penny *et al.*, 1963; Smith and Robertson, 1971) or severe foot damage (sheep, dairy cows: Wierenga and Peterse, 1987).

Comfort and freedom from injury constitute two of the 'five freedoms' (Webster, 1984, 1989a) which underpin the MAFF Codes of Welfare for Livestock. The designers of farm buildings have always given great attention to the control of air temperature. They have also sought to avoid injurious fixtures and fittings because these things can be seen by the producer to have direct influence on productivity and therefore on income. Other creature comforts, like access to a secure bed with a good mattress, have been given a low priority because they are seen by the producer as a net cost rather than a net gain. If the priorities for comfort were set by the dairy cow, the 'good bed' would probably rank first.

This chapter first defines the criteria for comfort and freedom from injury as perceived by the animal and illustrates these general principles by examples only. The most important problems of discomfort and injury for each of the farm species are then briefly described. More comprehensive details of housing solutions to these problems are given in subsequent chapters.

In the first analysis, it is possible to distinguish thermal, physical and psychological comfort. Thermal comfort implies an environment that is neither excessively too cold nor too hot in extent or duration. This is not necessarily synonymous with the thermal zone for optimal productivity (see below). Physical comfort cannot be defined so precisely but must include access to a resting area suitable to the species and freedom to perform maintenance activities such as feeding, drinking and excreting. Psychological comfort implies both a sense of security and an absence of frustration. This depends on a proper balance between the reassuring presence of familiar animals, probably, although not necessarily, of the same species, and the opportunity to create personal space and so avoid harmful contact with others, whether malevolent or accidental.

Criteria for Comfort and Freedom from Injury

Thermal comfort

Much of this book is concerned with heat exchanges of animals within farm buildings. In this and most such reviews (e.g. Monteith and Mount, 1974; Curtis, 1983a) optimal standards for the thermal environment are variously described as 'the thermoneutral zone, the zone of thermal comfort or the zone of optimal productivity'. Furthermore, it is often assumed incorrectly that these three expressions are synonymous.

The zone of thermal neutrality is defined by the classical curves relating air temperature to metabolic heat production (Monteith and Mount, 1974). Figure 3.1 (from Webster, 1983a) illustrates how the effects of air temperature on metabolic heat production (H_p, $\mathrm{W\,m^{-2}}$), sensible (H_n) and evaporative (H_e) heat losses of farm animals may be categorized within two groups. Group I includes species such as pigs and poultry which have limited ability to regulate H_e, especially from the skin surface. In 'natural' conditions, i.e. those experienced by wild or feral pigs and poultry living out of doors in temperate environments, these species maintain homeothermy by regulating H_p to keep body temperature *up* to the set point. Group II includes ruminants, horses (and clothed man) which have considerable ability to regulate H_e at negligible cost by sweating and/or thermal panting. In most 'natural' environments these species maintain homeothermy by regulating H_e to keep body temperature *down* to the set point.

In Group II species, there is a clearly defined thermoneutral zone wherein H_p is independent of air temperature (T_a). Some definitions further state that H_p is elevated during acute exposure to heat stress by the work of thermal panting, etc., in chronic experiments and in practical farm situations the natural response of an animal to heat stress is to reduce H_p usually, although not invariably, by reducing food intake.

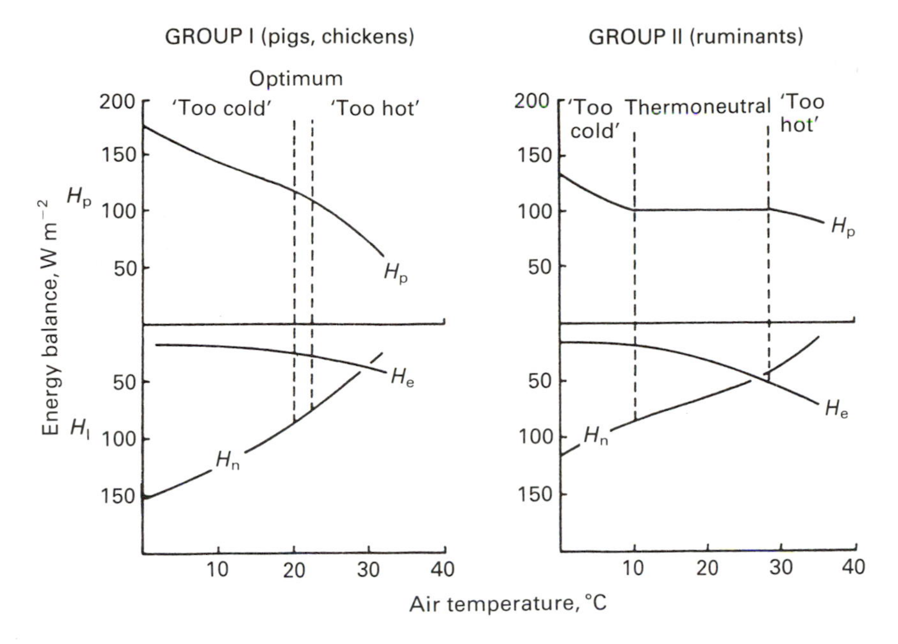

Fig. 3.1. Patterns of heat exchange in farm animals.
Heat production (H_p) = Heat loss (H_l) = $H_n + H_e$
Group I, e.g. pigs and chickens, species which maintain homeothermy principally by regulating H_p. Group II, e.g. sheep and cattle, species which maintain homeothermy principally by regulating H_e (from Webster, 1983a).

The extent of the thermoneutral zone for any individual animal is defined by physiological factors, e.g. thermoneutral metabolic rate, coat depth and variations in microclimate (convection and radiation). Effects of microclimate on the thermal exchanges of animals will be considered in detail elsewhere. The most important physiological factors are as follows:

1. *Food intake relative to maintenance requirement.* The more food any animal eats the greater is its H_p. This applies particularly to horses and ruminants for which the heat increment of feeding may range between 0.3 and 0.7 kJ per kJ increment in ME intake (Webster, 1983b). Thus the thermoneutral H_p of a high-yielding dairy cow (W m^{-2}) is more than twice that of an animal on a maintenance ration. It follows that the animal that eats the most (relative to maintenance) is the most tolerant of cold and the most sensitive to heat.
2. *Coat depth.* A thick coat obviously reduces sensible heat loss but also impairs the evaporation of moisture.
3. *Acclimatization to heat and cold.* This may involve changes in thermoneutral H_p, coat depth and blood flow through the superficial tissues of the body. In extreme cases this has been shown to reduce the lower critical temperature of cattle by as much as 20°C (Webster *et al.*, 1970).

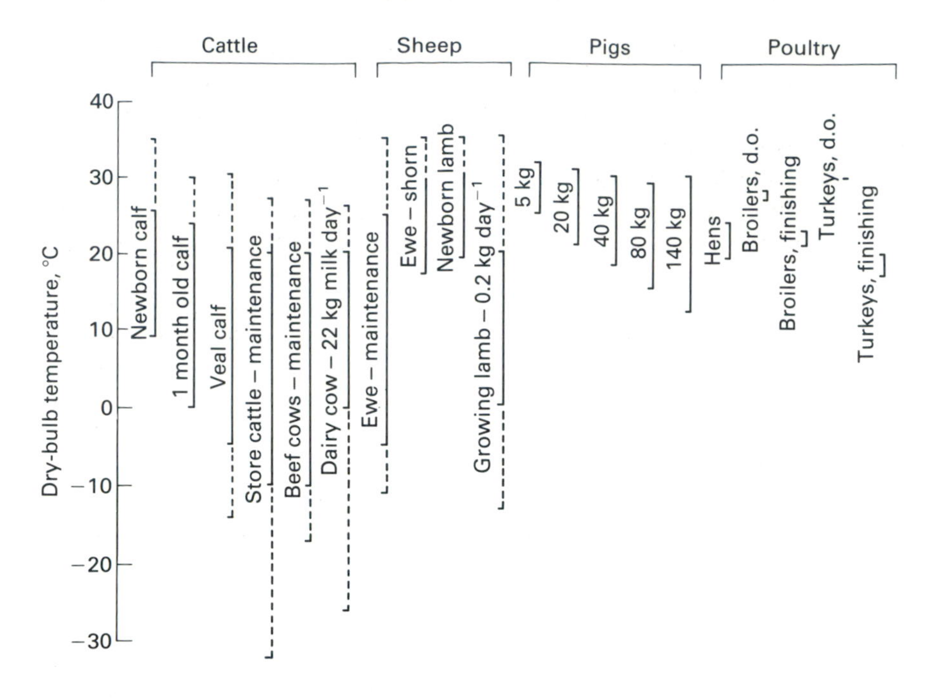

Fig. 3.2. Recommended air temperatures within livestock buildings. Solid lines indicate ideal temperatures for optimal productivity. Dotted lines show the range over which an acclimatized animal can adapt (from Wathes *et al.*, 1983).

Approximate ranges for the thermoneutral zone for farm animals are shown in Fig. 3.2 (Wathes *et al.*, 1983). The wide ranges for Group II animals do not necessarily imply optimal productivity throughout the range. Lactating dairy cattle, for example, have a lower critical temperature close to −20°C (by virtue of a high H_p) but milk yield declines (MacDonald and Bell, 1958) and mastitis incidence may increase at air temperatures below 0°C, in both cases linked perhaps to a reduced blood flow to the mammary gland (Thompson and Thomson, 1977). This is because the udder is sensitive to local cooling. Similarly a horse in full winter coat (or clipped and rugged) may have a lower critical temperature of −10°C but be more affected by tendon strains and other leg problems at air temperatures close to 0°C when blood flow to those regions is restricted.

The zone of thermal comfort can be described experimentally as the thermal state which the animal will select for itself given the chance (Curtis, 1983a, b). This is undoubtedly narrower than the thermoneutral zone. However, anyone who has watched a cat before a fire should accept that an animal's concept of thermal comfort may at times be hedonistic. For Group II species most environments within the thermoneutral zone may be considered acceptable on welfare grounds unless there are problems associated with local cooling (e.g. dairy cows) or if the animal is sick.

The zone of optimal productivity for Group I species (pigs and poultry) is extremely narrow (Fig. 3.2). For example, the optimal temperature for laying hens is accepted to be 21°C (Emmans and Charles, 1977). However, it would be ridiculous to suggest that a well-feathered, well-fed hen strutting in a farmyard at 15°C was suffering cold stress. Such a bird would, however, have a greater appetite than one in a cage at 21°C, thus an elevated thermoneutral H_p, greater cold tolerance but a poorer efficiency of conversion of chicken feed to eggs. The same principle applies to the growing pig. Thus the recommended air temperatures in intensive pig and poultry houses constitute the upper limit of the zone of thermal comfort. At an air temperature modestly below the economic optimum (say, 8°C), pigs and poultry (other than neonates) will only feel cold if food intake is restricted. At an air temperature 8°C above the economic optimum, pigs and poultry may experience intolerable heat stress unless alternative means are available for increasing heat loss by convection or evaporation. It is an interesting paradox that the farm species most susceptible to heat stress (pigs and poultry) by virtue of their limited capacity to regulate H_e are confined in houses designed to maintain T_a well above ambient by a combination of high stocking density, high insulation and restricted ventilation. For most of the year in cool temperate zones this is a perfectly satisfactory arrangement but as ambient temperature rises progressively above 20°C it becomes at first difficult and then impossible to prevent intolerable heat stress simply by increasing ventilation. It cannot be denied that some intensive houses for (especially) broilers are potentially lethal in conditions that may reasonably be expected to occur during a normal English summer.

Shock, exhaustion and fever

Optimal air temperatures for housed animals given throughout this book only apply so long as the animals are healthy and properly fed. If not, the rules change. An animal such as a calf in shock (peripheral circulatory failure following loss of extracellular fluid through diarrhoea) typically has a low rectal temperature and cold extremities; metabolic rate and cardiac output are both abnormally low. Such a calf is obviously more susceptible to the direct stress of cold and to bacterial pneumonia as a secondary consequence of partial pulmonary anoxia (Webster, 1990).

Calves that have been on lorries and through markets may have spent many hours with little, if any, rest, food or sleep. In these circumstances they are, like us, more susceptible to cold.

Fever, or an upward re-setting of the body thermostat, is a normal, if somewhat baffling, response to infection. Initially this involves an increase in H_p and reduction in H_e. The animal shivers, rectal temperature (T_r) rises but the extremities feel cold. When T_r has stabilized, the extremities (e.g. ears) may feel hot but the animal may continue to shiver to maintain T_r at the elevated rate. Fever is usually accompanied by inappetence and increased loss of fluid, electrolytes and nitrogen in the urine (Blood and Radostits, 1989). These factors, in combination, can lead to exhaustion and rapid loss of body condition. In very rare cases, T_r may be elevated so far as to constitute a threat to life. If so, it may be necessary to cool the animal down, e.g. with cold water. What is far more common is the calf or young pig with a moderate, persistent fever who lies in a cold box shivering prodigiously to maintain T_r at (say) 39.5°C.

In shock, exhaustion and all but the most extreme forms of fever, heat loss can be reduced by the use of a rug, deep straw bedding or an infrared lamp. The designer of animal houses should provide hospital pens to ensure these and other facilities for the individual care of sick animals.

Comfort at rest

It is essential to the welfare of any animal that it should have unrestricted access to an area where it can rest and sleep without discomfort or disturbance. Optimal conditions for the resting area are species specific. Table 3.1 (from Webster, 1992) assesses the needs of different farm animals for a resting area according to the following properties: dryness, hygiene, warmth, 'give' (in the sense that a mattress has 'give') and security. Poultry naturally perch and sleep in branches which are dry, good for the feet and provide some security against terrestrial predators. They do not require a bed as such. Provision of sufficient perching space in intensive units meets all these needs, although the sense of security may be misplaced when the predator is another hen. A deep litter bed of wood shavings does not, however, match the specifications for a suitable resting area for poultry (Table 3.1). Feet and leg strength would probably both be improved if birds had access to perches. Moreover, recent evidence has shown that poultry are relatively reluctant to use wood shavings for grooming (i.e. dust bathing) and prefer sand (Liere *et al.*, 1990).

The resting area for an adult sow should possess all the properties of a good 'bed', as we understand the word. The spacious covered yard which gives a sow room to find her own secure bed in deep, clean straw is just about ideal. The sow stall provides security (if only the security of solitary confinement). Concrete floors deny thermal and physical comfort. The dry sow, isolated in a stall, has a lower critical temperature of 18°C. Insulating the floor under the concrete to reduce conductive heat loss is relatively ineffective because of lateral heat transfer (Bruce, 1979). Giving sows on concrete access to small amounts of straw may help them to pass the time but it is unlikely to have much effect on physical comfort.

Weaner pigs are lighter, less dangerous but more prone to infection

Table 3.1. A ranking of the properties of the resting area according to the needs of different farm animals.

Animals	Dryness	Hygiene	'Give'	Warmth	Security*
Poultry					
broilers	+++	+	0	+	(+)
layers	++	+	0	0	(++)
Pigs					
weaners	++	++	+	+	+
dry sows	++	+	+	++	++
Cattle					
calves	+++	++	+	+	+
beef, fatteners	+	0	++	0	+
dairy cows	++	+++	++	0	++
Neonates (general)	+++	+++	+/0	+++	(+++)

Source: Webster, 1992.

*Pluses in brackets indicate that security is important but usually achieved by other means.

than sows. Security and 'give' thus assume less importance than hygiene which is why perforated floors are popular for weaners (Robertson and Anderson, 1979). At their best (e.g. plastic coated expanded metal) they are dry, clean, non-abrasive and difficult to criticize on grounds of comfort alone. Thus flat deck systems, where the perforated floor constitutes the piglet's entire living space, may be healthy and cost effective, but they are not strictly necessary since pigs, given the chance, will discriminate between areas for resting, feeding and excreting. The barren environment of the flat deck may also predispose to behavioural disorders such as tail biting (Fraser and Broom, 1990). Ideally, the perforated floor should be restricted to the area of the pen where the pigs choose (or are persuaded) to excrete.

The cubicle or free stall provides dairy cows with a secure resting area which they may enter or leave as they please. Hygiene is also of paramount importance to minimize the incidence of environmental mastitis usually associated with the ubiquitous organism *Escherichia coli* (Blowey, 1985). Until recently, there has been little incentive to provide dairy cows with a mattress because it confers no obvious economic advantage. When given the choice, however, cows show an overwhelming preference for beds which have the property of 'give' (Daelemans *et al.*, 1983) which is hardly surprising given their weight and the design of their limbs.

The criteria listed in Table 3.1 raise doubts as to the welfare of large animals such as finishing cattle housed entirely on concrete slatted floors. Undoubtedly slatted floors are acceptably dry, warm and hygienic for beef cattle when housed at high stocking density. Feet are usually in good condition although abrasions and bursitis are common around knees and hocks. Plastic covers for slats may provide a little more physical comfort, at a price (Gracie and Kelly, 1990). However, young bulls, in particular, densely stocked in a barren environment are prone to injury from aggressive or sexual encounters. Perhaps the most distressing form of animal housing that I have seen involved bull calves raised for veal to weights approaching 400 kg in groups of four on concrete slats. This was practised as a (cynical) response to public criticism of the individual stall for veal calves. These pubertal calves on essentially all-liquid diets were still orally frustrated and thus persisted in stereotypic licking or tongue rolling, but, in addition, spattered each other and the slats with wet faeces and slipped and slithered when attempting, or failing to avoid, mounting behaviour. If legislation to free veal calves from individual crates leads only to this, the calves will be worse off than before.

The newborn animal has special needs for the properties of dryness, warmth, hygiene and security. Because it is relatively light it has less need than the adult for a bed with 'give'. However, the delicate skin of the newborn is particularly prone to abrasion. Far too many piglets have scabby knees.

Behavioural freedom

The fifth freedom is to 'express normal, socially acceptable patterns of behaviour' (Webster, 1984). Certain activities, usually called maintenance behaviour, are deemed to be essential for survival and physical comfort. The list includes not only eating, drinking and excreting but also the original five freedoms of the Brambell Committee (1965), namely the opportunity to 'stand up, lie down, turn round, groom itself and stretch its limbs'. The major criticism of intensive systems for sows, laying hens and veal calves has been that they fail to meet even these minimal standards.

Social, sexual and parental behaviour, while not essential to the life and physical comfort of the individual, do constitute powerful behavioural needs. A free licence to sex and aggression, for example, would be as chaotic in a population of farm animals as in a population of humans and, in both cases, exacerbated by high stocking density. I repeat, however, that the use of solitary confinement to control undesirable social behaviour does not solve the welfare problem. It removes the consequences of social interaction, but does not (initially at least) remove the motivation. This illustrates a most important principle in welfare evaluation. Our assessment of animal welfare is usually based on observations of behaviour, i.e. what they *do*, whereas theirs is based on *perception* of the quality of life within a spectrum from suffering to pleasure, i.e. how they *feel*. It is possible to devise ways of asking animals how they feel, e.g. by measuring strength of motivation

(Dawkins, 1983; see also this volume, Chapter 4). However, it really does not need further research to justify the conclusion that a sentient animal like the pig experiences frustration when confined in such a way as to deny much maintenance and nearly all social behaviour. One long-term consequence of frustration is the development of stereotypies, or the prolonged performance of apparently purposeless behaviour. Stereotypies may help an animal to cope with frustration, although even this is uncertain (Fraser and Broom, 1990). However, their existence in pigs, calves, horses or zoo animals must be taken as evidence that the housing environment is unsatisfactory.

Farm animals also display, to a varying degree, advanced patterns of behaviour such as exploration and play. Some exploration, e.g. foraging may be motivated simply by the expectation of reward in the form of food. Some play may simply be for fun. Exploration and play are both highly educational. Animals use these activities to build up within their own minds a map of their environment and an autobiography of their experience (Ristau, 1991). The more they learn, the more their perception of any novel experience (e.g. new food, social contact, travel, etc.) will be modulated by memory previously stored and processed in the mind.

The question 'how much education do farm animals need?' is not one that can be pursued too far. Nevertheless I will cite two examples where improved educational opportunities for animals may be of benefit not only to them but also to the stockman. The first involves controlled (and humane) preconditioning of animals to conditions similar to those experienced during transport and handling before slaughter. The second involves engineering into housing systems facilities which permit animals to make constructive choices as to their own welfare. A sow, for example, wearing a transponder, could control not only her own access to a feeding station but also access to her piglets or her own thermal comfort, e.g. by turning on a sprinkler. My personal belief that such developments rate a high priority within welfare research is based on a somewhat heretical view of stockmanship. The stockman is traditionally viewed as the provider of food and creature comfort. By this definition the better the stockman the less the contribution made by the animal to its own welfare. This well-meaning paternalism has led to systems of housing and management where the animal has no option but servile dependence on the stockman and the automated systems which *he* controls. Simple, reliable systems controlled by the animals themselves would help to reduce frustration (and the aggression consequent upon frustration) by allowing animals to make a more constructive contribution to the quality of their own life, provided, of course, that these decisions do not conflict with their own best interests or those of their immediate neighbours.

Freedom from injury

Injury, or physical damage to body tissue, occurs when single or repeated stresses (usually mechanical but possibly chemical or thermal) overcome the capacity of the tissues (skin, hoof, bone, etc.) to absorb them. This rather ponderous definition is needed for a proper analysis of the incidence of injury to animals in different housing systems, since it recognizes that the system may determine not only the intensity and frequency of the shocks to which the animals are exposed but also their capacity to resist them. Thus, for example, Gregory *et al.* (1990) showed that laying hens in battery cages may have more fragile bones than those in percheries (through less activity), fewer breaks during life (less trauma) but more breaks during harvesting and transport (fragile bones plus catching method).

Injuries to housed animals may be separately classified into those which are self-inflicted (e.g. foot damage) and those inflicted by other animals (e.g. tail biting in pigs). In the first case the structure of the building may be at fault, in the second case its design and management.

Foot injuries

Injuries to the feet of housed animals may be caused or precipitated by excessive pressure, shear forces, softening or chemical erosion of the hoof or skin, or internal damage due to improper nutrition. The problem of foot lameness is particularly important and particularly complex in the dairy cow kept in a cubicle house over winter (Wierenga and Peterse, 1987). The most important predisposing factors are:

1. *Conformation of the cow.* Over 70% of all cases of injury to the hoof occur in the outer claw of the hind foot and many cases occur in early lactation. This can be attributed to a change in load on the outer claw as the udder expands and is controlled by appropriate foot trimming prior to parturition (Wierenga and Peterse, 1987).
2. *Floor condition.* The hardness of the concrete used for passageways is unavoidable and does not constitute a problem in itself. Indeed the wall of the cow's hoof grows at a rate that is well suited to moderate exercise on hard ground. In a cubicle house, cows may get insufficient exercise to ensure even wear, may stand in wet slurry which softens their hooves and slip on floors which are too smooth or too slimy. All these things predispose to foot injuries, in particular separation of the sole from the wall along the 'white line'.
3. *Nutrition.* Overfeeding of starchy concentrates probably induces laminitis which can progress to a solar ulcer (Greenough *et al.*, 1981). However, the extent to which nutritional laminitis contributes to the clinical problem of lameness in housed dairy cattle is by no means clear. The indirect

consequence of eating large amounts of wet silage (i.e. passageways covered in wet faeces) may be far more important.

4. *Behaviour.* The feet of cattle may become bruised and more prone to injury if cattle are forced to stand for excessively long periods in concrete passageways. Newly-calved heifers in particular may suffer if they are bullied, unused to cubicles or if there are insufficient cubicles for all animals.

Orthopaedic injuries

Orthopaedic injuries may involve bones (fractures), joints (dislocations and arthritis), tendons (bursitis) or nerve/muscle paralysis (the downer cow syndrome).

Fractures may be caused by direct trauma (hitting something) or sudden, abnormal movement (slipping). Septic arthritis ('joint-ill') in calves and lambs may be due to infection via the navel with *E. coli* from dirty bedding. Aseptic arthritis in sows in stalls may be attributed to the length of time that they spend lying on concrete (Penny *et al.*, 1963). This effect itself may be further analysed into effects of prolonged pressure, enforced inactivity and low blood supply to cold limbs.

Bursitis ('big knees and hocks') is commonly seen in cattle on slatted floors (Cermak, 1983a). This excessive secretion of synovial fluid is due to chronic pressure and rubbing. It may not be particularly painful but it is a very conspicuous indicator of the fact that concrete slats cannot be considered comfortable for cattle.

Weakness or paralysis in farm animals can result from nerve damage. The 'downer cow', which fails to get up after calving, may or may not have damaged the obdurator nerve during delivery. In any event if she remains in one position for too long, even in a well-strawed box, the constant pressure on a single site will cause severe destruction of nerve and muscle tissue within 3–4 hours. The management of the downer cow is not within the scope of this chapter (see Blowey, 1985). This example merely serves to indicate the severity of the discomfort and injury that can arise when large animals like cattle and adult pigs are made to lie for long periods on hard surfaces. No one who has ever spent a night in a sleeping bag without a mattress or felt their leg 'go to sleep' after sitting or lying in one position for perhaps one hour should feel complacent about the physical comfort of large farm animals forced to lie on concrete.

Injuries from other animals

Animals may injure one another by accident (e.g. tramping on a teat), by deliberate acts of aggression, or through activities such as feather pecking which may not be strictly aggressive yet are decidedly antisocial. Housing solutions to problems of accidental injury and aggression can be relatively straightforward, in both cases animals need both sufficient space and an escape route. The problem of 'mindless' mutual destruction like feather pecking in poultry or tail biting in pigs is more difficult. Outbreaks of feather pecking have variously (but dubiously) been blamed on poor ventilation, high humidity and other deficiencies in the physical environment (Moss, 1980; Fraser and Broom, 1990). Bright light, especially shafts of sunlight entering the building at a particular time of day can also act as a trigger. Control of feather pecking through subdued lighting is not possible in free-range systems. In these circumstances it is probably more constructive to offer hens other things to peck at but we need to know more about what motivates the hens to peck (Hughes, 1984; see also this volume, Chapter 4).

Tail biting in growing pigs begins with gentle chewing, which is tolerated but becomes progressively destructive. Despite this, the recipients tend to remain submissive although the condition is clearly painful (Fraser and Broom, 1990). The condition is most common when early weaned pigs are reared in a barren environment. It may be exacerbated by heat, cold and other sources of discomfort. For practical purposes it may be assumed that tail biting arises through frustration of normal oral activity (sucking, foraging and investigatory behaviour) and becomes worse when the frustrated animals cannot get comfortable.

Priorities for Comfort

This chapter began by examining the principles that determine comfort and freedom from injury in housed animals, the intention being to create a logical sequence of questions to address these problems in any housing situation. It concludes with a very brief review of the most serious problems of discomfort and injury in the various species and suggestions as to how they might be avoided, or at least ameliorated, by improvements to housing.

Laying hens

For the laying hen, the most serious problems of discomfort and injury are:

1. *Foot injuries and deformities.* These can be controlled in cages by attention to floor design and by provision of perches (Moss, 1980).
2. *Bone weakness leading to fractures during life.* As indicated earlier, this can be reduced by providing birds with more space, better quality space (e.g. perches and nest boxes) but less risk of bumping into hard objects (e.g. perches and nest boxes) at speed (Wokac, 1987; Gregory *et al.*, 1990).
3. *Restricted maintenance behaviour (grooming, stretching, wing flapping) due to insufficient space.* The Farm Animal Welfare Council, in its report on colony

systems for laying hens, has recommended at least 1425 cm^2 per bird (i.e. seven birds per m^2) except in multi-tier systems where overhead perches/platforms provide space for at least 25% of the hens when the stocking rate shall not exceed 9.3 hens per m^2 (Farm Animal Welfare Council, 1992a). If this recommendation becomes law it will become difficult to maintain hen houses at 21°C, the temperature for optimal productivity rather than optimal thermal comfort.

4. *Lack of facilities for highly motivated patterns of behaviour.* For example, sand for dust bathing, objects for 'investigatory' pecking and (of course) a preferred site for egg laying.

5. *Lack of security.* This covers two aspects: attack from other hens in all units and lack of real and perceived security from predators out of doors. The former can be controlled by attention to lighting, selection of birds or (if all else fails) de-beaking. The latter requires provision of surrogate bushes out of doors under which hens may hide when faced by a real or imagined threat from the air.

Broilers

Over 60% of broilers have some evidence of injury or abnormality of development in the bones and joints of their legs when examined after commercial slaughter (Whitehead, 1992). This leg damage is clearly associated with loss of mobility and we must assume it to be a source of chronic pain. In any event, the Farm Animal Welfare Council (1992b) concluded that it is unacceptable. The immobility of broilers in their last days of life has been attributed to high stocking density (17 2-kg birds per m^2) but is equally likely to be because it hurts the birds to move. Orthopaedic problems in broilers can be controlled if growth rate is reduced by reducing daylength and thus access to food (Pierson and Hester, 1982). 'Hock burn' is usually associated with factors that cause the litter to deteriorate but this condition is hardly ever seen in birds which are grown more slowly and stand normally on their toes.

There is a pressing need for good research into housing and management systems for broilers which can help to overcome the problem of chronic orthopaedic pain. At present we are able to point to deficiencies within existing systems but are not able to suggest alternatives with any confidence.

Adult sows

There are many options for sow housing within a spectrum that ranges from the individual sow stall to the outdoor paddock with arks. The sow stall is uncomfortable, boring, sometimes cold and does predispose to skin sores and injuries to feet and legs. Deep, dry straw yards are warm and comfortable but fighting is always a possibility. The outdoor sow with access to an ark roofed with corrugated iron may be able to escape the problems of frustration and aggression but will experience both cold and heat stress. The latter is more serious (even in UK conditions) because the modern white-skinned sow is not only unable to sweat efficiently but also prone to sunburn. Sows outdoors in summer should have access both to wallows and to shade.

The farrowing crate is undeniably uncomfortable and frustrates normal maternal behaviour. It does help to prevent crushing of piglets but this is only a problem during the first 48 hours of life; thereafter the crate becomes unnecessary. More humane (but expensive) alternatives to the farrowing crate have been developed (Baxter, 1991). In my opinion, however, it would be more logical to develop a radically different approach to the rearing of pigs to weaning whereby sows go into a hygienic maternity suite (perhaps involving a farrowing crate) for as short a time as possible and then proceed to nursing accommodation which is less restrictive and less expensive.

Growing pigs

Growing pigs are well fed and reasonably fit, by virtue of youth rather than environment. Their main problems arise from injury or threat of injury from their active, frustrated and aggressive compatriots. Genuine aggression at feeders and elsewhere can be reduced by providing solid partitions between individual pigs or even popholes in the walls into which pigs may stick their heads (Baxter, 1987). It might be assumed that such ostrich-like behaviour would render pigs more rather than less vulnerable. It may be, however, that the pig that hides its head no longer constitutes a challenge and is therefore not attacked.

Tail biting cannot be controlled by this method, presumably because the motivation to tail-bite is not aggressive. The provision of chewing toys or balls may eliminate tail biting in many cases. Pigs may, however, tire of such 'toys' because they offer so limited a reward. The welfare interests of the animals would be better served by engineering into their environment the opportunity to forage constructively for the occasional reward in the form of food.

Sheep

Sheep are relatively light, well-insulated, non-aggressive, unambitious animals, all of which make it relatively easy for us to house them in comfort. There are two main problems. Pregnant ewes may suffer heat stress when brought off the hill into poorly ventilated accommodation in mid-winter. Since sheep thermoregulate by panting, respiration rate provides an excellent indicator of heat stress. If respiration rate exceeds $60\,min^{-1}$ in sheep at rest indoors they are unnecessarily warm; if it exceeds 100 min^{-1} they are far too hot. Moderate heat stress reduces appetite which predisposes to low lamb weights or, in severe cases, pregnancy ketosis or twin-lamb disease. The practice of shearing ewes at housing, originally done to reduce the amount of trough space required by each sheep, has led in some circumstances to increases in lamb weights and viability but probably only because the winter accommodation was insufficiently well ventilated and unshorn ewes became too hot. In a well-ventilated building, shearing at housing probably confers no welfare advantages and may predispose to cold stress, especially if the ewes are turned out immediately after lambing.

The second problem for sheep is wet ground. Their fleece provides excellent insulation from cold unless it becomes saturated, e.g. while lying in a sodden field that once contained turnips. Their feet are especially vulnerable to overgrowth, injury and infectious foot rot if they are forced to stand permanently on soft, wet ground, indoors or out. Perforated floors, being hard and dry, may be preferable to straw bedding for housing store lambs or ewes prior to lambing in some circumstances, e.g. when the dry matter content of the diet is low (silage, roots) and the sheep are passing large amounts of urine and wet faeces.

Calves and beef cattle

The thermoneutral zone of cattle is so wide that thermal comfort can be ensured (under UK conditions) in any well ventilated building so long as it is dry and free from draughts (Webster, 1983a). It is now illegal, in the UK although not in the rest of Europe, to confine a veal calf in an individual crate that denies it the opportunity to turn round, groom itself or adopt a comfortable sleeping position. Probably the greatest source of discomfort to the young, artificially reared calf is that of feeling thoroughly ill with diarrhoea and pneumonia. I have discussed the special housing requirements of the sick calf already.

Well-grown beef cattle will not be entirely comfortable if housed entirely on concrete slatted floors or on straw. Solid, sloped concrete floors (Paterson, 1981) may be worse than slats because they are dirtier and the slope forces animals to lie on one side with their legs pointing downhill. This has to be less comfortable than a system which does not restrict cattle from shifting from one side to another when their limbs become stiff (Webster, 1987). It is a fallacy to assume that there is a single, ideal floor surface for cattle (even a field!) since it must variously be warm and yielding, dry, hygienic, non-abrasive but non-slip and easy to clean (Webster, 1987). It is better for all cattle to provide a separate lying area from that where the animals eat, drink and pass much, but regrettably not all, their excreta. The lying area should have the warmth, security and 'give' of a good bed. The passageways should be hard but dry to ensure proper wear on the feet. Deep, damp straw bedding predisposes to overgrowth and softening of the hoof and increases the risk not only of injury to the sole but also of infectious interdigital necrobacillosis ('foul of the foot').

Dairy cattle

Many of the welfare problems of intensively housed farm animals can be attributed to boredom, through having too little to do, and the physical consequences of lying around doing nothing.

In absolute contrast, the main welfare problem of the dairy cow is that she has too much to do. The energy demands of lactation exceed those of any other form of animal production or hard manual labour in man (Webster, 1989b). To meet this demand for energy and other nutrients the cow is compelled to eat for long periods. Finally, she is usually expected to stand around in collecting yards for perhaps two hours a day awaiting entry to the milking parlour. We must assume that her first priority is for a comfortable bed in which she can rest secure for as long a time as possible.

The free stall or cubicle, when properly designed (Cermak, 1983b) and given a comfortable, hygienic bed, does constitute for most housed cattle within the UK the best compromise between the needs of comfort, hygiene, economics and ease of management. The free stall is undoubtedly superior to the tie-stall in terms of comfort and injury (Ekesbo, 1966). It is possible that the incidence of environmental mastitis and lameness in dairy cattle has increased since the development of cubicle housing but this may be attributed to the simultaneous switch from dry hay to wet (but more nutritious) silage.

No cow should be denied access to a cubicle and forced to stand in the dunging passage by virtue of an absolute shortage of cubicles, passageways which restrict freedom of movement and encourage bullying, or simply through timidity and inexperience. This requires not only proper design in the cubicle house but proper training of heifers prior to calving down for the first time.

Another source of discomfort and potential injury to the dairy cow is the extreme distension of the udder. The beef cow normally feeds its calf 5–7 times per day. The dairy cow, producing perhaps six times as much milk is conventionally restricted to two milkings per day. Udder distension certainly predisposes to injury in the outer claws of the hind feet and probably predisposes to mastitis (Blowey, 1985; Webster, 1987). Milking three times a day at regular intervals will decrease udder distension and increase milk yield. However, in a conventional parlour system this increases by 50% the time each cow has to stand in a collecting yard and further erodes the time available for feeding and rest. The development of robotics may permit the design of service stations for dairy cows which they can enter freely, and without prolonged waiting, say 4–6 times per day, to feed, drink and be milked as necessary. The problems of such systems lie not only in the design of the robotics but also in creating the proper incentives for cows to enter them. However, at best they could improve resting time and milk yield and reduce both the physical discomfort of a distended udder and the consequent risk of injury and infection.

Horses

The horse has an excellent ability to regulate both sensible heat loss – by adjusting coat depth – and evaporative heat loss – by sweating. It is able to acclimatize (given time) to extremes of both heat and cold. In the UK the horse is usually expected to perform as an athlete and should be housed accordingly. To ensure that the animal becomes neither overheated during exercise nor too cold in the stable the owner or trainer usually clips the hair coat and then provides alternative, removable insulation in the form of a stable blanket. This is perfectly acceptable, although sometimes dictated more by fashion than necessity. It is certainly preferable to provide local insulation than to attempt to keep the house warm by restricting ventilation since this can predispose to chronic obstructive pulmonary disease (Clarke, 1987).

The competition horse is particularly prone to injuries of the tendons, distal bones and joints of the limbs. Blood supply to these extremities is reduced when the animal feels cold. This can reduce the rate of healing and probably prolongs the discomfort of tendon strains, sore shins, etc. Once again the obvious solution is to increase blood flow by the use of stable bandages for the legs. The ancient practice of firing horses' tendons was based on the assumption that healing could be stimulated by doing more damage to create inflammation and more blood flow. This absurd extrapolation from sound physiology has now been banned by the Royal College of Veterinary Surgeons.

As legs and feet are so important to a valuable horse, they are usually given a sufficient depth of dry bedding to ensure dryness, hygiene and comfort. Wood shavings probably make the best bedding on grounds of both comfort and hygiene (Clarke, 1987). Other features essential to comfort and freedom from injury for horse and man include sufficient space, at least $12\,m^2$ for a 15-hand thoroughbred, the absence of projecting fixtures and fittings and, especially for large horses, some provision to ensure that they do not become 'cast' in their stable (trapped in a lying position and unable to rise). Anti-casting measures include the use of a 'roller' worn over the stable rug which prevents the horse rolling over in the stable, or building one course of recessed blocks into the walls on which the horse may get a purchase with its feet as it struggles to right itself.

Boredom is probably the greatest problem for the fit, highly-trained performance horse isolated in a stable box for 22 hours each day. Many stable accessories are available which purport to control stereotypies or stable vices such as weaving, crib biting and wind sucking. Devices such as anti-weaving bars may prevent the performance of this exhausting form of neurotic behaviour but they do not eliminate the motive, thus causing the horse to become even more frustrated. The welfare of a gregarious, restless species such as the thoroughbred horse is best ensured if the animals have plenty of social contact and plenty to do.

References

Baxter, M.R. (1987) Implications of behavioural studies on the development of housing systems. In: *Pig Housing and the Environment.* British Society of Animal Production, Occasional Publication No. 11, pp. 99–102.

Baxter, M.R. (1991) The 'Freedom farrowing system'. *Farm Building Progress* 104, 9–15.

Blood, D.C. and Radostits, O.M. (1989) *Veterinary Medicine,* 7th edn. Baillière Tindall, London.

Blowey, R.W. (1985) *A Veterinary Book for Dairy Farmers.* Farming Press, Ipswich.

Brambell, F.W.R. (1965) Report of the technical committee to enquire into the welfare of animals kept under intensive livestock husbandry systems (Cmnd. 2836). HMSO, London.

Bruce, J.M. (1979) Heat loss from animals to floors. *Farm Building Progress* 55, 1–4.

Cermak, J.P. (1983a) Review of injuries in cattle housing. MAFF, Farm Buildings and Structures. RD/FBS/16.

Cermak, J.P. (1983b) Cubicle design and dimensions: an assessment of spatial requirements of the dairy cow as related to body weight and body dimensions. MAFF, Farm Buildings and Structures. RD/FBS/08.

Clarke, A.F. (1987) Stable environment in relation to the control of respiratory diseases. In: Hickman, J. (ed.), *Horse Management.* Academic Press, London, p. 137.

Curtis, S.E. (1983a) *Environmental Management in Animal Agriculture.* Iowa State University Press, Iowa.

Curtis, S.E. (1983b) Perception of thermal comfort by farm animals. In: Baxter, S.H., Baxter, M.R. and MacCormack, J.A.C. (eds), *Farm Animal Housing and Welfare.* Martinus Nijhoff, The Hague, pp. 59–68.

Daelemans, J., Maton, A. and Lambrecht, J. (1983) Appraisal of some cubicle floors by cows. *Farm Buildings Digest* 18, 19–22.

Dawkins, M. (1983) Battery hens name their price: consumer demand theory and the measurement of animal needs. *Animal Behaviour* 31, 1195–1205.

Ekesbo, I. (1966) Disease incidence in tied and loose housed dairy cattle. *Acta Agricuturae Scandinavica,* Suppl. 15.

Emmans, G.C. and Charles, D.R. (1977) Climatic environment and poultry feedings in practice. In: Haresign, W., Swan, H. and Lewis, D. (eds), *Nutrition and the Climatic Environment.* Butterworths, London, pp. 31–50.

Farm Animal Welfare Council (1992a) Welfare of laying hens in colony systems. MAFF, Tolworth.

Farm Animal Welfare Council (1992b) Report on the welfare of broiler chickens. MAFF. Tolworth.

Fraser, A.F. and Broom, D.M. (1990) *Farm Animal Behaviour and Welfare*, 3rd edn. Baillière Tindall, London.

Gracie, D.I. and Kelly, M. (1990) Rubber matting on slats to increase cattle comfort. *Farm Building Progress* 100, 15–18.

Greenough, P.R., MacCallum, F.J. and Weaver, A.D. (1981) *Lameness in Cattle*. Wright Scientechnica.

Gregory, N.G., Wilkins, L.J., Eleperuma, S.D., Ballantyne, A.J. and Overfield, N.D. (1990) Broken bones in domestic fowls: effect of husbandry system and stunning method in end-of-lay hens. *British Poultry Science* 31, 59–70.

Hughes, B.O. (1984) Feather pecking and cannibalism in domestic fowls. *Hohenheimer Arbeiten* 121, 138–146.

Liere, D.W. van, Kooijman, J. and Wiepkema, P.R. (1990) Dust bathing behaviour of laying hens as related to quality of dust bathing material. *Applied Animal Behaviour Science* 26, 127–142.

MacDonald, M.A. and Bell, J.M. (1958) Influence of temperature on milk yield and milk composition. *Canadian Journal of Animal Science* 38, 160–170.

Monteith, J. and Mount, L.E. (1974) *Heat Loss from Animals and Man*. Butterworths, London.

Moss, R. (1980) *The Laying Hen and its Environment*. Martinus Nijhoff, Dordrecht, Netherlands.

Paterson, K.H. (1981) Minimal bedding cattle court development in Orkney. *Farm Building Progress* 64, 9–10.

Penny, R.H.C., Osborne, A.D. and Wright, A.I. (1963) The causes and incidence of lameness in store and adult pigs. *Veterinary Record* 75, 1225–1235.

Pierson, F.M. and Hester, P.Y. (1982) Factors influencing leg abnormalities in poultry. A review. *World Poultry Science Journal* 38, 5–17.

Ristau, C.A. (1991) *Cognitive Ethology, the Minds of Other Animals*. Lawrence Erlbaum, London.

Robertson, A.M. and Anderson, A.W.F. (1979) Perforated floors for pig housing. *Farm Building Progress* 57, 9–12.

Smith, W.J. and Robertson, A.M. (1971) Observations on injuries to sows in part slatted stalls. *Veterinary Record* 89, 531.

Thompson, G.E. and Thomson, E.M. (1977) Effect of cold exposure on mammary circulation, oxygen consumption and milk secretion in the goat. *Journal of Physiology. London* 272, 187–196.

Wathes, C.M., Jones, C.D.R. and Webster, A.J.F. (1983) Ventilation, air hygiene and animal health. *Veterinary Record* 113, 554–559.

Webster, A.J.F. (1983a) Nutrition and the thermal environment. In: Rook, J.A.F. and Thomas, P.C. (eds), *Nutritional Physiology of Farm Animals*. Longman, London, pp. 639–669.

Webster, A.J.F. (1983b) Energetics of maintenance and growth. In: Girardier, L. and Stock, M.J (eds), *Mammalian Thermogenesis*. Chapman & Hall, London, pp. 178–207.

Webster, A.J.F. (1984) *Calf Husbandry, Health and Welfare*. Collins, London.

Webster, A.J.F. (1987) *Understanding the Dairy Cow*. Blackwell Scientific Publications, London.

Webster, A.J.F. (1989a) Animal housing as perceived by the animal. *Veterinary Annual* 29, 1–8.

Webster, A.J.F. (1989b) Bioenergetics, bioengineering and growth. *Animal Production* 48, 249–269.

Webster, A.J.F. (1990) Housing and respiratory disease in farm animals. *Outlook on Agriculture* 19, 31–35.

Webster, A.J.F. (1992) Problems of feeding and housing: their diagnosis and control. In: Moss, R. (ed.), *Livestock Health and Welfare.* Longman, London, pp. 293–333.

Webster, A.J.F., Chumlecky, J. and Young, B.A. (1970) Effects of cold environments on the energy exchanges of young beef cattle. *Canadian Journal of Animal Science* 50, 89–100.

Whitehead, C.C. (1992) *Bone Biology and Skeletal Disorders in Pathology.* Butterworth Heinemann, London.

Wierenga, H.K. and Peterse, J. (1987) *Cattle Housing Systems, Lameness and Behaviour.* Martinus Nijhoff. Dordrecht, Netherlands.

Wokac, R.M. (1987) Skeletal deformations in laying hens in battery and deep litter husbandry. *Berliner und Munchener Tierarztliche Wochenschrift* 100, 191–198.

4 Behaviour and Welfare

C.J. NICOL
Department of Clinical Veterinary Science,
University of Bristol, UK

Introduction

There have been a number of attempts to define the term 'welfare'. Most recognize the importance of considering both the physical and mental health of the animal, but there are nuances in the definitions of different authors. Duncan and Poole (1990) state that 'although physical health and freedom from injury are important, ultimately it is how the animal "feels" about its bodily state, how it "perceives" its environment and how "aware" it is of these feelings and perceptions that are crucial for its welfare'. The implication here is that the welfare of an injured or stressed individual is not compromised so long as that individual is not aware that it is injured or stressed; for example because it is unconscious or narcotized. Fraser and Broom (1990) would disagree. They define the welfare of an individual as 'its state as regards its attempts to cope with its environment', and would prefer the term 'well-being' to refer to the way the animal feels about that state. Using Fraser and Broom's definition the welfare of an unconscious but injured animal would be reduced. Semantics aside, it becomes obvious that animals' feelings about themselves and their environments are of great importance. Feelings, unfortunately, are not amenable to direct study but it is hoped to show that by observing behaviour and designing behavioural experiments some insight is gained into the private mental world of farm animals.

When we choose to house animals, and take over responsibility for their physical needs for food, water and shelter, we may feel that our duties have been discharged. We may even feel that these animals are leading an easy, almost luxurious, life compared with their counterparts braving climatic extremes, seasonal food shortages and risks of the outside world. However, unless a lot of thought is put into designing the house from the animals' point of view, we are likely to be under a delusion about their welfare. Housing animals confronts them with a range of new problems, not least of which is how to reallocate their time when their basic physiological needs are so easily satisfied (Hughes and Duncan, 1988). Of course, not all farm livestock are kept under conditions of plenty – sows and broiler chickens kept for breeding purposes are often fed severely restricted food rations, and I shall return to their problems later – but many farm animals are kept on *ad libitum* rations and no longer need to look for their food, water or shelter. European wild boar spend 85% of their active time foraging and feeding (Briedermann, 1971; cited by Simonsen, 1990), yet pregnant sows housed under intensive conditions may consume their daily rations in 30 min or less (Appleby and Lawrence, 1987). Horses in the Camargue spend 60% of their time grazing and browsing (P. Duncan, 1980), while Carson and Wood-Gush (1983) estimate an overall average of 66% of a horse's day on pasture is spent grazing. Even in a stable or stall horses spend 60% of their time feeding if provided with loose hay (Marsden, 1993). However, when hay of exactly the same fibre content is pelleted the time spent feeding falls to just 10% (Marsden, 1993). It is possible that genetic selection for improved production and docility in domestic breeds has resulted in animals that are no longer motivated to forage or explore. However, this cannot be assumed without further investigation because selection programmes have not attempted to alter motivation for these particular behaviour patterns. Domestic animals may be content to sleep or they may be even more strongly motivated to forage or explore than more reactive animals.

Differences in time budgets may also matter for some species more than others. Domestic fowl, for example, do not appear to adapt easily to a ready food supply by performing other behaviours. On the contrary, Dawkins (1989) discovered that junglefowl hens at Whipsnade Park Zoo, England, spent the majority of their day foraging in leaf litter, even though they were fed three times a day by keepers. Hens will also choose to work to obtain food by pecking a key even when the same food is presented freely in a dish in front of them (Duncan and Hughes, 1972). It seems that, for chickens at least, foraging behaviour itself is important, and not simply the means to a full stomach. Chickens may consequently find it very difficult to readjust their time budgets, and perhaps some opportunity should be provided to allow them to forage or work for their food. It is also known that hens (Hughes *et al.*, 1989) and sows (Arey *et al.*, 1991) are strongly motivated to show nesting behaviour even when they are provided with a perfect ready-made nest. Taken together these findings refute Baxter's (1983) general proposition that it is the environmental endpoint of any behaviour which is important, and not the performance of the behaviour itself. It is still possible, of course, that *some* behaviours will not be motivated if their usual consequences are already provided. We need to consider the likelihood that gluts in food supply, or the fortuitous appearance of suitable shelters or nest sites, may have occurred frequently enough during the evolution of each domestic species for adaptive behavioural responses to have been selected. Animals which have evolved to respond to serendipitous conditions in the wild may be better equipped to deal with the frustrations of overprovision by man.

In some cases then, satisfying the immediate physiological needs of an animal may stimulate it to find a mate, extend a territory or search further afield than usual for good feeding sites, in an attempt to increase its reproductive success. In other situations, perhaps as winter approaches, a safe physiological state may be the cue to hibernate (McFarland, 1989). If pigs, cattle or horses have been selected to respond to the ready availability of food, water and shelter by exploring, reproducing or even sleeping then, so long as we give them the chance to behave in these ways, it may not matter that their budgets differ from their feral relatives. Unfortunately, most housed animals are not provided either with the opportunity to forage, or the chance to reproduce or explore. Indeed, if we compare the behaviour of animals in wild or semi-natural environments with the behaviour of animals in typical productive animal houses there are striking differences, not just in overall time budgets, but also in the types of behaviour being performed. The complete range of behaviours a given species is capable of performing is called an ethogram (Tinbergen, 1951), but this complete range is unlikely to be observed when animals are housed under different conditions from those in which the behaviours evolved. None the less, where seminatural conditions are provided a wide range of behaviours may be seen. For example, 60 behaviours were commonly observed in a study of blue-breasted quail (*Coturnix chinensis*) housed in pairs in laboratory enclosures containing sand, turf, shrubs and rocks (Schleidt *et al.*, 1984). I.J.H. Duncan (1980) has compiled an ethogram for the domestic hen based on an amalgamation of behaviours observed in different environments. He describes a complex range of sexual, parental and anti-predator behaviour, in addition to normal maintenance activities. Although not necessarily a fair comparison, since the aims of the authors were different, studies of broiler chickens in high density sheds have listed only 11 (Murphy and Preston, 1988) or 19 (Newberry *et al.*, 1987) behaviours, while Nicol (1987a) recorded only 18 behaviours in a study of caged hens. There certainly appear to be many behaviours which these housed birds were not performing.

The job of the ethologist trying to answer questions about the welfare of animals in modern housing systems is to discover why animals are not performing certain behaviour patterns, and under what conditions non-performance becomes so frustrating that the animals actually suffer. As well as this, the ethologist needs to keep an eye on the activities that are being performed. Is wobbling, defined as a brief but distinct loss of balance while upright (Newberry *et al.*, 1987), an activity to encourage in broiler houses? What about feather pecking or agonistic interactions? Far from advocating that animals should be allowed to perform every behaviour of which they are capable (Thorpe, 1965) we need to establish which behaviours are important to the animal, which are unimportant, which are indicative of disease, pain or pathology, and which may harm others.

Rather than simply sit back and wait for this detailed information, many attempts have been made to design housing systems which allow animals a greater freedom of behavioural expression. Some of the approaches that have been taken have led to housing designs that go some considerable way to improving the welfare of farm animals. However, there are drawbacks and uncertainties associated with all the new systems that have been proposed.

Current Approaches to Housing Design

Extensification

The degree of spatial restriction, confinement or restraint has often been the focus for criticisms of intensive animal housing (Thorpe, 1965; Animal Welfare Institute, 1987; Ryder 1989). Battery cages, sow tethers and veal crates often prevent animals from performing the simplest movements. They may be unable to lie down, turn around, stretch limbs or groom themselves. At first sight the obvious solution is simply to break down the cage walls or remove the tethers. But this is to forget that there were *some* important reasons compatible with welfare for introducing these restrictions in the first place. A battery cage isolates a bird from its own droppings so disease is minimized. Tethered sows are unable to injure each other by fighting. This is no defence of the systems as a whole, but attempts to improve welfare by simply removing physical barriers and letting large groups of animals 'get on with it' are liable to go very wrong. Disease, aggression and mortality are often higher in free-range or extensive units (Swarbrick, 1986; Matter and Oester, 1989). In the UK the use of veal crates was banned in 1990, and the tethering of dry sows is currently being phased out. It is essential that alternatives are carefully designed to promote good welfare.

Behavioural key features

Stolba and Wood-Gush (1984) pioneered the idea of ethologically minimal housing by observing pigs in a natural environment and identifying the features that were required for certain frequent behaviour patterns to be performed. Their main assumption was that welfare would not be compromised if the motivational and functional requirements of each behaviour were satisfied separately, e.g. the exploratory elements of foraging with dummy materials, and the nutrient requirements with a well-balanced food mixture. The environmental features identified during the initial observations were then honed down to the simplest form still recognized by the pigs: the 'key features'. One problem with this approach is the unstated assumption that behaviour observed in a natural setting is the ideal to be aimed for. Dawkins (1980) has discussed this general issue and concludes that 'there is too much suffering in wild animals for a comparison between them and captive ones to be used as a standard for welfare unless there is a great deal of other supporting evidence'. The other, more pedestrian, problem is that the family pig pen system that resulted from this approach has yet to be widely adopted by commercial producers, despite favourable reports in experimental trials (Kerr *et al.*, 1988; Wechsler *et al.*, 1991). This seems to be largely because the system is still viewed as overcomplicated with, for example, higher labour costs (Kerr *et al.*, 1988). But if alterations to cut costs are attempted, a knowledge of the pigs' own priorities and preferences becomes essential to ensure welfare. Their highest priority behaviours will not necessarily be those observed most frequently in a natural environment.

Trial and error

Some very successful housing designs have been arrived at by successive modifications of an initial idea. On a small scale, Simonsen (1990) describes how he was able to modify a multi-activity pen for fattening pigs to encourage more even use of the available space. In the first version the pigs spent most of their time in the straw and feeder sections, but in the second version they were encouraged into the underutilized corridor sections by the addition of logs hung from the corridor walls.

On a larger scale this approach is exemplified by the search for alternatives to the battery cage for laying hens. Fifteen years ago both aviary systems for large flocks, and 'get-away' cages for much smaller groups of hens, were being tested (reviewed by Elson, 1986). The development of the aviary into a tiered wire floor system and multi-tiered percheries for large flocks has been achieved by systematic modification of a series of prototypes over the past decade at Spelderholt, The Netherlands (Centre for Poultry Research and Extension, 1988) and at ADAS, Gleadthorpe, UK, while get-away cages for 15–60 hens have been modified and improved in a similar series of trials at Celle, Germany (Wegner, 1990). It is notable that initial differences in design between these two systems, in group size for example, have persisted despite the process of trial and modification undergone by each. A danger with this approach is that the initial idea may not be fully justified, but it may be difficult to change course after substantial investment of time and money. Provision for important behaviours may continue to be overlooked if it did not feature in the original plan, and even ultimately successful designs may be overcomplicated in comparison with designs arrived at from first principles.

Environmental enrichment

Two rather different, although partially overlapping, aims are often subsumed under the heading of environmental enrichment. One approach concentrates on keeping animals occupied by the provision of a variety of objects, often with the aim of reducing feather pecking or tail biting (Fig. 4.1) (e.g. Braastad, 1990; Blokhuis and van der Haar, 1992). Aggression also appears to be reduced if newly weaned gilts are provided with tyres (Schaefer *et al.*, 1990) and a reduction in inactive or apathetic lying has been noted in piglets provided with an earth trough (Wood-Gush and Beilharz, 1983; Appleby and Wood-Gush, 1988), and sows allowed access to straw (Fraser, 1975). The second approach concentrates on altering developmental patterns by increasing the complexity of the neonatal environment (Jones, 1989). Benefits include a reduction in fearfulness in young chicks (Jones, 1989; Gvaryahu *et al.*, 1989), laying hens (Reed *et al.*, 1993) and pigs (Pearce *et al.*, 1989). Environmental enrichment can also result in improved growth efficiency in chicks (Jones *et al.*, 1980) and broilers (Gvaryahu *et al.*, 1989).

Despite these advantages there are a number of pitfalls to environ-

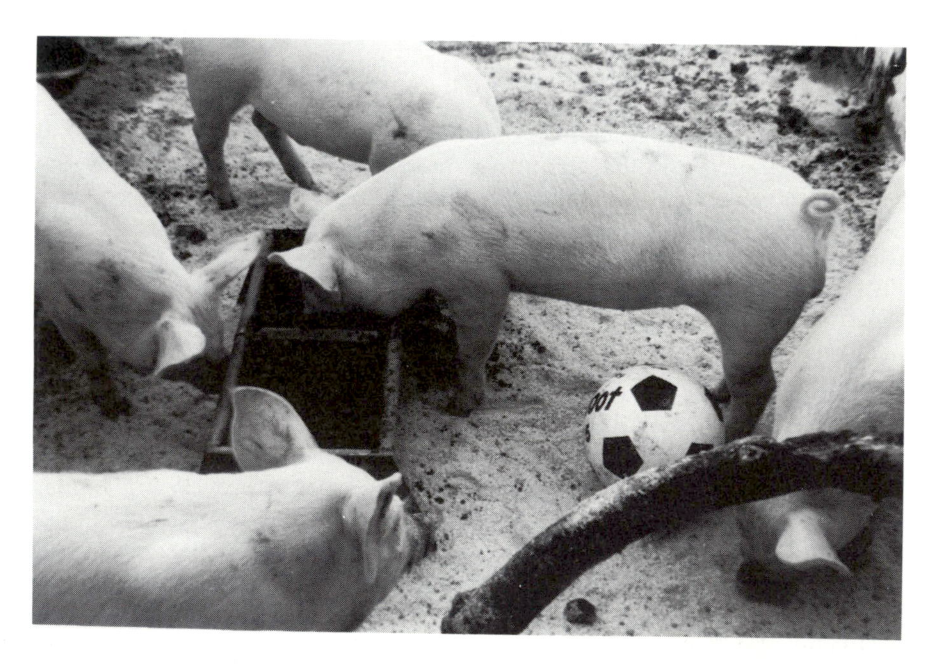

Fig. 4.1. Growing pigs in an enriched environment with earth trough, branches and balls.

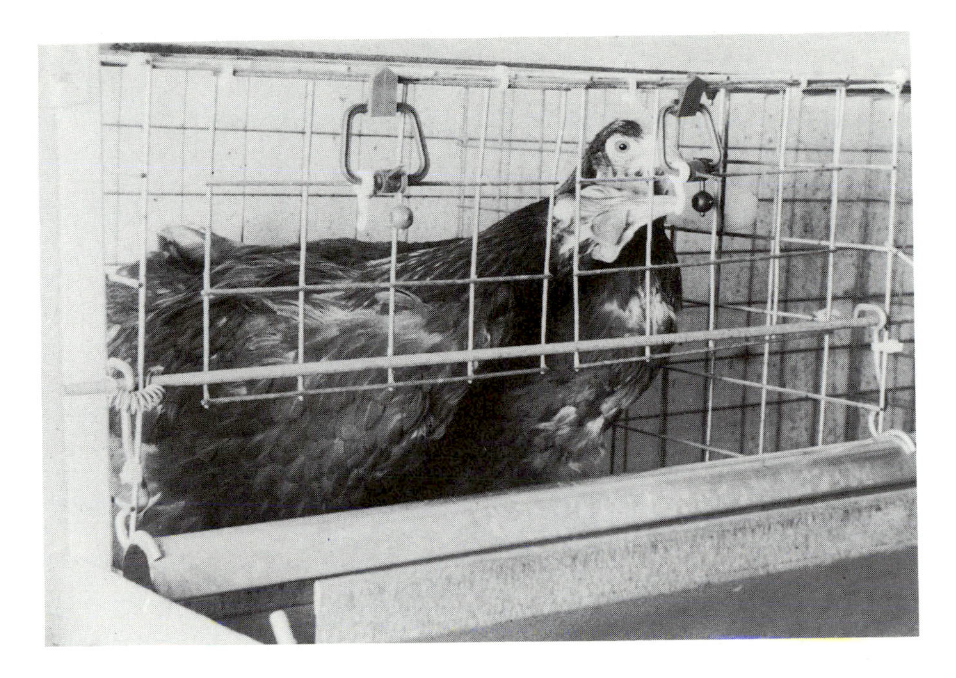

Fig. 4.2. Caged hens peck at simple coloured objects at a high initial rate, but (with objects similar to these shown) this declines rapidly as the hens habituate.

mental enrichment programmes that illustrate the need for fundamental behavioural studies. One problem is that providing extra objects may motivate territorial behaviour or resource-defence, and result in increased aggression (McGregor and Ayling, 1990). Some individuals within a social group may be denied access to the new features and suffer greater frustration as a result. Animals may also habituate rapidly to novel objects. Piglets, for example, gradually lose interest in earth troughs (Appleby and Wood-Gush, 1988), and are likely to work for access to earth once they have had some experience with it (Hutson, 1989). Hens habituate very rapidly to simple and 'motorized' pecking objects hung from the cage front (Sherwin, 1991, 1993) (Fig. 4.2). Lastly, there is often no clear rationale for the choice of objects provided. Shepherdson (1989) has argued that animals may simply redirect stereotypic or other 'abnormal' behaviour towards the new objects.

The five freedoms

Recognizing the importance of conjoint consideration of physical and mental well-being Webster (1984) proposed that housing systems should be evaluated according to the degree that the animals housed within them are free: (i) from hunger and malnutrition; (ii) from thermal and physical discomfort; (iii) from injury and disease; (iv) from fear and stress; and (v) to express normal behaviour. Commercial rearing of calves in crates fails to protect any of these freedoms (Webster *et al.*, 1986), and the conventional battery cage subjects birds to chronic discomfort and restricts the performance of normal behaviour (FAWC, 1985). The five freedoms provide a useful framework for evaluating existing systems. But the idea that animals should be able to perform normal behaviour begs many questions when it comes to designing improved housing systems. What is normal behaviour and what are the consequences of preventing it? Webster *et al.* (1986) state that the 'access' system for group rearing calves with controlled access to milk and dry food does not compromise any of the five freedoms. Yet the calves are still separated from their mothers and have to suckle from a teat rather than the udder. A literal reading of the five freedoms would overturn deep seated agricultural practices, such as weaning. A calf may or may not suffer from loss of maternal contact if it is housed with others, but we will need evidence one way or the other if we want to alter commercial practice so radically.

The approaches outlined above have all contributed to the improvement of animal housing, but it is clear that further information about behavioural priorities is still needed to answer lingering doubts about welfare, and to overcome practical problems. This information must primarily come from experiments.

Experiments in Animal Behaviour

Motivation – identification of causal factors

In order to behave an animal must have a body to behave with and an environment to behave in. It is therefore a truism to say that all behaviour depends on both internal and external factors. Toates and Jensen (1991) argue, however, that variations in the appearance of different behaviours may depend on either internal or external factors. Given a relatively constant environment in an animal house and an *ad libitum* balanced ration, the appearance of bouts of feeding behaviour might be explained almost entirely in terms of variations in internal state. On the other hand, feeding behaviour might be initiated in an apparently full animal if a particularly tasty morsel (external factor) is presented. Some behaviours may very rarely be elicited by anything other than internal factors, while others may be almost totally dependent on external factors for their appearance. Welfare implications of preventing behaviour performance will depend on these differences in causation, and on the strength of the animal's resultant motivation.

External factors have been postulated as of primary importance in the occurrence of behaviours such as aggression, fear and sheltering (Hughes and Duncan, 1988). If animals do not encounter aggressive rivals, predators or extreme weather conditions they may not be motivated to perform the appropriate adaptive behaviours, and their welfare will not be compromised if they are housed in conditions where aggressive or fearful behaviours are difficult to perform. Even behaviours which the animal finds it pleasurable to perform, sunbathing perhaps, or wallowing (Stolba and Wood-Gush, 1989) may not be missed if the relevant external cues (unfiltered sunlight or high ambient temperatures) are never encountered. However, welfare problems may arise if an animal is prevented from performing a behaviour when the relevant external causal factor is present. Such situations are often referred to as frustrating (Duncan, 1970). A caged rabbit unable to move out of sight of an excited dog, or a tethered sow unable to reach some food spilt nearby are two hypothetical examples. Usually, in these cases there will be two different ways of reducing frustration: either allowing the animal to perform the relevant behaviour or removing the causal factor. The welfare of

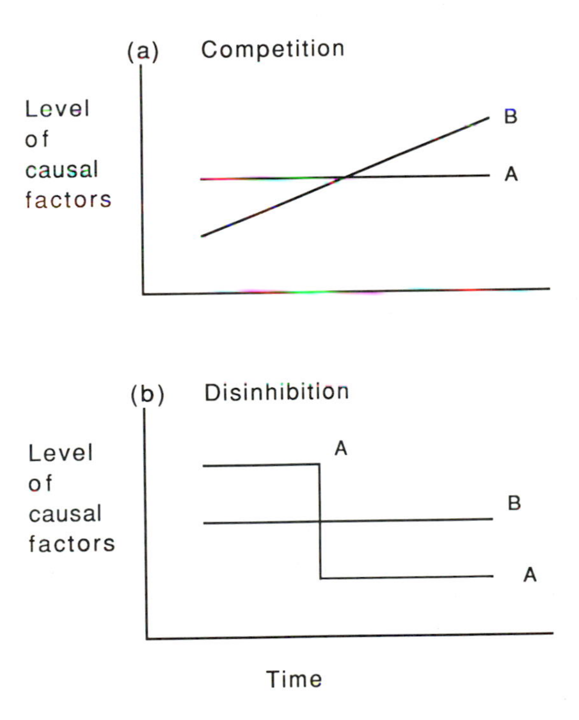

Fig. 4.3. (a) Behaviour B is expressed because the level of its own causal factors rises. (b) Behaviour B is expressed only when the level of causal factors for behaviour A falls (after McFarland, 1985).

a tethered animal unable to shake rain off its head, for example, might be equally improved either by loosening the tether or by mending the roof. However, where *internal* factors are of primary importance in the appearance of a behaviour we will be able to do little to reduce motivation by environmental manipulation. We still may need to know whether the behaviour normally appears in response to a rise in strength of its internal causal factors relative to others (appearance by competition) or only in response to falls in the strength of other causal factors (appearance by disinhibition) (Fig. 4.3). Suffering will be particularly likely where competitive internal factors are involved because animals will have been selected to pay attention to rises in the strengths of these factors and act upon them, perhaps by ceasing other ongoing behaviour or by initiating a search for the necessary consummatory stimuli (such as food, mates or even novelty). We should therefore allow animals the opportunity to perform these behaviours, particularly if motivation is high.

Despite the importance of understanding motivation there have been few detailed attempts to discover the relative contribution of internal and external causal factors in the motivation of farm animal behaviour. It is not easy to ascertain the nature and strength of internal causal factors. Detailed physiological investigations can be undertaken and have, for example, helped to elucidate the basis of drinking behaviour in goats (Thornton and Baldwin, 1985). Occasionally animals may display visible and reliable markers of their internal state. Baerends *et al.* (1955) found that the tendency of male guppies to behave sexually towards females could be gauged from the colour of their skin. But such markers will only be seen if communication of information about its motivational state is evolutionarily advantageous to the displaying individual (Krebs and Dawkins, 1984). However, much can still be learnt about internal state by careful behavioural experiments. For example, behavioural sequences can be interrupted by presenting a stimulus or 'probe' which allows the animal to perform an alternative behaviour without preventing it from continuing with its current behaviour (McFarland, 1989). This type of experiment has not so far been widely used by applied ethologists, although Culshaw and Broom (1980) have assessed the effects of interruptions at different points during bouts of feeding or preening behaviour in domestic chicks. The results provide evidence about changes in motivational state during each bout.

To date, however, most inferences about internal state have been drawn from observations of behaviour after a period of deprivation. It is often found that animals show a greatly increased tendency to perform certain behaviours once the restrictions on performance have been lifted. Lying in dairy cows (Metz and Wierenga, 1984) and wing flapping in hens (Nicol, 1987b) provide good examples of this rebound effect in farm animals. In fact rebound behaviour may occur at rates higher than those ever observed before deprivation (Nicol, 1987b) (Fig. 4.4). Rebound behaviour has often

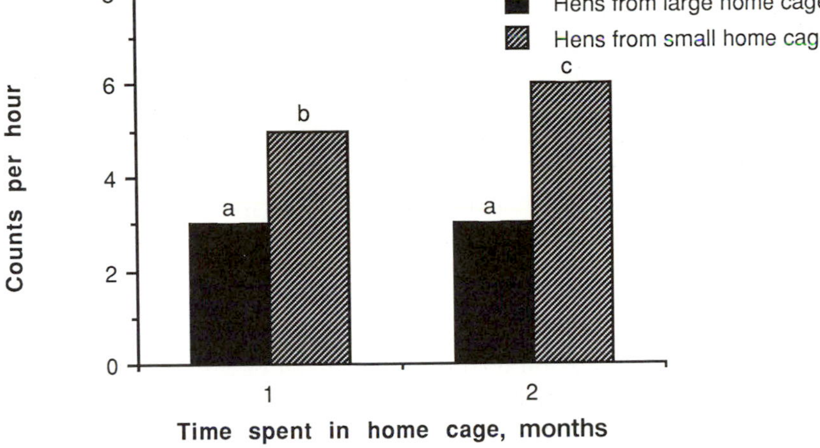

Fig. 4.4. A rebound in wing flapping is seen when hens are moved after one month from small home cages to large test cages. The rebound in wing flapping is even more pronounced after two months' confinement in a small home cage. Control hens are simply moved between large home and test cages (after Nicol, 1987b).

been interpreted as evidence for a rise in strength of internal causal factors during the deprivation period, and hence as a potential source of suffering. However, McFarland (1989) has emphasized that rebound after deprivation might sometimes be explicable as a response to renewed novelty. He imagines a child playing with a new toy at a high level but gradually reducing the level of play as the toy becomes more familiar. If the toy is then removed for some time, the child may show an increased level of play when the toy is returned. In order to distinguish between these possibilities we need evidence that internal causal factors rise during the period of deprivation itself, before external stimuli are re-presented. Van Liere and Wiepkema (1992) have recently shown that the amount of dustbathing without litter (sham dustbathing) by hens kept on a wooden slatted floor increased steadily during a 21 week period of sand deprivation. Initially, in the presence of weak external cues provided by the slatted floor, the overall motivation to dustbath was low, and little sham bathing was seen. But, as the weeks passed, sham dustbathing began to appear and was performed in an increasingly complete form. The authors infer that the motivation to dustbathe increased during the period of sand deprivation. Another way of investigating motivational state during deprivation is to ask whether the animal (or child) makes any attempt to search for the missing resource (or toy). Bell (1991) gives examples of searching behaviour initiated in the absence of external stimulation, e.g. by birds for their migratory destinations, and by squirrels for hidden acorns. Nicol and Guilford (1991) found that both food-deprived and litter-deprived hens spent more time engaged in unrewarded searching activity than non-deprived controls. That birds should search for food is not surprising. That they should search for litter is perhaps less obvious, as it is easy to imagine activities such as dustbathing only being performed when the hen stumbles across the appropriate stimulus. These results, however, do suggest that hens may be motivated to obtain litter during periods of deprivation. At this point it may be important to note that battery hens are deprived not just of litter but also of the opportunity to search for it. Exploratory behaviour may be reinforcing in itself (Wood-Gush and Vestergaard, 1989) and important in giving animals a feeling of control over their environment (Wiepkema, 1990).

It is perhaps easier to ascertain the nature and strength of any external causal factors, provided proper account is taken of the animals' perceptual abilities. Experimental animals may simply be exposed to different environments (which must not restrict the performance of the behaviour in question) or to rewards of differing quality, and conclusions drawn according to the behaviours observed. The visibility and proximity of other hens, for example, appears to be an external cue for the performance of stretching and preening behaviour in hens (Nicol, 1989). External causal factors may, of course, act over a longer period of time as, for example, seasonal changes in daylength which affect reproductive behaviour in most farm animals.

Increasing information in this area means that ethologists are now able to construct accurate models that show how internal and external causal factors are integrated in the motivation of specified behaviour patterns in farm animals. Jensen (1993) for example, has shown that the initial preparation of the nest site in sows is controlled largely by internal factors, whereas the later gathering and nest-building site is largely dependent on external cues.

Motivation strength

Once the relative contribution of internal and external causal factors in the motivation of behaviour has been ascertained we need to establish just how strong the animal's motivation now is. The standard way of doing this has been to get the animal to 'work' to obtain the opportunity to behave. This can be done by spatial separation of the factors needed for a particular behaviour, so that the animal has to move to obtain access. The animal may be allowed free access between two or more environments, or may be required to make an initial choice in a T-maze and then confined for a period of time in its chosen environment before being required to choose again. The motivation of hens to obtain litter has been assessed in this way (Dawkins, 1981). Access can be made more difficult by requiring the animals to squeeze through narrow gaps (Nicol, 1986) or push through weighted doors (Duncan and Kite, 1987; Petherick and Rutter, 1990). Sometimes the aim is not to assess the animal's motivation to perform any particular behaviour, but simply to examine its preferences for varying designs of environmental features such as floor types (Hughes and Black, 1973), nest boxes (Huber *et al.*, 1985), or farrowing sites (Baxter, 1990). It is obviously important to consider the influence of position preferences, period of deprivation (Vestergaard, 1988), experience with each alternative offered (Dawkins, 1983), and exploratory 'monitoring' behaviour shown during the test (Nicol, 1986).

Animals can also be trained to make an operant response such as pressing a bar or pecking a key to receive the relevant reward. Preferences for quantitative changes in the intensity of positive reinforcers such as heat and light have traditionally been assessed in this way, but diverse studies of food preferences and milking plant design in cattle, social contact and access to earth in pigs, and litter and cage size in hens have also been undertaken using operant conditioning. The use of operant technology in these contexts has recently been reviewed by Kilgour *et al.* (1991). Access can be made more difficult in operant tests by increasing the number of responses the animal must make to obtain the same reward. Dawkins (1990) has argued that strength of demand can be assessed by examining the elasticity of response when the animal has to work harder for the same amount of reward. If the animal shows that it has an inelastic demand for a particular environment or reward by continuing to work even when access is made progressively more difficult, and when there are no suitable substitutes available (Matthews, 1991), then that environment or reward can be defined as a necessity. Pigs and hens appear to show an inelastic demand for food (Matthews and Ladewig, 1987; Dawkins, 1990). Indeed, increasing concern about the welfare of animals kept on restricted food rations, such as sows and broiler parents is underlined by operant studies of food demand (Lawrence and Illius, 1989). In some cases it appears that individual sows are so hungry that they will actually sustain an energy deficit to gain additional food (Hutson, 1991). Inelastic demand for access to a nest box has been demonstrated in hens (Duncan and Kite, 1987), although demand for social contact is more elastic (Dawkins, 1990). This implies that a suitable nest is a necessity for a hen but other features may be luxuries whatever their motivational basis. Further work is obviously required for all farm livestock (studies so far have tended to concentrate on laying hens and pigs) before a list of housing priorities could be compiled for each species.

It is important not only to consider motivation to perform particular behaviour patterns or obtain different resources, but also the motivation of animals to escape from housing conditions or other situations which they find aversive. Preference and operant conditioning tests can be used again in this context, but extra problems can arise if the animals exhibit incompatible

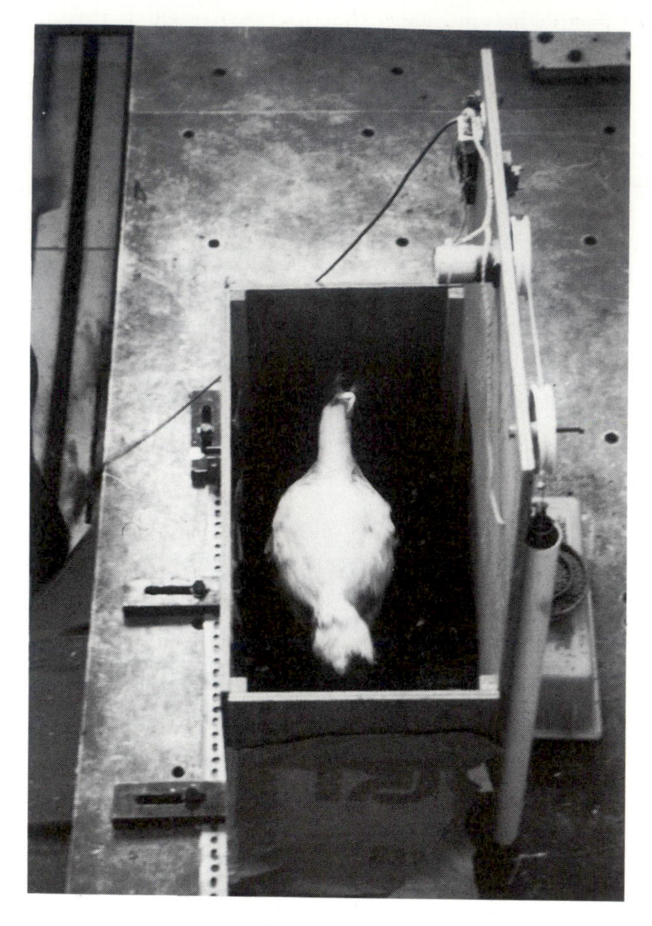

Fig. 4.5. Chickens in an operant chamber on a movement simulator quickly learn not to peck the key for food if they find the subsequent contingent motion aversive (Nicol *et al.*, 1991).

innate reactions. Highly fearful birds, for example, may 'freeze', thus affecting their ability both to walk away from the situation or to perform an operant response. Rutter and Duncan (1992) have shown that aversion can be better measured in chickens by training them to avoid responding (for some pre-set reward) in order to avoid exposure to an aversive stimulus. An operant passive avoidance technique of this type has been used to assess the aversiveness of different types of motion to broiler chickens (Nicol *et al.*, 1991) (Fig. 4.5). Rushen (1986) has discussed the general problems of validating behavioural measures of aversion.

Observing the Behaviour of Housed Animals

Although well-designed experiments are the backbone of behavioural welfare assessment, it is often helpful to have some reliable indicators which can be used to assess a housing system *in situ*. Redirected behaviours, stereotypies and agonistic interactions are all commonly observed in farm animals. What do they tell us about welfare?

Redirected behaviour

Outbreaks of behaviours such as feather pecking, tail biting or cannibalism are all causes for concern because of the physical pain or injury suffered by the victims (Fig. 4.6). It is less clear whether the perpetrators also suffer. It may be that pecking another chicken is an adequate substitute for deprived nesting, foraging or dustbathing activity, but the question is somewhat superfluous. However, where the redirection of behaviour does not damage another animal the same question is more important. Fraser and Broom (1990) cite examples of animals eating their own hair or feathers, wood, earth or dung. Often deleterious effects on health will be noticed, but where they are not, it is difficult to argue a priori that welfare is reduced. Indeed,

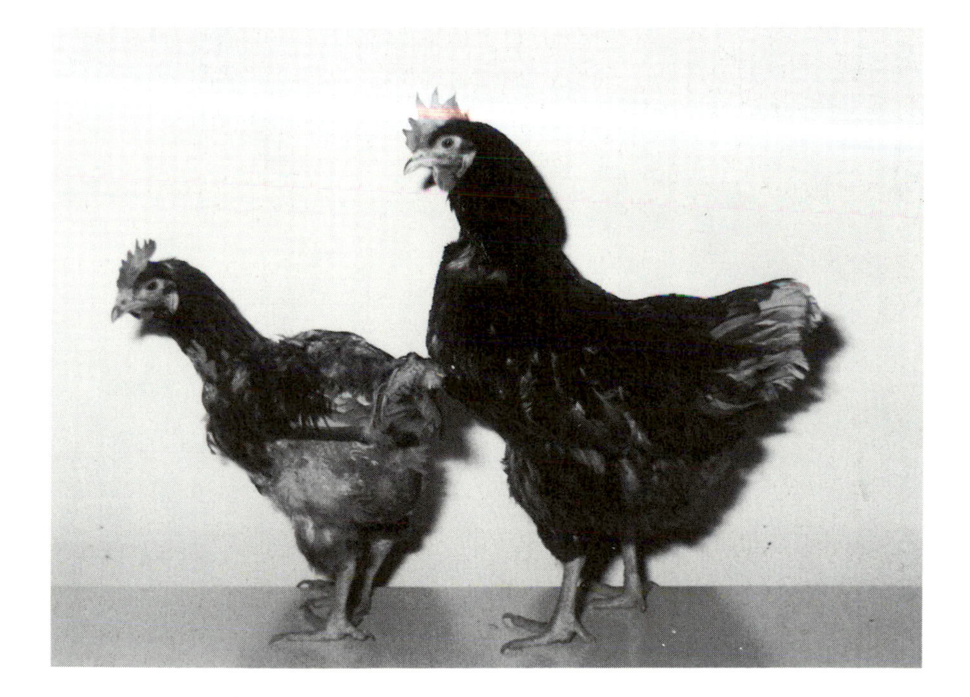

Fig. 4.6. The results of feather pecking are painful denuded areas of flesh.

the explicit aim of many environmental enrichment programmes is to redirect oral behaviour towards artificial substrates of one kind or another.

Stereotypies

Stereotypies, defined as repeated, relatively invariant sequences of movements with no obvious purpose (Fraser and Broom, 1990), are common in confined livestock, and include bar biting and sham chewing in pigs, pre-egg-laying pacing in hens, and weaving and crib biting in horses. The diversity in appearance of stereotypies is reflected by diversity in their causes and effects (Mason, 1991). Some stereotypies may be associated with stress, or negative feelings such as aversion, but this may not be a universal feature (Duncan *et al.*, 1993). A number of studies have shown that stereotypies arise when the normal expression of a motivational state is blocked. The blocked motivation may be to move or escape from restrictive housing. Blocked feeding motivation also appears to be an important cause of stereotypies in many species. Strong experimental evidence, reviewed in Rushen *et al.* (1993), links an increased incidence of stereotypies in pigs, sheep and poultry with the feeding of restricted rations.

A controversial issue is whether the performance of stereotypies might

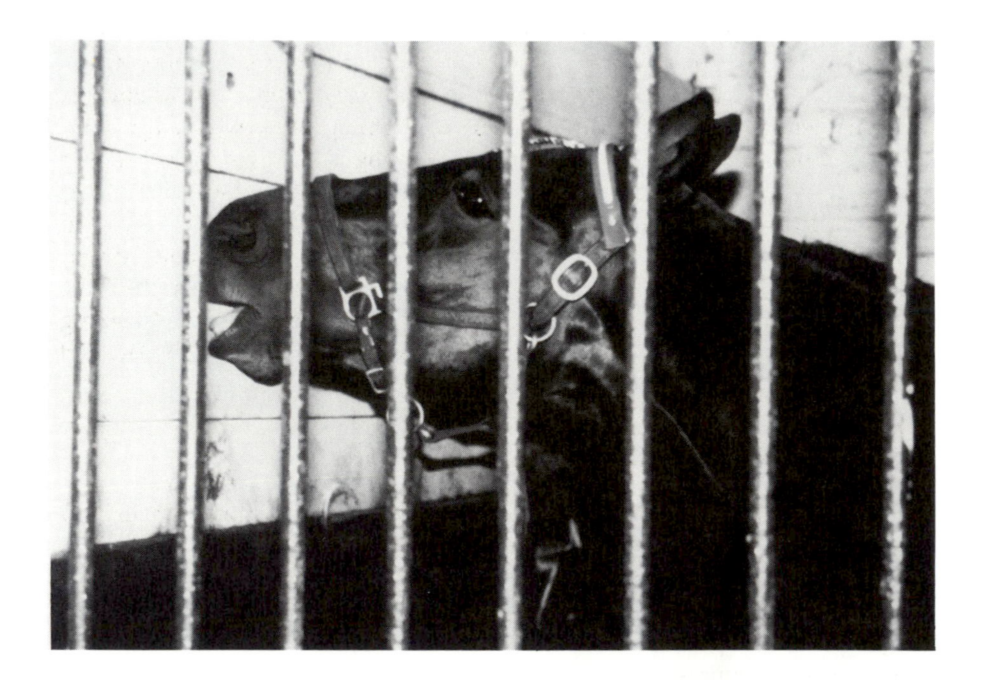

Fig. 4.7. Owners often attempt to prevent horses from showing stereotypies such as cribbing and weaving. This may compromise welfare still further (photo A. Clarke).

in any way help an animal cope with deprivation or aversion (Odberg, 1989). In voles, preventing the performance of stereotypies by erecting physical barriers results in an increase in corticosteroids associated with stress (Kennes and De Rycke, 1988). It also appears that previously robust environmental preferences diminish as stereotypies develop (Cooper and Nicol, 1991), suggesting that stereotypic individuals become less aware of, or less concerned about, their external environment. An unpleasant environment may correspondingly be perceived as less aversive. A healthy debate currently surrounds this area of research (Cooper and Nicol, 1993; Rushen 1993). However, if it turns out that some stereotypies cause (rather than are simply associated with) a reduction in feelings of aversion then preventing stereotypies by erecting anti-weaving bars in stables, for example, can only reduce welfare further (Fig. 4.7). Such measures simply attempt to disguise the symptoms of a complex, underlying problem.

Aggression

Huntingford and Turner (1987) find no substantial evidence that aggression is mediated by competitive internal causal factors, i.e. that aggressive motivation increases as a function of the time since it was last performed. There are also few well-documented cases of animals working hard for the opportunity to fight. In general, if animals are kept in stable social groups in conditions where pain, frustration and competition for resources are minimized, aggression does not appear to be actively sought. The welfare of animals which are injured as a result of fighting is undoubtedly compromised but aggressors may also suffer. Fighting is often defensive and an indicator of a strong state of fearfulness. In some species, the parts of the brain which control offensive and defensive fighting overlap, whereas in other species these parts of the brain are separate (Huntingford and Turner, 1987, p. 146). It may therefore be highly species specific whether the aggressor actually suffers from fear or frustration during an attack. Avoiding the environmental conditions which may provoke aggression is the desired course.

Indicators of good welfare

It is something of an indictment that this section is so short. Fraser and Broom (1990) state that 'the recognition of good welfare ... depends, principally, on the absence of indicators of poor welfare ...'. Yet behaviours such as play or laughter would seem to be indicators of positive enjoyment in people. Perhaps we have not looked closely enough for analogous behaviours in animals.

Putting Animals in Control

Ethologists have recommended that automated systems should be designed to give animals more control over their own environments (Appleby and Hughes, 1993). The advent of electronic feeders operated via implanted or attached transponders mean that pigs and cows are increasingly provided with the opportunity to choose their own feeding times. Advances in robotic milking (Frost, 1990) mean that in future dairy cows may also be able to choose when to be milked. Operant conditioning has also been used to grant animals more control over their own heating and lighting in experimental studies (Baldwin and Start, 1981; Curtis, 1983; Morrison *et al.*, 1987). More work is needed to evaluate the commercial possibilities of extending this approach, and to avoid problems of agonistic encounters arising from competition for access (Hunter *et al.*, 1988) or too rare or too frequent use of the resource (Metz and Ipema, 1990). Differences in the needs of individuals within the group must also be considered (Appleby and Hughes, 1993). Wiepkema (1990) points out that on modern farms animals may well be able to predict changes in their environment (the arrival of food, lighting changes, etc.) but are often not in a position to control these changes. He argues that a reduction in predictability may matter more to relatively 'passive' individuals, while a reduction in controllability will have a more adverse effect on relatively 'active' animals.

Future Research

The goal of high-welfare housing is an important one, and will not be achieved simply by abandoning intensive systems. Duncan (1993) believes that many of the mistakes made in designing animal housing in the 1970s and 1980s stemmed from an attempt to design housing that people imagined would suit the animals rather than allowing the animals to choose what was most important to them. A new approach is to work from first principles, designing a husbandry system that caters for the animals' highest priority needs first, and then adding features of lower priority in a methodical and controlled way (Duncan, 1993). This approach is exemplified by work on modified cages for hens (Sherwin and Nicol, 1992; Appleby, 1993). In many cases this approach will inevitably result in giving farm animals more freedom to move around, to control their environment and to interact with others. Our understanding of farm animal behaviour will have to become more detailed if we are to understand fully how they react to these less restricted environments. Rather than concentrating just on simple responses we will need to investigate their cognitive abilities in some depth.

Most farm animals are descended from group-living ancestors, with complex and subtle social lives. It is salutary to realize that we do not yet fully understand how individuals recognize each other (Ryan, 1982; Bradshaw and Dawkins, 1993). One potential advantage to living in a group is the opportunity to learn new and advantageous patterns of behaviour by observing or imitating others. Hens (Nicol and Pope, 1992, 1993) and cattle (Veissier, 1993) have been shown to learn new responses from each other, but much remains for further study. More information about the reaction of animals to pain and distress in their companions would be valuable in the humane design of housing systems and slaughterhouses. We do not know, for example, how the sight, sound or smell of a shackled chicken or a stunned pig affects waiting animals, although exposure to blood or conspecific tissue has been shown to be aversive to rats (Stevens and Gerzog-Thomas, 1977) and frightening to chickens (Jones and Black, 1979). Lastly, we should tackle the question of whether animals are able to think back or anticipate future events. The welfare of an animal that cannot think about the past or the future will depend entirely on its current state. Although this could prevent it worrying about future aversive events or possibilities, its welfare may be compromised if it is unable to foresee the end of a period of pain or discomfort (Duncan and Petherick, 1991).

References

Animal Welfare Institute (1987) *Factory Farming: the Experiment that Failed.* The Animal Welfare Institute, Washington.

Appleby, M.C. (1993) Should cages for laying hens be banned or modified? *Animal Welfare* 2, 67–80.

Appleby, M.C. and Hughes, B.O. (1993) The future of applied ethology. *Applied Animal Behaviour Science* 35, 389–395.

Appleby, M.C. and Lawrence, A.B. (1987) Food restriction as a cause of stereotypic behaviour in tethered gilts. *Animal Production* 45, 103–110.

Appleby, M.C. and Wood-Gush, D.G.M. (1988) Effect of earth as an additional stimulus on the behaviour of confined piglets. *Behavioural Processes* 17, 83–92.

Arey, D.S., Petcher, A.M. and Fowler, V.R. (1991) The preparturient behaviour of sows in enriched pens and the effect of pre-formed nests. *Applied Animal Behaviour Science* 31, 61–68.

Baerends, G.P., Brouwer, R. and Waterbolk, M.J. (1955) Ethological studies of *Lebiste reticulatis.* 1. An analysis of the male courtship pattern. *Behaviour* 8, 249–334.

Baldwin, B.A. and Start, I.B. (1981) Sensory reinforcement and illumination preference in sheep and calves. *Proceedings of the Royal Society, London* series B, 211, 497–507.

Baxter, M.R. (1983) Housing and welfare from first principles. In: Baxter, S.H., Baxter, M.R. and MacCormack, J.A.C. (eds), *Farm Animal Welfare and Housing.* Martinus Nijhoff, The Hague.

Baxter, M.R. (1990) Confounded preference tests: sow choices around farrowing. *Applied Animal Behaviour Science* 28, 295–296.

Bell, W.J. (1991) *Searching Behaviour: the Behavioural Ecology of Finding Resources.* Chapman & Hall, London.

Blokhuis, H.J. and van der Haar, J.W. (1992) Effects of pecking incentives during rearing on feather pecking of laying hens. *British Poultry Science* 33, 17–24.

Braastad, B.O. (1990) Effects on behaviour and plumage of a key-stimuli floor and a perch in triple cages for laying hens. *Applied Animal Behaviour Science* 27, 127–139.

Bradshaw, R.H. and Dawkins, M.S. (1993) Slides of conspecifics as representatives of real animals in laying hens (*Gallus domesticus*). *Behavioural Processes* 28, 165–172.

Carson, K. and Wood-Gush, D.G.M. (1983) A review of the literature on feeding, eliminative and resting behaviour in horses. *Applied Animal Ethology* 10, 179–190.

Centre for Poultry Research and Extension (1988) *The Tiered Wire Floor System for Laying Hens,* The Netherlands.

Cooper, J.J. and Nicol, C.J. (1991) Stereotypic behaviour affects environmental preference in bank voles. (*Clethrionomys glareolus*). *Animal Behaviour* 41, 971–977.

Cooper, J.J. and Nicol, C.J. (1993) The coping hypothesis of stereotypic behaviour: a reply to Rushen. *Animal Behaviour* 45, 616–618.

Culshaw, A.D. and Broom, D.M. (1980) The imminence of behavioural change and startle responses of chicks. *Behaviour* 73, 64–76.

Curtis, S.E. (1983) Perception of thermal comfort by farm animals. In: Baxter, S.H., Baxter, M.R. and MacCormack, J.A.C. (eds), *Farm Animal Welfare and Housing.* Martinus Nijhoff, The Hague, pp. 59–66.

Dawkins, M.S. (1980) *Animal Suffering. The Science of Animal Welfare.* Chapman & Hall, London.

Dawkins, M.S. (1981) Priorities in the cage size and flooring preferences of domestic hens. *British Poultry Science* 22, 255–263.

Dawkins, M.S. (1983) The current status of preference tests in the assessment of animal welfare. In: Baxter, S.H., Baxter, M.R. and MacCormack, J.A.C. (eds), *Farm Animal Welfare and Housing.* Martinus Nijhoff, The Hague, pp. 20 26.

Dawkins, M.S. (1989) Time budgets in Red Junglefowl as a baseline for the assessment of welfare in domestic fowl. *Applied Animal Behaviour Science* 24, 77–80.

Dawkins, M.S. (1990) From an animal's point of view: motivation, fitness and animal welfare. *Behavioural and Brain Sciences* 13, 1–61.

Duncan, I.J.H. (1970) Frustration in the fowl. In: Freeman, B.M. and Gorden, R.F. (eds), *Aspects of Poultry Behaviour.* British Poultry Science, Edinburgh, pp. 15–31.

Duncan, I.J.H. (1980) The ethogram of the domesticated hen. In: Moss, R. (ed.), *The Laying Hen and its Environment.* Martinus Nijhoff, The Hague, pp. 5–16.

Duncan, I.J.H. (1993) Designing environments for animals – not for public perceptions. *British Veterinary Journal* 148, 475–477.

Duncan, I.J.H. and Hughes, B.O. (1972) Free and operant feeding in domestic fowls. *Animal Behaviour* 20, 775–777.

Duncan, I.J.H. and Kite, V.G. (1987) Some investigations into motivation in the domestic fowl. *Applied Animal Behaviour Science* 18, 387–388.

Duncan, I.J.H. and Petherick, J.C. (1991) The implications of cognitive processes for animal welfare. *Journal of Animal Science* 69, 5017–5022.

Duncan, I.J.H. and Poole, T.B. (1990) Promoting the welfare of farm and captive animals. In: Monaghan, P. and Wood-Gush, D. (eds), *Managing the Behaviour of Animals.* Chapman & Hall, London, pp. 193–232.

Duncan, I.J.H., Rushen, J. and Lawrence, A.B. (1993) Conclusions and implications for animal welfare. In: Lawrence, A.B. and Rushen, J. (eds), *Stereotypic Animal Behaviour: Fundamentals and Applications to Welfare.* CAB International, Wallingford.

Duncan, P. (1980) Time budgets of Camargue horses. *Behaviour* 72, 26–47.

Elson, H.A. (1986) Poultry management systems – looking to the future. *World's Poultry Science Journal* 44, 103–111.

Ewbank, R. (1988) Animal welfare. In: *Management and Welfare of Farm Animals,* 3rd edn. Ballière Tindall, London.

Farm Animal Welfare Council (1985) *Assessment of Egg Production Systems.* FAWC, Tolworth, Surrey.

Fraser, A.F. and Broom, D.M. (1990) *Farm Animal Behaviour and Welfare,* 3rd edn. Ballière Tindall, London.

Fraser, D. (1975) The effect of straw on the behaviour of sows in tether stalls. *Animal Production* 21, 59–68.

Frost, A.R. (1990) Robotic milking: a review. *Robotica* 8, 311–318.

Gvaryahu, G., Cunningham, D.L. and Van Tienhoven, A. (1989) Filial imprinting, environmental enrichment and music application effects on behaviour and performance of meat-strain chickens. *Poultry Science* 68, 211–217.

Huber, H.U., Folsch, D.W. and Stahli, U. (1985) Influence of various nesting materials on nest site selection of the domestic hen. *British Poultry Science* 26, 367–374.

Hughes, B.O. and Black, A.J. (1973) The preference of domestic hens for different types of battery cage floor. *British Poultry Science* 14, 615–619.

Hughes, B.O. and Duncan, I.J.H. (1988) The notion of ethological 'need', models of motivation and animal welfare. *Animal Behaviour* 36, 1676–1707.

Hughes, B.O., Duncan, I.J.H. and Brown, M.F. (1989) The performance of nest building by domestic hens: is it more important than the construction of a nest? *Animal Behaviour* 37, 210–214.

Hunter, E.J., Broom, D.M., Edwards, S.A. and Sibly, R.M. (1988) Social hierarchy and feeder access in a group of 20 sows using a computer-controlled feeder. *Animal Production* 47, 139–148.

Huntingford, F.A. and Turner, A.K. (1987) *Animal Conflict.* Chapman & Hall, London.

Hutson, G.D. (1989) Operant tests of access to earth as a reinforcement for weaner pigs. *Animal Production* 48, 561–569.

Hutson, G.D. (1991) A note on hunger in the pig: sows on restricted rations will sustain an energy deficit to gain additional feed. *Animal Production* 52, 233–235.

Jensen, P. (1993) Nest building in domestic sows: the role of external stimuli. *Animal Behaviour* 45, 351–358.

Jones, R.B. (1989) Development and alleviation of fear in poultry. In: Faure, J.M. and Mills, A.D. (eds), *The Proceedings of the Third European Symposium on Poultry Welfare.* French Branch of the World's Poultry Science Association.

Jones, R.B. and Black, A.J. (1979) Behavioural responses of the domestic chick to blood. *Behavioral and Neural Biology* 27, 319–329.

Jones, R.B., Harvey, S., Hughes, B.O. and Chadwick, A. (1980) Growth and the plasma concentrations of growth hormone and production in chicks: Effects of 'environmental enrichment', sex and strain. *British Poultry Science* 21, 457–462.

Kennes, D. and De Rycke, P.H. (1988) Influence of the performance of stereotypies on plasma corticosterone and leucocyte levels in the bank vole (*Clethrionomys glareolus*). In: Unshelm, J., Van Putten, G., Zeeb, K. and Ekesbo, I. (eds), *Proceedings of the International Congress on Applied Ethology in Farm Animals.* Darmstadt, pp. 238–240.

Kerr, S.C.G., Wood-Gush, D.G.M., Moser, H. and Whittemore, C.T. (1988) Enrichment of the production environment and enhancement of welfare through the use of the Edinburgh family pen system of pig production. *Research and Development in Agriculture* 5, 171–186.

Kilgour, R., Foster, T.M., Temple, W., Matthews, L.R. and Bremner, K.J. (1991) Operant technology applied to solving farm animal problems: an assessment. *Applied Animal Behaviour Science* 30, 141–166.

Krebs, J.R. and Dawkins, R. (1984) Animal signals: mind reading and manipulation. In: Krebs, J.R. and Davies, N.B. (eds) *Behavioural Ecology,* 2nd edn. Blackwell Scientific Publications, Oxford, pp. 380–402.

Lawrence, A.B. and Illius, A.W. (1989) Methodology for measuring hunger and food needs using operant conditioning in the pig. *Applied Animal Behaviour Science* 24, 273–286.

McFarland, D. (1985) *Animal Behaviour.* Longman, Harlow.

McFarland, D. (1989) *Problems of Animal Behaviour.* Longman, Harlow.

McGregor, P.K. and Ayling, S.J. (1990) Varied cages result in more aggression in male CFLP mice. *Applied Animal Behaviour Science* 26, 277–281.

Marsden, M.D. (1993) Feeding practices have greater effect than housing practices on the behaviour and welfare of the horse. In: *Proceedings of the Fourth International Livestock Symposium.* American Society of Agricultural Engineers, Coventry (in press).

Mason, G.J. (1991) Stereotypy: a critical review. *Animal Behaviour* 41, 1015–1037.

Matter, F. and Oester, H. (1989) Hygienic and welfare implications of alternative husbandry systems. In: Faure, J.M. and Mills, A.D. (eds), *Proceedings of the Third European Symposium on Poultry Welfare.* French Branch of the World's Poultry Science Association.

Matthews, L.R. (1991) Behavioural deprivation: are there substitutes for the real thing? In: Appleby, M.C., Horrell, R.I., Petherick, J.C. and Rutter, S.M. (eds), *Applied Animal Behaviour: Past, Present and Future.* Universities Federation for Animal Welfare, Potters Bar, pp. 125–129.

Matthews, L.R. and Ladewig, J. (1987) Stimulus requirements of housed pigs assessed by behavioural demand functions. *Applied Animal Behaviour Science* 17, 363–383.

Metz, J. and Ipema, A.H. (1990) Behavioural problems associated with robot milking. *Applied Animal Behaviour Science* 26, 298–299.

Metz, J.H.M. and Wierenga, H.K. (1984) Spatial requirements and lying behaviour of cows in loose housing systems. In: Unselm, J., van Putten, G. and Zeeb, K. (eds), *Proceedings of the International Congress of Applied Ethology of Farm Animals.* Kiel, Darmstadt, pp. 179–183.

Morrison, W.D., Bate, L.A., Amyot, E. and McMillan, I. (1987) Performance of large groups of chicks using operant conditioning to control the thermal environment. *Poultry Science* 66, 1758–1761.

Murphy, L.B. and Preston, A.P. (1988) Time budgeting in meat chickens grown commercially. *British Poultry Science* 29, 215–222.

Newberry, R.C., Gardiner, E.E. and Hunt, J.R. (1987) Behaviour of chickens prior to death from sudden death syndrome. *Poultry Science* 66, 1446–1450.

Nicol, C.J. (1986) Non-exclusive spatial preference in the laying hen. *Applied Animal Behaviour Science* 15, 337–350.

Nicol, C.J. (1987a) Effect of cage height and area on the behaviour of hens housed in battery cages. *British Poultry Science* 28, 327–335.

Nicol, C.J. (1987b) Behavioural responses of laying hens following a period of spatial restriction. *Animal Behaviour* 35, 1709–1719.

Nicol, C.J. (1989) Social influences on the comfort behaviour of laying hens. *Applied Animal Behaviour Science* 22, 75–81.

Nicol, C.J., Blakeborough, A. and Scott, G.B. (1991) The aversiveness of noise and motion to broiler chickens. *British Poultry Science* 32, 243–254.

Nicol, C.J. and Guilford, T. (1991) Exploratory activity as a measure of motivation in deprived hens. *Animal Behaviour* 41, 333–341.

Nicol, C.J. and Pope, S.J. (1992) Food deprivation during observation reduces social learning in hens. *Animal Behaviour* 45, 193–196.

Nicol, C.J. and Pope, S.J. (1993) Social learning in small flocks of laying hens. *Animal Behaviour* (in press).

Ödberg, F.O. (1989) Behavioural coping in chronic stress conditions. In: Blanchard, R.J., Brain, P.J., Blanchard, D.C. and Parmgiani, S. (eds), *Ethoexperimental Analysis of Behaviour.* Kluwer Academic Press, Dordrecht.

Pearce, G.P., Paterson, A.M. and Pearce, A.N. (1989) The influence of pleasant and unpleasant handling and the provision of toys on the growth and behaviour of male pigs. *Applied Animal Behaviour Science* 23, 27–37.

Petherick, J.C. and Rutter, S.M. (1990) Quantifying motivation using a computer-controlled push-door. *Applied Animal Behaviour Science* 27, 159–167.

Reed, H.J., Wilkins, L.J., Austin, S.D and Gregory, N.G. (1993) The effect of environmental enrichment during rearing on fear reactions and depopulation trauma in adult caged hens. *Applied Animal Behaviour Science* 36, 39–46.

Rushen, J. (1986) The validity of behavioural measures of aversion. *Applied Animal Behaviour Science* 16, 309–323.

Rushen, J. (1993) The coping hypothesis of stereotypic behaviour. *Animal Behaviour* 45, 613–615.

Rushen, J., Lawrence, A.B. and Terlouw, E.M.C. (1993) The motivational basis of stereotypies. In: Lawrence, A.B. and Rushen, J. (eds), *Stereotypic Animal Behaviour: Fundamentals and Applications to Welfare.* CAB International, Wallingford.

Rutter, S.M. and Duncan, I.J.H. (1992) Measuring aversion in domestic fowl using passive avoidance. *Applied Animal Behaviour Science* 33, 53–62.

Ryan, C.M.E. (1982) Concept formation and individual recognition in the domestic chicken. *Behaviour Analysis Letters* 2, 213–220.

Ryder, R.D. (1989) *Animal Revolution: Changing Attitudes Towards Speciesism.* Blackwell Publishers, Oxford.

Schaefer, A.L., Salomons, M.O., Tong, A.K.W., Sather, A.P. and Lepage, P. (1990)

The effect of environmental enrichment on aggression in newly weaned pigs. *Applied Animal Behaviour Science* 27, 41–52.

Schleidt, W.M., Yakalis, G., Donnelly, M. and McGarry, J. (1984) A proposal for a standard ethogram, exemplified by an ethogram of the blue-breasted quail (*Coturnix chinensis*). *Zeitschrift fur Tierpsychology* 64, 193–220.

Shepherdson, D. (1989) Environmental enrichment. *Ratel* 16, 4–9.

Sherwin, C.M. (1991) The preference of hens for pecking simple objects of different colours. In: Appleby, M.C., Horrell, R.I., Petherick, J.C. and Rutter, S.M. (eds), *Applied Animal Behaviour: Past, Present and Future.* Universities Federation for Animal Welfare, Potters Bar, pp. 153–156.

Sherwin, C.M. (1993) Pecking behaviour of laying hens provided with a simple motorised environmental enrichment device. *British Poultry Science* 34, 235–240.

Sherwin, C.M. and Nicol, C.J. (1992) Behaviour and production of laying hens in three prototypes of cages incorporating nests. *Applied Animal Behaviour Science* 35, 41–54.

Simonsen, H.B. (1990) Behaviour and distribution of fattening pigs in the multi-activity pen. *Applied Animal Behaviour Science* 27, 311–324.

Stevens, D.A. and Gerzog-Thomas, D.A. (1977) Fright reactions in rats to conspecific tissue. *Physiology and Behaviour* 18, 47–51.

Stolba, A. and Wood-Gush, D.G.M. (1984) The identification of behavioural key features and their incorporation into a housing design for pigs. *Annuale de Recherches Veterinaires* 15, 287–298.

Stolba, A. and Wood-Gush, D.G.M. (1989) The behaviour of pigs in a semi-natural environment. *Animal Production* 48, 419–425.

Swarbrick, O. (1986) Clinical problems in 'free range' layers. *Veterinary Record* 118, 363.

Thornton, S.N. and Baldwin, B.A. (1985) Drinking in the goat in response to simultaneous peripheral and central infusions of angiotensin. *Physiological Behaviour* 35, 753–755.

Thorpe, W.H (1965) The assessment of pain and distress in animals. In: Brambell, F.W.R. (Chairman) *Report of the Technical Committee to Enquire into the Welfare of Animals kept under Intensive Livestock Systems.* HMSO, London.

Tinbergen, N. (1951) *The Study of Instinct.* Oxford University Press, London.

Toates, F.M. and Jensen, P. (1991) Ethological and psychological models of motivation – towards a synthesis. In: Meyer, J.A. and Wilson, S. (eds), *From Animals to Animats.* MIT Press/Bradford Books, Cambridge, pp. 194–205.

Van Liere, D. and Wiepkema, P.R. (1992) Effects of long term deprivation of sand on dust bathing behaviour in laying hens. *Animal Behaviour* 43, 549–558.

Veissier, I. (1993) Observational learning in cattle. *Applied Animal Behaviour Science* 35, 235–243.

Vestergaard, K. (1988) Deprivation choice tests – a new method to assess the relative strength of two motivational systems. In: Unshelm, J., Van Putten, G., Zeeb, K. and Ekesbo, I. (eds), *Proceedings of the International Congress on Applied Ethology on Farm Animals,* pp. 65–73.

Webster, A.J.F. (1984) *Calf Husbandry, Health and Welfare.* Collins, London.

Webster, A.J.F., Saville, C. and Welchman, D. (1986) *Improved Husbandry Systems for Veal Calves.* Animal Health Trust, Farm Animal Care Trust.

Wechsler, B., Schmid, H. and Moser, H. (1991) Der Stolba-Familienstall fur

Hausschweine. *Animal Management* 22, Birkhauser Verlag, Basel.

Wegner, R-M. (1990) Experience with the get-away cage system. *World's Poultry Science Journal* 46, 41–47.

Wiepkema, P.R. (1990) Stress: ethological implications. In: Puglisi-Allegra, S. and Oliverio, A. (eds), *Psychology of Stress.* Kluwer Academic Publishers, The Netherlands, pp. 1–13.

Wood-Gush, D.G.M. and Beilharz, R.G. (1983) The enrichment of a bare environment for animals in confined conditions. *Applied Animal Ethology* 10, 209–217.

Wood-Gush, D.G.M. and Vestergaard, K. (1989) Exploratory behaviour and the welfare of intensively kept animals. *Journal of Agricultural Ethics* 2, 161–169.

Physical Principles

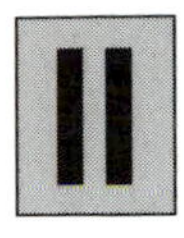

Thermal Exchanges 5

J.A. CLARK AND A.J. MCARTHUR
Department of Physiology and Environmental Science, Sutton Bonington Campus, University of Nottingham, UK

Introduction

The thermal environment in animal houses is important because of its direct thermal effects on the metabolic rate and the efficiency of production by the stock, and its indirect effects on their health and welfare. It is, therefore, important to understand the thermal interactions between stock and their building microclimate, and between the building microclimate and the weather outside, whether the stock are housed for climatic or management reasons. Poor building design and unsuitable microclimates can result in thermal stress on the stock, with consequent productivity losses and risks to welfare. Poor ventilation may also increase the risks to the stock of disease and damaging concentrations of atmospheric contaminants, particularly ammonia (Charles, 1981; Clark and Cena, 1981).

This chapter considers the processes which determine the heat balances of buildings and animals. It is important to distinguish between the two, although interactions between them are important. In particular, the heat input to animal houses in the UK is usually dominated by the non-evaporative heat released by the animals – which in turn is both determined by and is a major determinant of the house temperature. Similarly, the humidity in animal houses is determined by the interaction between the microclimate and evaporation due to the stock (both direct evaporation and that from urine and faeces). Control of the microclimate within houses is, therefore, complicated by the interactions between the animals and their environments. Control criteria are based on the relations between metabolic rate, food consumption and 'environmental temperature' (Clark and Cena, 1981; see also this volume, Chapter 1). Air temperature is the main variable controlled in animal houses, but the controlling variable is usually the ventilation rate or, for young stock in the cold, the heat input (this volume, Chapter 7; Vansteelant *et al.*, 1988).

The heat balance

The principles of heat balance are well established, both for buildings (e.g. Esmay, 1969) and for animals and other living organisms (e.g. Monteith and Mount, 1974; McArthur, 1981a; Monteith and Unsworth, 1990). The heat balance *is* the current state of the particular building or animal. The heat balance equation is the mathematical statement of this balance – which must obey the First Law of Thermodynamics, the law of mass and energy conservation. Fundamentally, we are concerned with the exchange of enthalpy (total heat content) in the system, and the section of this chapter concerned with the heat balance of buildings will consider mainly the enthalpy changes in the ventilating air. However, to facilitate understanding, most treatments of the heat balance of animals separate the transport of non-evaporative heat (often termed sensible (dry) heat) by convection, conduction and radiation, from that of latent heat, due to changes in atmospheric humidity (Cena, 1974; McLean, 1974; Mitchell, 1974).

Thermal Exchanges of Livestock Houses

Ventilation

Ventilation transports heat, respiratory gases and contaminants between buildings and their surroundings, and is the key environmental variable both in the control of livestock housing and in our understanding of the house heat balance. However, both the specification and measurement of ventilation are prone to error and ambiguity. The ventilation rates of buildings, whether by forced or natural means (Vant' Ooster and Both, 1988) are usually specified as air changes per hour (h^{-1}). Fans for mechanical ventilation of buildings are bought in terms of their volume capacity against a known resistance ($m^3 s^{-1}$, or cubic feet per minute in imperial units), and ventilation rates can be measured in volumetric units by monitoring the air velocity in fan-ducts and multiplying the cross-section area of the duct by the mean velocity. However, ventilation rates are ambiguous when expressed in either air change or volume units, because the volume of air changes with its temperature, pressure and humidity. For example, $1\,m^3 s^{-1}$ of air entering a building at 0°C becomes $1.07\,m^3 s^{-1}$ when leaving at 20°C, even without any change in water content. The fundamental quantity is mass transfer: the *masses* of air entering and leaving the building must be equal. The rate at which a material is transported into or out of a building, Q_m (kg s^{-1}), is the product of the difference between the mixing ratios for the particular material inside and outside the building with the ventilating air mass. Thus:

$$Q_m = \theta(\psi_o - \psi_i) \quad (1)$$

where θ is the ventilation rate (kg s^{-1}) and ψ_o and ψ_i are the mixing ratios (kg of the material per kg of air) of the particular material outside and inside the building, respectively. Ventilation rates are best estimated from measurements of tracer gas concentration, using either quasi-steady state or transient methods, rearranging Equation (1) to give θ (Clark and Cena, 1981).

Equation (1) can be rearranged to show how the concentration of a contaminant in the house atmosphere depends on ventilation rate:

$$\psi_i = \psi_o - \frac{Q_m}{\theta} \quad (2)$$

because in steady state the source strength in the building Q_m must equal the quantity transferred from the building by ventilation. Equation (2) shows that contaminant concentrations in animal houses can be controlled by 'diluting' the contaminant with ventilation air. Concentrations of materials such as ammonia will be proportional to the source strength in the house and inversely proportional to ventilation rate, when the external concentration is close to zero.

Equations (1) and (2) assume perfect mixing of the house atmosphere, i.e. that the condition of air in the house is the same as that leaving it. This is rarely true, and many of the practical problems of environmental control in animal houses are concerned with the pattern of air mixing (Carpenter, 1981; see also this volume, Chapter 6).

Heat balance equation

The energy *gains* by animal houses are the heat released by animal metabolism M, supplementary heating F and, in houses with windows or open panels, the net radiation R_n. Here, R_n is the net gain of radiant energy by the space enclosed within the building (not the flux from the environment to the external surface, which influences the house microclimate via the wall heat transfer). The (usual) heat *losses* (although, in principle, all terms can be of either sign) are the enthalpy transferred to the ventilation air flow Q_H, the heat conducted through walls and roof of the building G_w, through the floor G_f and the heat stored due to temperature changes of the stock and building structure J. The heat balance equation is:

$$M + F + R_n = Q_H + G_w + G_f + J \quad (3)$$

This equation can be analysed in terms of a whole building (W), a standard number of animals (e.g. W per 10,000 chickens) or unit area of building ($W m^{-2}$). Except where specified, in this chapter all terms in the house heat balance are expressed as an energy flux density ($W m^{-2}$), based on the area of building floor A (m^2). Over extended periods $G_f \simeq J \simeq 0$, and ventilation is the main route of heat exchange in well-insulated buildings where G_w is close to zero.

Heat gains

The metabolic heat input M is determined mainly by the stocking rate, species and size of animal, feeding level and house temperature (see later). Values of M range from a few $W m^{-2}$ for our own dwellings to about 200 $W m^{-2}$ for intensive poultry units (Charles, 1981; see also Chapter 7).

Heat inputs originating from the burning of fuel may arise both directly, from energy used to raise the temperature within the house, and indirectly, from the heat dissipated by machinery such as ventilation equipment. In temperate climates like that of the UK, supplementary heating is used to control house temperature only for cold-sensitive animals (e.g. newly hatched chicks and piglets) and at low ventilation rates. In these conditions fuel heat inputs will always be either zero or positive. Cooling by 'air conditioning' is seldom an economic option for animal houses, but when used in hot weather it 'pumps' heat against the temperature gradient, resulting in a *negative* heat input for the house.

Net radiation should be close to zero within windowless animal (e.g. poultry) houses, and will be low in those with small windows (e.g. pig units). However, in strong sunshine R_n may be several hundred $W m^{-2}$ in the polythene houses used to shelter sheep for winter lambing. When R_n is an important factor in the heat gain the influence of the external conditions is through the solar irradiance, which is determined by weather, by the shadow geometry of the site, by building window area and building orientation.

Heat losses

VENTILATION HEAT EXCHANGE

Most analyses separate the enthalpy transfer via ventilation into dry heat (C_v) and latent heat (λE_v) components. The dry component is obtained by dividing the product of volumetric ventilation rate v ($m^3 s^{-1}$), the volumetric specific heat of air ρc_p ($\simeq$ 1300 $J m^{-3} K^{-1}$ at 20°C) with the difference between the air temperatures inside and outside the building (T_i and T_o, respectively) by the floor area. Thus, $C_v \simeq v\rho c_p(T_i - T_o)/A$. Similarly, λE_v is estimated from the product of the latent heat of vaporization λ ($J kg^{-1}$) with the mass flux density of water E_v ($kg m^{-2} s^{-1}$). Hence, $\lambda E_v = \lambda v(\chi_i - \chi_o)/A$, where χ_i and χ_o are the water vapour concentrations ($kg m^{-3}$) inside and outside the building, respectively.

The above treatment facilitates our understanding of the processes involved, but is inaccurate. As noted earlier, errors may arise in the estimation of the heat balance because we measure volume rather than mass flow rates, and of humid rather than dry air. Potential errors are often in the range ±5%. A further error can arise in the estimation of house heat balances if we neglect the specific heat of the water vapour in humid air.

The rate of enthalpy (total heat) transfer ($J s^{-1}$) by ventilation is the product of the mass flux θ ($kg s^{-1}$) of (dry) air in the ventilation stream with the difference in enthalpy per unit mass ΔH ($J kg^{-1}$) between the air entering (H_o) and leaving (H_i) the building (Esmay, 1969; Mangold *et al.*, 1983). The equivalent of the ventilation term Q_H in Equation (3) is obtained by dividing by the house floor area, A. It follows that:

$$Q_H = \frac{\theta \Delta H}{A} = \frac{\theta (H_i - H_o)}{A} \tag{4}$$

In a conventional animal house, without 'air conditioning', $\theta \Delta H$ must always represent a loss of energy, i.e. the enthalpy of the exhaust air is higher than that at the intake. The processes involved in ventilation control of house heat balance in representative conditions can be understood best in the context of the psychrometric chart (Fig. 5.1). Readers are likely to be familiar with psychrometric charts used for measurement of atmospheric humidity, which have vapour pressure on the ordinate. In Fig. 5.1 the ordinate is the mixing ratio of humid air, the mass of water vapour associated with each kg of *dry* air. The diagonal lines represent loci of constant enthalpy, the slopes of which correspond to the 'psychrometer constant' (here in units of K^{-1}).

Representative UK operating conditions correspond to the example shown in Fig. 5.1(a). In this example air enters a house at 10°C (T_o), 40% relative humidity (RH) and mixing ratio 3.0 g $H_2O kg^{-1}$ dry air, corresponding to point **A** in Fig. 5.1(a). If the house set temperature T_i is 20°C, then (ideally) the control system will adjust the ventilation rate to maintain the set temperature by balancing heat losses with the heat input. The dry heat to be removed is approximately $C_v \simeq v\rho c_p(T_i - T_o)/A$. When $T_o = 10°C$ and $T_i = 20°C$, it follows that:

$$\theta = \frac{C_v A}{10\, c_p} \tag{5}$$

However, C_v is always less than the metabolic heat production of the animals, because even in the cold a minimum of about 10% of M is lost as latent heat, partly by vapour loss to the air breathed and partly by diffusion through the skin (see later). In addition, most animal houses contain wet surfaces (particularly faeces, bedding and drinking troughs) from which evaporation takes place, converting some of the dry heat lost by *the animals* to latent heat which must be lost from *the building*. Consequently, the total

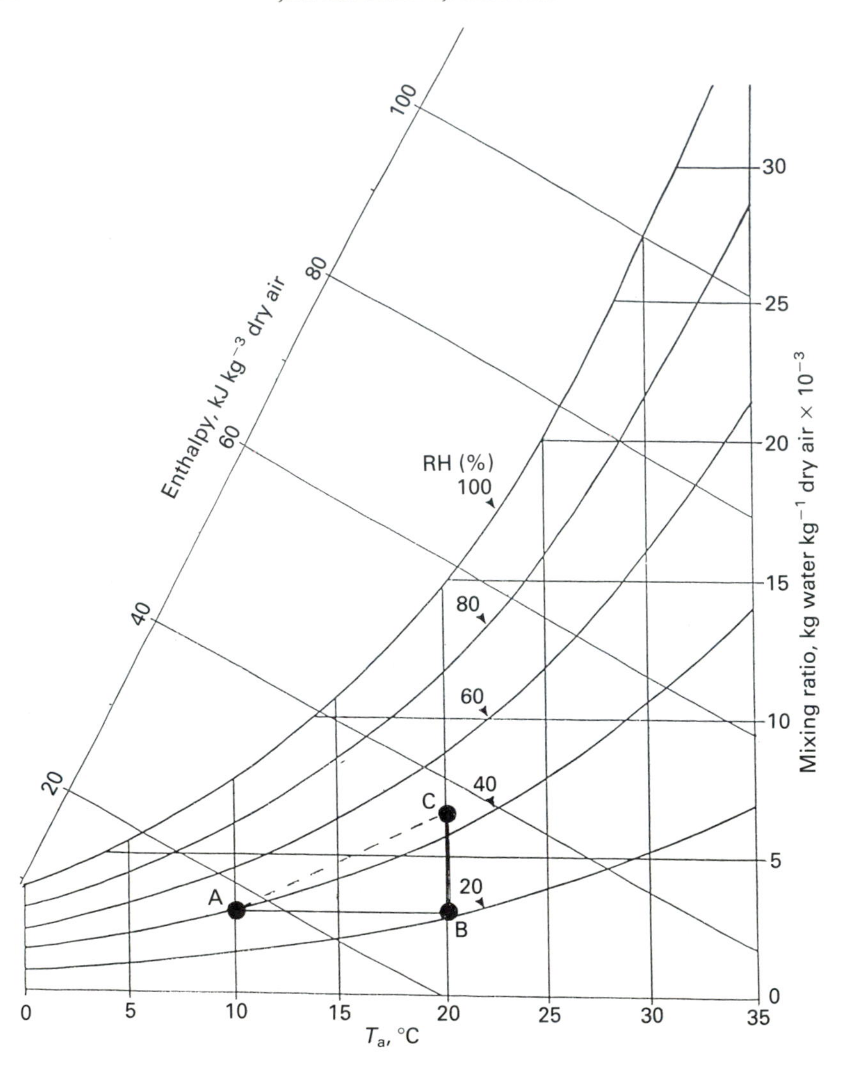

Fig. 5.1. (a) Psychometric chart for the temperature range 0–35°C, in terms of mixing ratio plotted against air temperature T_a. Mixing ratio curves are shown for saturated air (100% RH), 80, 60, 40 and 20% RH. The diagonal lines are loci of equal enthalpy, expressed relative to dry air at 0°C. Diagram represents enthalpy changes in the ventilatory air of an animal house in average conditions in a cool temperate climate.

change in enthalpy of the ventilating air is that due to the changes of the temperature of the air plus that due to changes in water content, **A→C** in Fig. 5.1(a), with the components C_v and λE_v indicated by lines **A→B** and **B→C**, respectively. For steady conditions the total enthalpy transfer (including wall losses) must equal the sum of the sources in the building.

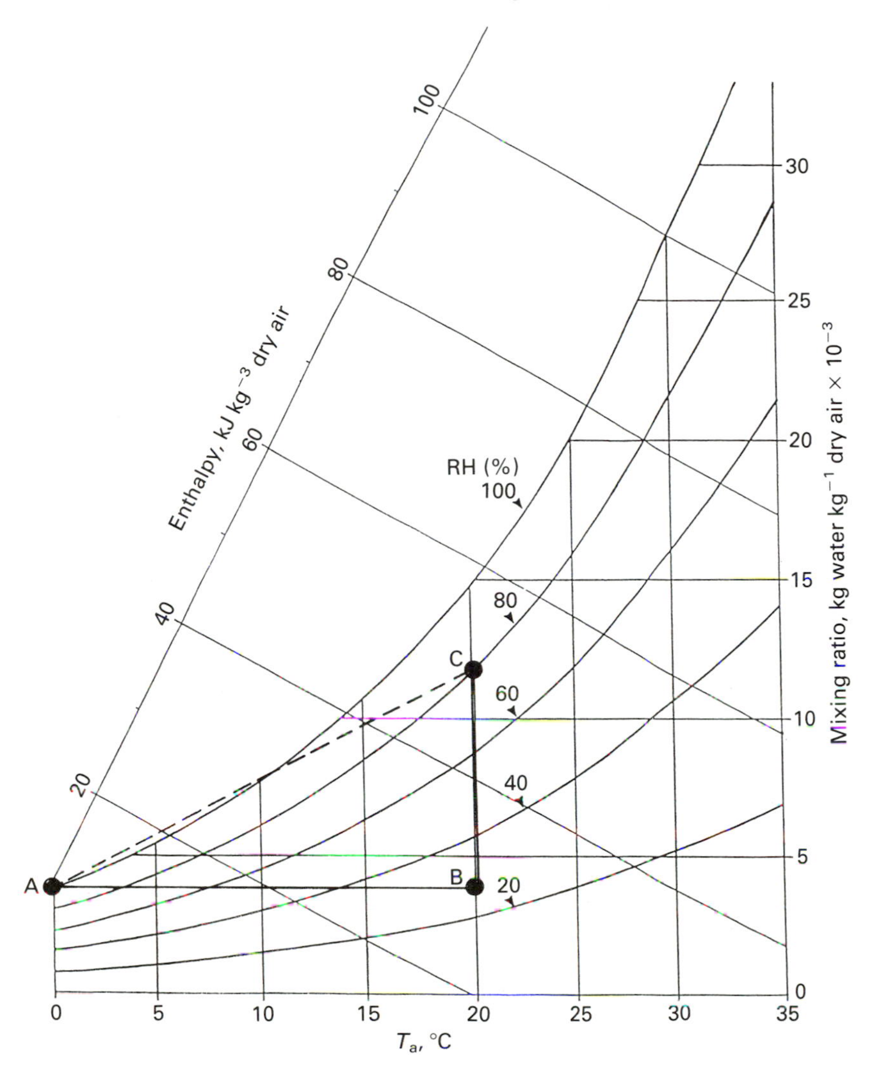

Fig. 5.1. (b) Enthalpy changes in the ventilatory air in cold conditions in a temperate climate.

A specimen calculation will suffice to illustrate the enthalpy changes in the ventilating air corresponding to the conditions shown in Fig. 5.1(a). The example is for a poultry house, using $M = 10$W per bird for poultry (Charles, 1981), with 20 birds per m^2 of floor, the losses from the building total 200 W m^{-2}. When the outside air and building surface temperatures are 10°C, assuming a mean wall/roof conductance of 0.5 W m^{-2}K^{-1} (Wathes, 1981) and a 'wall'/floor area ratio of 1.3, approximately 7 W m^{-2} (of floor) will be lost through the walls. The remaining heat must be lost by ventilation,

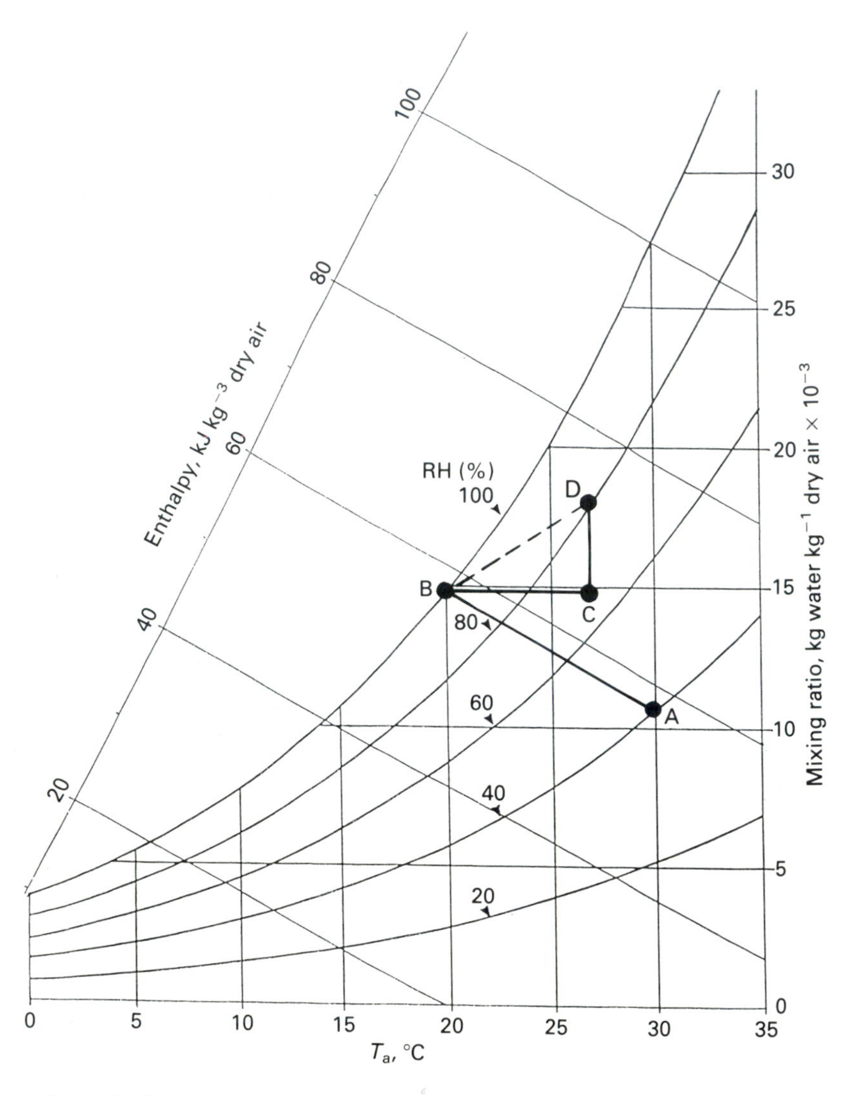

Fig. 5.1. (c) Enthalpy changes in the ventilating air when wet pad cooling is employed in a warm but dry climate.

193 W m^{-2}. The required mass ventilation rate is about 10 g s^{-1} of air per m^2 of building floor, equivalent to approximately 4 m^{3}s^{-1} per 10,000 birds. This ventilation rate should produce a house temperature T_i of 20°C with a humidity increment of about 3.7 g water per kg dry air, indicated by the line **B→C** in Fig. 5.1(a), and about 45% RH (at 20°C) in the exhaust air. The increase in the enthalpy of the ventilating air from inlet to outlet is about 19 kJ kg^{-1}. The diagram would correspond to wet conditions in the poultry

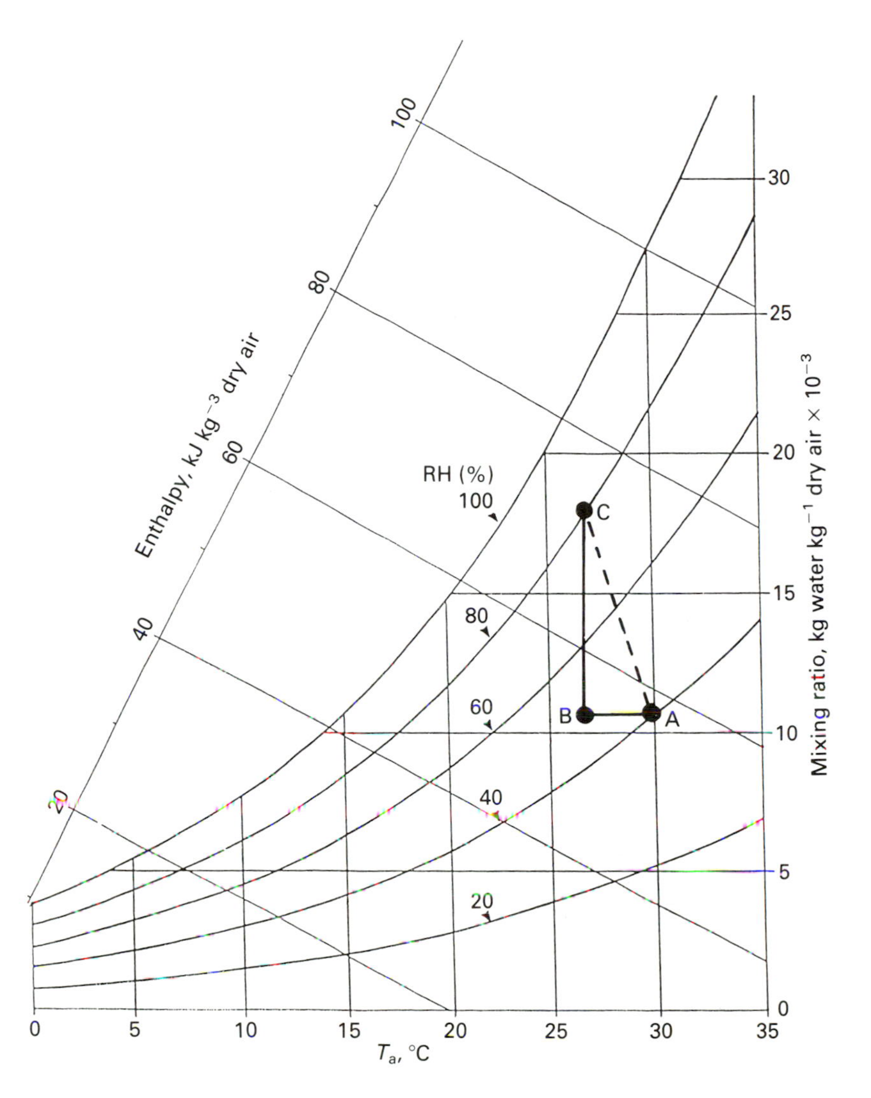

Fig. 5.1. (d) The same net enthalpy transfer as in Fig. 5.1.(c), but without wet pad cooling.

house, for example where some of the heat produced by the birds was used to evaporate water from damp bedding.

Wall heat fluxes

The insulation provided by the 'walls' (wall and roof) is an important determinant of the thermal environments in animal houses, just as coat insulation is in the energy balance of the animals.

The rate of heat transfer by conduction through unit area of a wall, the wall heat flux density G_{wa} ($W m^{-2}$), is simply the product of the temperature difference across the wall with the wall conductance U ($W m^{-2} K^{-1}$):

$$G_{wa} = U(T_i - T_o) \qquad (6)$$

The conductance U is determined by the construction materials and wall thickness (Wathes, 1981; see also this volume, Chapter 8). The lowest values of U provided by animal house structures (at least when new) are $0.4 W m^{-2} K^{-1}$ or less, and correspond to insulation thicknesses in excess of 150 mm of fibreglass. In contrast, the conductance of a single skin of asbestos or glassfibre-cement sheet is a factor of 15 higher, about $6 W m^{-2} K^{-1}$. Design, therefore, plays a large part in the building heat balance, both because it determines U and because the effective value of the wall flux density G_w in the heat balance (Equation 3) exceeds G_{wa} by the ratio of the total 'wall' area A_w to the floor area A of the house: i.e.

$$G_w = G_{wa} \frac{A_w}{A} \qquad (7)$$

The ratio A_w/A depends on house geometry, with minimum values of about 1.2 for flat roofed buildings.

The climatic determinant of G_w is the temperature difference across the wall. In well-insulated buildings, the temperature at the inner surface will be close to the inside air temperature, but may differ from it significantly if U is large. The outside wall temperature is determined by the climate and weather of the site, the main factors being air temperature and radiant heat exchanges. In consequence, for poorly insulated buildings the wall flux is one of the largest and least predictable components of the house heat balance. In such buildings, at night low air temperatures and radiative cooling can cause cold stress to housed stock. In contrast, during sunny days the internal temperature of a poorly insulated roof can exceed 50°C even in the UK, and may cause heat stress.

Problems at low temperatures

At low temperatures, environmental problems arise when the ventilation rate required falls below the controllable range. This problem is most likely in buildings with low stocking rates (low M) and/or poor wall/roof insulation. When most of the heat produced by animal metabolism is lost from the building through the walls and roof, the target ventilation rate for temperature control may become insufficient to remove water which evaporates from the stock and other sources. Removal of contaminants such as ammonia may also be inadequate at low ventilation rates. With computer-controlled systems it is possible to override temperature control to give priority to other environmental criteria, e.g. to prevent some set ammonia concentration being exceeded (Clark and Cena, 1981).

Humidity can cause more subtle problems, one of which is illustrated by Fig. 5.1(b). In this example, air enters a house at 0°C and close to saturation (point **A**). The stock lose dry heat (corresponding to the change **A** → **B**) and water vapour (**B** → **C**) to the air, which leaves the house at 20°C and 80% RH (point **C**). The house heat balance appears well under control. However, there would be a risk of condensation in the house, even though condensation on solid surfaces is expected only when RH exceeds about 85%. In Fig. 5.1(b) the line connecting the initial and final points on the psychrometric chart is above the 85% RH locus for most of its length, and above the saturation vapour pressure (svp) versus temperature curve between 0°C and about 10°C. Consequently, condensation would occur both as the cold outside air mixed with the air in the house and on any relatively cool surfaces within the house, e.g. due to 'thermal bridges' in the structure (Baxter, 1984).

Additional problems occur when condensation within the building structure degrades its insulation and causes damage. Condensation is most likely when the humidity of the house air is high. In general, diffusion of water vapour through a structure takes place in parallel with heat transfer through the wall by conduction (Wathes, 1981). In a wall of uniform properties, a reasonable approximation for the insulation of most animal houses, conductive heat exchange and the diffusion of water vapour should produce linear gradients of temperature and humidity, respectively, between the internal and external surfaces. When the outside temperature is lower than that inside, the linear fall of temperature through the wall will result in a relatively more rapid drop in saturation vapour pressure, because of the approximately exponential relation between svp and temperature (°C). Condensation will occur within a wall structure if the vapour pressure and svp loci intersect, a frequent occurrence in cold and temperate regions in winter. We again base an example on Fig. 5.1(b). Line **A** → **C** is below the svp curve at temperatures under about 10°C. When temperatures within the wall are below this value, moisture would accumulate as the result of condensation. Prevention of condensation requires increased ventilation rates, to decrease the mixing ratio of the air in the house and lower point **C** until the line **A** → **C** lies below the svp curve throughout the path of vapour transfer. This measure involves the abandonment of temperature control. Alternatively, prevention is better than cure: the wall structures of animal houses for cool climates should incorporate vapour barriers at the *inner* surface (Wathes, 1981).

Problems at high temperatures

In hot conditions (even in the UK!) control of house temperature will be lost when outside air temperature T_o approaches or exceeds the target house temperature T_i. The maximum ventilation rates for animal houses are designed to produce an acceptable temperature lift above ambient, usually of about 3 K (Charles, 1981). In hot weather, latent heat loss may cool house air temperatures below those outside, in one of the two ways illustrated in Figs 5.1(c) and (d). For simplicity, we will consider only changes to the ventilating air, without specifying the class of stock involved. The examples use the same basic diagram as in Figs 5.1(a) and (b), and therefore illustrate the principles of evaporative cooling, but at the low end of the temperature range in which it is important. In each case the ventilation air leaves the house cooler and more humid than at the intake, at 27°C and 80% RH compared with 30°C and 40% RH, but with a net enthalpy increase of about 15 kJ kg^{-1}.

Figure 5.1(c) represents the processes involved in *wet pad cooling* of the intake air, a method often exploited in hot climates to cool animal houses (and greenhouses). When air passes over a wet pad it can be cooled to the wet bulb temperature if the change takes place under (ideal) adiabatic conditions, i.e. with no change in the enthalpy content of the air. In Fig. 5.1(c) the adiabatic cooling of (the outside) air entering the house, which is initially at point **A**, corresponds to the line (**A**→**B**). Point **B** represents the wet bulb temperature, 20°C and 100% RH. The heat lost by the *stock* would then add dry heat and latent heat to the *air*, the heat increments corresponding to lines (**B**→**C**) and (**C**→**D**), respectively, in Fig. 5.1(c). Point **D** represents the state of the air leaving the house, 27°C and 80% RH. An alternative route *for the same net enthalpy increase of the air* (and loss by the stock) is indicated in Fig. 5.1(d). In this case, without wet pad cooling, the stock lose about twice as much latent heat (and therefore water) as in the previous case, the corresponding enthalpy (and water) added to the air being represented by the line (**B**→**C**) in Fig. 5.1(d) (for comparison see (**C**→**D**) in Fig. 5.1(c)). In the case without wet pad cooling the stock therefore themselves cool the air by evaporation.

The choice of whether to adopt wet pad cooling to alleviate heat stress on stock must depend both on the conditions and the class of animals housed. In dry, hot climates the wet bulb temperature is lower and wet pad cooling is more effective than in hot humid conditions. Animals with the ability to sweat at high rates (e.g. cattle, horses and man) and with free access to water are likely to cope with heat stress better without than with wet pad cooling. However, wet pad cooling will usually alleviate heat stress in non-sweating animals (e.g. pigs and poultry).

Thermal Exchanges of Animals

Common farm animals are homeothermic: they maintain their body-core temperatures within fairly narrow limits despite large changes in the temperature of their environment. The 'normal' body-core temperature depends on species, and to some extent on size and breed, with values for livestock ranging from about 38°C (e.g. cattle) to 41°C (e.g. poultry). Body temperatures within this range are consistent with the requirements of the heat balance, in particular the need to minimize energy expenditure in the cold and to conserve water in hot conditions (McArthur and Clark, 1988). Small variations in body-core temperature occur, associated with time of day, activity, feeding and environmental conditions. Although it is the temperature of the hypothalamus which is regulated (Bligh, 1966), temperature differences between organs within the central core are usually small. However, it has long been recognized that the outer body tissues can be considerably cooler than the core and, when environmental temperature is low, that large temperature differences can exist between the skin surface of the trunk and that on the extremities (Whittow, 1962).

Continuous exchange of heat between an animal and its environment is an inevitable consequence of the temperature and humidity differences between the body-core and the surroundings. To maintain a steady body-core temperature, the rate at which the body gains heat must balance the rate at which heat is dissipated. Failure to achieve this balance would change the heat content of the body and, hence, its temperature.

Homeotherms *gain* heat mainly from their own metabolic activity: they generate heat by the oxidative metabolism of protein, fat and carbohydrate within the body. The rate of metabolism depends on the level of food (metabolizable energy) intake (Graham *et al.*, 1959; Webster *et al.*, 1976), but the rate is also influenced by muscular activity (Tucker, 1970; Hoyt and Taylor, 1981) and by the thermal environment (Bianca, 1976; Blaxter, 1977). Although animals outdoors can also gain substantial amounts of heat during the day by absorption of solar radiation (Cena, 1974), this heat input is usually negligible indoors.

Heat *loss* to the environment occurs by two main routes: firstly, non-evaporative heat transfer to the air and surrounding surfaces by convection, conduction and thermal radiation exchange; secondly, evaporative heat transfer associated with the loss of water vapour from the body surface and respiratory system.

Heat balance equation

We can write the steady state heat balance equation for any animal as:

$$M = C + G_{\mathrm{k}} + L_{\mathrm{n}} + \lambda E \tag{8}$$

where M is the rate of metabolic heat production, here for the particular animal. The quantities C, G_{k} and L_{n} are the rates of non-evaporative heat loss by convection, conduction and longwave radiation exchange, respectively, and λE is the rate of evaporative heat loss (the quantity E is the total rate of water loss from the animal by evaporation). As for buildings, the terms in Equation (8) can be expressed in several ways. For a single animal the relevant units are W or MJ day^{-1} (previously kilocalories per day). However, in an analysis of the mechanisms of heat exchange it is more convenient to express each term as the corresponding heat flux density ($W m^{-2}$), based on the surface area of the body.

Equation (8) is often simplified to:

$$M = G + \lambda E \quad (9)$$

where $G = (C + G_k + L_n)$ is the total non-evaporative heat loss. Many animal scientists refer to G as the sensible heat loss although, strictly, the sensible heat loss is that by convection C only. The thermal exchanges of animals indoors will now be described.

Convection

Most of the heat transfer by convection occurs between the outer surface of the body and the surrounding air, the rate being governed by two factors: the temperature difference between the surface and the air, and the thermal insulation provided by the boundary layer of air around the body. In wind, the heat is removed by 'forced convection' at a rate dependent on speed and direction of air movement (Wiersma and Nelson, 1967; Mitchell, 1985). In still air, the movement of air around the body is a consequence of buoyancy forces and 'free convection' is the mechanism involved (Mitchell, 1974). The equivalent processes for buildings are ventilation due to wind and to the 'chimney' effect. The rates of air movement close to stock inside animal houses are usually between 0.1 and 1.0 $m s^{-1}$, conditions in which heat will be removed by 'mixed' free and forced convection (Wathes and Clark, 1981). Usually, the surface temperature of the body is warmer than the surrounding air and the heat transfer by convection represents a loss of energy. However, in some circumstances the body surface cools below the air temperature, so that heat is gained by convection from the air. This reversal of the temperature gradient can occur as a result of radiative cooling during nights outdoors with clear skies (McArthur, 1991a), but also indoors as a result of evaporative cooling when the body surface is wet (McArthur and Ousey, 1994).

Animals also lose heat by convection from their respiratory systems, because the expired air is usually warmer than the inspired air. The heat added to the air by breathing depends on the ventilation rate of the respiratory system (measured by animal scientists as minute volume), as well as the increase in temperature. Strictly, as for buildings, one should consider the change in enthalpy of the air breathed. However, because the volumetric specific heat of air is low ($\simeq$ 1300 $J m^{-3} K^{-1}$), the rate at which housed stock dissipate heat by this route is a small fraction (about 3%) of their total heat loss at normal air temperatures. Consequently, the error incurred by neglecting heat loss by convection from the respiratory system is usually negligible.

Conduction

Heat transfer by conduction takes place between an animal and any surface (in particular the floor) with which it is in contact. Animals which are standing lose insignificant amounts of heat by conduction because the area of contact is small. However, conductive heat losses from a lying animal can be significant when the floor is made of a relatively good conductor such as concrete (Mount, 1967; Bruce, 1979).

Radiation

Most natural surfaces, including animal coats, behave as black body emitters of longwave radiation (Hammel, 1956). The flux density of radiant energy emitted from such a surface is proportional to the fourth power of its absolute temperature (K) and increases, for example, from 316 W m^{-2} at 0°C (273 K) to more than 600 W m^{-2} at 50°C (323 K). Animals receive several hundred W m^{-2} from their environment, in a building from the walls, floor, etc., and the other animals. The emission of longwave radiation from the outer surface of an animal's body usually exceeds the receipt of radiation from the (cooler) surfaces in a building, resulting in a net loss of radiant energy. At the low air speeds typical of the environments in animal houses (and our own dwellings) the rate of heat loss by radiative exchange is just as important as convection, especially for large animals. Typically, about 50% of the non-evaporative heat loss from a housed animal exposed to slowly moving air in an isothermal environment will occur by radiation (Gates, 1962). However, a poorly insulated roof in sunny weather can result in a significant radiative heat gain on the backs of the animals.

The thermal insulation provided by the boundary layer around the body decreases with increasing air speed, as does the coat insulation, increasing the proportion of non-evaporative heat loss carried by convection. Consequently, convection is dominant at high windspeeds – hence, much of the environmental advantage of shelter from wind. Conversely, air speeds must be low for infrared heating to be effective (e.g. for young stock).

Evaporation

The latent heat of vaporization of water λ is high, about 2400 J g^{-1}. Like most homeotherms, farm animals rely on the evaporation of water as a means to dissipate metabolic heat in warm conditions, when the non-evaporative loss is limited by small temperature differences between the body and its surroundings. In particular, the rate of evaporative heat loss increases progressively when the air temperature is raised above the lower critical value (see below). Some species respond to heat by panting, thereby increasing the rate of water vapour loss from their respiratory systems; some species sweat freely in response to heat, and the subsequent evaporation of this moisture carries heat from the skin surface; some both sweat and pant (see below).

The metabolic diagram

The literature contains a wealth of information describing how the heat balance of livestock depends on air temperature. Figure 5.2 shows the metabolic diagram, the general relationship between the rate of metabolic heat production and air temperature. The values shown are adapted from Mount (1979) for a shorn sheep with only a few millimetres of fleece. This

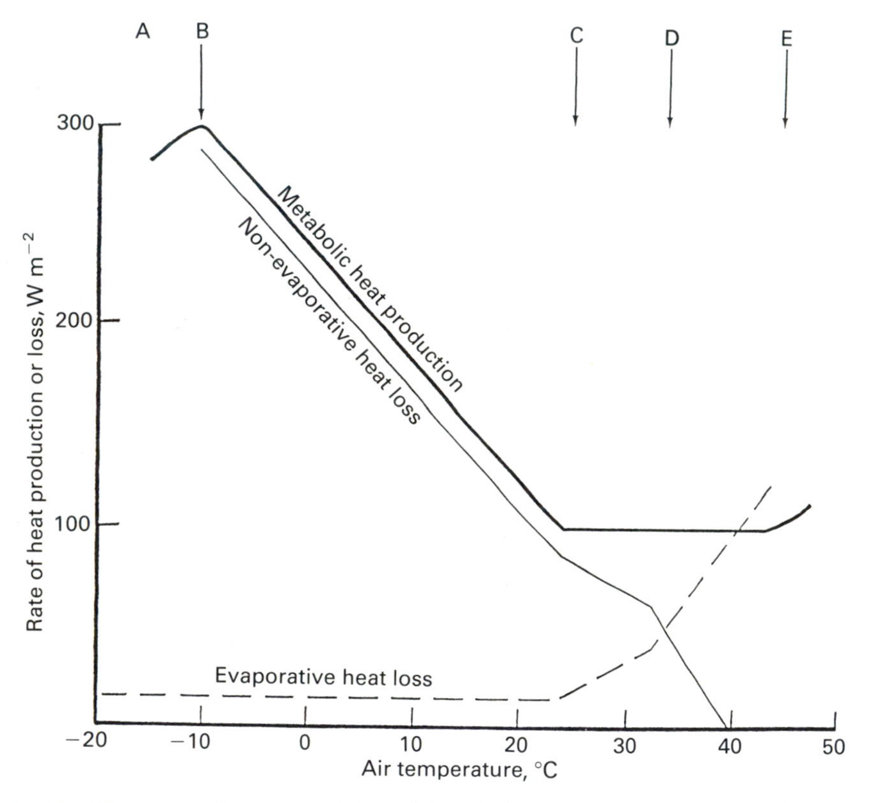

Fig. 5.2. Diagrammatic representation of the relations between environmental temperature, heat production and the evaporative and non-evaporative heat losses for a poorly insulated sheep (adapted from Mount, 1979). The symbols A to E are defined in text.

diagram, which also shows the non-evaporative (G) and evaporative (λE) components of heat loss, can be divided into different zones in terms of the animal's response.

When the levels of food intake and activity are fixed, the rate of metabolic heat production is minimal and independent of air temperature in the 'thermoneutral zone' between lines **C** and **E**. This level of heat production, termed the resting metabolic rate M_{tn}, is shown in Fig. 5.2 as $100\,W\,m^{-2}$. The narrow zone, between lines **C** and **D**, is termed the 'zone of least thermoregulatory effort'. Within this zone the metabolic rate is minimal, the evaporative heat loss is only slightly above the minimum value, and the animal regulates its heat balance mainly by altering peripheral blood flow and, hence, body insulation. Ideally, the temperature in an animal house should be within the zone **CD** to maximize production efficiency (Van Kampen, 1981). Outwith the zone **CD** production efficiency is depressed by the consequences of thermal stress (Chapter 1).

Problems at low temperatures

In environmental conditions below the lower critical temperature (**C** in Fig. 5.2), an animal must increase its metabolic rate above the resting value (e.g. by shivering) in order to balance the rate at which heat is lost to the surroundings. In these conditions, heat loss occurs mainly by the non-evaporative routes, evaporative heat loss is minimal, body insulation is maximal, and the rates of non-evaporative heat loss G and metabolism M both increase almost in proportion to the temperature difference between the body-core and the air. The rate of metabolic heat production required for homeothermy in the cold is given by:

$$M = \rho c_p(T_b - T_i)/r_{tot} + [(r_c + r_e)\lambda E_s/r_{tot} + (\lambda E_r + C_r)] \qquad (10)$$

where the volumetric specific heat of air $\rho c_p (= 1300\,J\,m^{-3}K^{-1})$ is introduced as a dimensional constant, T_b is the body-core temperature (°C), λE_s is the evaporative heat flux density from the skin surface ($W\,m^{-2}$), and λE_r and C_r are the evaporative and convective heat losses ($W\,m^{-2}$), respectively, from the respiratory system (McArthur, 1991b). The quantities r_c and r_e are the thermal resistances ($s\,m^{-1}$) of the coat and air (for convection plus thermal radiation exchange), respectively. The total body resistance r_{tot} ($s\,m^{-1}$) is the resistance to non-evaporative heat flow between the body-core and the environment. This resistance is provided by the body tissue, coat and air in series, and is simply:

$$r_{tot} = r_s + r_c + r_e \qquad (11)$$

where r_s is the thermal resistance of the body tissue ($s\,m^{-1}$). Vasoconstricted values of r_{tot} for livestock range from about $180\,s\,m^{-1}$ (e.g. for newborn piglets) to more than $1000\,s\,m^{-1}$ (e.g. for fully-fleeced sheep). Animal scientists who are more familiar with the traditional units of thermal insulation (Km^2W^{-1}) should note that a thermal resistance of $100\,s\,m^{-1}$ is equivalent to an insulation of $0.078\,Km^2W^{-1}$ (Cena and Clark, 1978; Monteith and Unsworth, 1990). Building scientists should note that the thermal resistance is inversely proportional to conductance U, and that a resistance of $100\,s\,m^{-1}$ is equivalent to $U = 12.9\,W\,m^{-2}K^{-1}$.

Below thermoneutrality, the term $[(r_c + r_e)\lambda E_s/r_{tot} + (\lambda E_r + C_r)]$ in Equation (10) is usually minimal and fairly constant, at about $10\,W\,m^{-2}$. Consequently, the slope of the line relating the metabolic rate of an animal (with constant insulation) to air temperature below thermoneutrality depends on its total body resistance (i.e. slope = $\rho c_p/r_{tot}$). For the sheep (T_b = 39.0°C) illustrated in Fig. 5.2, the chosen value of r_{tot} is $230\,s\,m^{-1}$ and its metabolic rate increases by $5.6\,W\,m^{-2}$ for each 1K drop in air temperature

Table 5.1. Values of lower critical temperature T_{lc} for different classes of stock.

Animal	Mass (kg)	Additional comments	T_{lc} (°C)	Source
Chick	0.036	Age 2–6 days	34	Poczopko (1981)
Chicken	2.4	Age 1 year	16	Poczopko (1981)
Newborn calf	35	Coat depth 1.2 cm	9	Webster (1981)
Calf	50	Age 1 month, coat depth 1.4 cm	0	Webster (1981)
Friesian cow	*c.*500	Peak lactation	−30	Webster (1987)
Piglet	2	Individual	30	Holmes and Close (1977)
Pig	100	Intake twice maintenance	19	Holmes and Close (1977)
Sow	140	Intake twice maintenance, thin, pregnant (112 days)	15	Holmes and Close (1977)
Sheep	50	Maintenance, coat depth 1 mm	28	Blaxter (1967)
Sheep	50	Maintenance, coat depth 10 cm	−3	Blaxter (1967)
Foal	31	Age 2–4 days	22	Ousey *et al.* (1992)
Horse	*c.*500	Mature quarter horse gelding	−10	McBride *et al.* (1983)

below the lower critical value of 23°C. When T_i = 5°C the metabolic rate required for homeothermy by this animal is 200 W m^{-2}, double the thermoneutral value.

It is generally assumed that the straight line relating M to T_i in the cold extrapolates to intercept the temperature axis at body-core temperature T_b. However, this assumption is incorrect. Equation (10) indicates that the line intercepts the temperature axis at a value above the body-core temperature, at about T_i = 40.5°C for the shorn sheep. In contrast, the corresponding line for a fully-fleeced sheep with r_{tot} = 1000 s m^{-1} would have a slope of only 1.3 W m^{-2}K^{-1}, and would intercept the temperature axis at about T_i = 50°C (McArthur, 1991b).

The lower critical temperature T_{lc} (C in Fig. 5.2) is the air temperature at which the heat emission from an animal with fully vasoconstricted skin, and with the skin and lungs losing minimal amounts of water vapour, is equal to its heat production in the thermoneutral zone (Blaxter, 1989). The value of T_{lc} is determined largely by total body resistance r_{tot} and resting metabolic rate M_{tn}. An expression for T_{lc} can be obtained by rearranging Equation (10) to give:

$$T_{lc} = T_b - r_{tot}[M_{tn} - (\lambda E_r + C_r) - (r_c + r_e)\lambda E_s/r_{tot}]/\rho c_p \qquad (12)$$

At the lower critical temperature, the combined rate of heat loss ($\lambda E_r + C_r + \lambda E_s$) is minimal, and r_{tot} is the maximum (vasoconstricted) value. To a good approximation, Equation (12) can be rewritten as:

$$T_{lc} = T_b - r_{tot}(M_{tn} - 10)/\rho c_p \qquad (13)$$

Table 5.1 presents values of T_{lc} for livestock exposed to the low rates of air movement typical in buildings (windspeed $\simeq$ 0.2 m s^{-1}). Most of these T_{lc} values have been calculated by the various authors from expressions in the form of Equation (13), by inserting appropriate figures for resting metabolic rate and insulation. The table shows a 64 K range of lower critical temperatures for livestock, from 34°C for young chicks to −30°C for high producing dairy cows.

The figures in Table 5.1 are a useful guide to the cold tolerance and thermal requirements of the different classes of livestock, and are of direct relevance to the target control temperatures for animal houses. However, the limitations of these figures should be recognized. Firstly, these values of T_{lc} apply to single animals rather than groups. Animals may modify their thermal environment by social cooperation. For example, Mount (1960) reported that the lower critical temperature of newborn pigs is reduced (by about 5 K) when they huddle, as is their metabolic response to temperatures below T_{lc}. Secondly, the common assumption that tissue insulation (and, hence, the value of r_{tot} in Equation (13)) is a maximum at the lower critical temperature may be invalid when this temperature is significantly less than 0°C. Below zero, cold-induced vasodilation may occur to prevent tissue damage on extremities such as the legs (e.g. Meyer and Webster, 1971), a physiological response which can cause unexpectedly large decreases in total body resistance (McArthur, 1981b). Consequently, calculated values of T_{lc} which are substantially below 0°C are likely to be too low. Thirdly, the values of T_{lc} in Table 5.1 apply to animals which are dry. Surface wetness can cause a large increase in heat loss. For example, Ousey *et al.* (1991) reported that the metabolic rates of newborn foals were above $200\,W\,m^{-2}$ during the first hour postpartum when they were wet with amniotic fluid and shivering. These metabolic rates are two to three times those when the foals were dry. It is likely that the lower critical temperature of the wet foals was close to 30°C, about ten degrees above the value expected when dry (McArthur and Ousey, 1994). The protection which housing affords to stock from wetting by rain eliminates a major cause of cold stress.

Equation (10) can be used to estimate an animal's rate of energy expenditure below thermoneutrality. To a reasonable approximation, this equation can be written as:

$$M = \rho c_p (T_b - T_i)/r_{tot} + 10 \tag{14}$$

For example, when $T_i = -13$°C a shorn sheep with $r_{tot} = 230\,s\,m^{-1}$ would need to produce heat by metabolism at a rate of about $300\,W\,m^{-2}$ (see Fig. 5.2) in order to maintain homeothermy. However, it is often unrealistic to assume that total body resistance remains constant when air temperature falls below T_{lc}. Several factors can increase r_{tot} below thermoneutrality, for example changes in posture, pilo-erection of the hair (or feathers), and reduction in peripheral blood flow. Competing processes may decrease r_{tot} in the cold. For example, shivering can cause a reduction in tissue resistance and the associated body movements may reduce the resistance provided by the coat and boundary layer. Indeed, it should not be assumed that a straight line relationship between M and T_i below thermoneutrality is indicative of constant insulation (McArthur, 1991b).

When the air temperature is in the zone **AB** (Fig. 5.2), the rate of metabolic heat production required for homeothermy exceeds the animal's maximum ability to generate heat (termed the summit metabolic rate, and shown in Fig. 5.2 as $300\,W\,m^{-2}$). Consequently, heat loss exceeds heat gain in this zone and body-core temperature declines. The decline in body-core temperature depresses the rate of heat production and causes hypothermia.

Problems at high temperatures

When air temperature increases above T_{lc} there is a natural decrease in the proportion of metabolic heat which an animal loses by non-evaporative routes to the building microclimate. For sheep, poultry and pigs, the corresponding increase in the rate of evaporative heat loss occurs mainly from the respiratory tract as a result of panting. For example, Blaxter *et al.*

(1959a) reported that the respiratory frequency (and the rate of water vapour loss) of closely-clipped sheep increased sharply when air temperature exceeded about 28(±3)°C, the actual value depending on feeding level. At lower temperatures, respiratory frequency was below 20 breaths per minute and the total evaporative heat loss was almost constant at about 15 W m^{-2}. For comparison, a fully-fleeced sheep (coat depth 10 cm) on a medium level of food intake had to raise respiratory frequency when air temperature exceeded about 9°C, and dissipated about 50% of its metabolic heat by evaporation (respiratory frequency about 90 min^{-1}) when T_i reached 28°C (Blaxter *et al.*, 1959b). Alexander (1974) reported that a panting adult sheep can lose up to 60 W m^{-2} by evaporation, equivalent to 80% of resting metabolic rate for a moderate food intake. 'First phase' panting in sheep involves shallow breathing, mainly through the nose, at rates up to about 320 breaths per minute (Hales and Webster, 1967). More severe heat exposure causes a change to a deeper and slower type of open-mouthed breathing, termed 'second phase' panting, often indicative of incipient hyperthermia. 'Second phase' panting, which results in a further increase in minute volume, has been observed in sheep and poultry during severe heat stress, but not in the pig (Ingram and Mount, 1975).

In contrast, cattle and horses rely much more on the evaporation of sweat from the skin surface as a means to remove excess heat. For example, Worstell and Brody (1953) found that E_s for Jersey cattle increased from 8 to nearly 40 mg m^{-2} s^{-1} (λE_s from 20 to 90 W m^{-2}) when T_i was raised from 0 to 40°C. The corresponding increase in E_r for these cattle was from about 4 to 10 mg m^{-2} s^{-1} (λE_r from 10 to 25 W m^{-2}), and in respiratory frequency from 20 to 120 breaths per minute. Cattle display second phase panting during severe heat exposure.

Figure 5.2 describes the acute response of a homeotherm to its thermal environment – there is a clearly defined 'thermoneutral zone' **CE** within which metabolic rate is independent of temperature. However, the metabolic response changes when adaptation takes place under chronic exposure. In particular, metabolic rate declines during prolonged exposure at high temperatures. This decline is associated with a decrease in food intake and thyroid activity. For example, Worstell and Brody (1953) kept Jersey cattle at various air temperatures for about two weeks. The metabolic rates of the cattle declined progressively with increasing temperature, from about 170 W m^{-2} when T_i = 15°C to about 110 W m^{-2} at 40°C.

Similarly, Van Kampen (1981) reported that the rate of heat production by the fowl decreases with increasing air temperature up to about 35°C, above which the rate increases. The upper limit of the thermoneutral zone (**E** in Fig. 5.2) is termed the upper critical temperature T_{uc}(°C), the value of which depends on metabolic rate, insulation and an animal's ability to dissipate heat by evaporation. The increase in metabolic rate above **E** is a consequence of the rise in body-core temperature and/or respiratory effort (e.g. Whittow and Findlay, 1968). Most species become hyperthermic when T_b exceeds about 42.5°C.

Most researchers use the same definition of *lower* critical temperature – the ambient temperature below which an animal must raise its rate of heat production to maintain homeothermy. In contrast, some confusion surrounds the definition of *upper* critical temperature. In their glossary of terms for thermal physiology, Bligh and Johnson (1973) preferred to define T_{uc} as 'the ambient temperature above which thermoregulatory evaporative heat loss processes (e.g. sweating) of a resting thermoregulating animal are recruited'. In this definition, it is assumed that evaporative heat loss remains constant and minimal within the zone of thermoneutrality, and that metabolic rate increases at some ambient temperature above T_{uc} when evaporative heat loss has reached its summit value (Bligh, 1985). However, Bligh and Johnson gave as a synonym the definition 'the ambient above which there is an increase in metabolic rate due to a rise in the core temperature of a resting thermoregulating animal'. Consequently, as Mount (1974) noted, the upper limit for the zone of thermal neutrality could refer to the temperature above which evaporative heat loss rises markedly (**D** in Fig. 5.2) or to the temperature (hyperthermic point) above which metabolic rate increases (**E** in Fig. 5.2). The latter definition is preferred by most animal scientists. For example, Yousef (1985) and Hahn and Hugh-Jones (1989) quote values of T_{uc}(**E** in Fig. 5.2) for cattle in the range 23–33°C, for sheep 25–31°C, and 28–32°C for sows.

Values of both T_{uc} and T_{lc} can be determined experimentally. However, values of T_{uc} cannot be calculated as easily as those of T_{lc} (Equation (13)) because the partition of heat loss from animals in hot environments is more difficult to quantify (McArthur, 1987).

Summary

To summarize, this chapter has considered the physical processes which govern the heat balances of buildings and the livestock they house. The major climatic influences on the house heat balance are the atmospheric temperature and humidity outside and, for poorly insulated houses, the net radiation (Chapter 8). Wind is also significant for most practical animal houses, because it interferes with the control of ventilation. Building design and husbandry influence the heat balance through the provision of insulation, the control system and the stock density. The other important variable in the house heat balance is the interaction between the metabolic heat production of the stock and the thermal microclimate provided by the building. The interaction between the physics of thermal exchange and the physiology of the animals is complex, but must be understood to a reasonable degree in order to design environments in which animals can be housed to meet both production and welfare requirements.

References

Alexander, G. (1974) Heat loss from sheep. In: Monteith, J.L. and Mount, L.E. (eds), *Heat Loss from Animals and Man.* Butterworths, London, pp. 173–203.

Baxter, S.H. (1984) Insulation and ventilation of pig buildings. In: Hsia, L.C. (ed.), *Environmental Housing for Livestock.* Pig Research Institute, Chunan, Taiwan.

Bianca, W. (1976) The significance of meteorology in animal production. *International Journal of Biometeorology* 20, 139–156.

Blaxter, K.L. (1967) *The Energy Metabolism of Ruminants,* 2nd edn. Hutchinson, London.

Blaxter, K.L. (1977) Environmental factors and their influence on the nutrition of farm livestock. In: Haresign, W., Swan, H. and Lewis, D. (eds), *Nutrition and the Climatic Environment.* Butterworths, London, pp. 1–16.

Blaxter, K.L. (1989) *Energy Metabolism in Animals and Man.* Cambridge University Press, Cambridge.

Blaxter, K.L., Graham, N.McC. and Wainman, F.W. (1959a) Environmental temperature, energy metabolism and heat regulation in sheep. II. The partition of heat losses in closely clipped sheep. *Journal of Agricultural Science, Cambridge* 52, 25–40.

Blaxter, K.L., Graham, N.McC. and Wainman, F.W. (1959b) Environmental temperature, energy metabolism and heat regulation in sheep. III. The metabolism and thermal exchanges of sheep with fleeces. *Journal of Agricultural Science, Cambridge* 52, 41–49.

Bligh, J. (1966) The thermosensitivity of the hypothalamus and thermoregulation in mammals. *Biological Review* 41, 317–367.

Bligh, J. (1985) Temperature regulation. In: Yousef, M.K. (ed.), *Stress Physiology in Livestock, Vol I, Basic Principles.* CRC Press Inc., Boca Raton, Florida.

Bligh, J. and Johnson, K.G. (1973) Glossary of terms for thermal physiology. *Journal of Applied Physiology* 35, 941–961.

Bruce, J.M. (1979) Heat loss from animals to floors. *Farm Buildings Progress* 55, 1–4.

Carpenter, S.A. (1981) Ventilation systems. In: Clark, J.A. (ed.), *Environmental Aspects of Housing for Animal Production.* Butterworths, London, pp. 331–350.

Cena, K.M. (1974) Radiative heat loss from animals and man. In: Monteith, J.L. and Mount, L.E. (eds), *Heat Loss from Animals and Man.* Butterworths, London, pp. 31–58.

Cena, K.M. and Clark, J.A. (1978) Thermal resistance units. *Journal of Thermal Biology* 3, 173–174.

Charles, D.R. (1981) Practical ventilation and temperature control for poultry. In: Clark, J.A. (ed.), *Environmental Aspects of Housing for Animal Production.* Butterworths, London, pp. 183–195.

Clark, J.A. and Cena, K.M. (1981) Monitoring the house environment. In: Clark, J.A. (ed.), *Environmental Aspects of Housing for Animal Production.* Butterworths, London, pp. 309–330.

Esmay, M.L. (1969) *Principles of Animal Environment.* Avi, Westport, Connecticut.

Gates, D.M. (1962) *Energy Exchange in the Biosphere.* Harper & Row, New York.

Graham, N.McC., Blaxter, K.L., Wainman, F.W. and Armstrong, D.G. (1959) Environmental temperature, energy metabolism and heat regulation in sheep. 1. Energy metabolism in closely clipped sheep. *Journal of Agricultural Science, Cambridge* 52, 13–24.

Hahn, G.L. and Hugh-Jones, M.E. (1989) Critical temperatures – a discussion. WMO Tech. note 191, *Animal Health and Production at Extremes of Weather,* Geneva, pp. 13–17.

Hales, J.R.S. and Webster, M.E.D. (1967) Respiratory function during thermal tachypnoea in sheep. *Journal of Physiology* 190, 241–260.

Hammel, J.T. (1956) Infrared emissivities of some arctic fauna. *Journal of Mammalogy* 37, 375–378.

Holmes, C.W. and Close, W.H. (1977) The influence of climatic variables on energy metabolism and associated aspects of productivity in the pig. In: Haresign, W., Swan, H. and Lewis, D. (eds), *Nutrition and the Climatic Environment.* Butterworths, London, pp. 51–73.

Hoyt, D.F. and Taylor, C.R. (1981) Gait and the energetics of locomotion in horses. *Nature, London* 292, 239–240.

Ingram, D.L. and Mount, L.E. (1975) *Man and Animals in Hot Environments.* Springer, New York.

McArthur, A.J. (1981a) Thermal insulation and heat loss from animals. In: Clark, J.A. (ed.), *Environmental Aspects of Housing for Animal Production.* Butterworths, London, pp. 37–60.

McArthur, A.J. (1981b) Thermal resistance and sensible heat loss from animals. *Journal of Thermal Biology* 6, 43–47.

McArthur, A.J. (1987) Thermal interaction between animal and microclimate: a comprehensive model. *Journal of Theoretical Biology* 126, 203–238.

McArthur, A.J. (1991a) Thermal radiation exchange, convection and the storage of latent heat in animal coats. *Agricultural and Forest Meteorology* 53, 325–336.

McArthur, A.J. (1991b) Metabolism of homeotherms in the cold and estimation of thermal insulation. *Journal of Thermal Biology* 16, 149–155.

McArthur, A.J. and Clark, J.A. (1988) Body temperature of homeotherms and the conservation of energy and water. *Journal of Thermal Biology* 13, 9–13.

McArthur, A.J. and Ousey, J.C. (1994) Heat loss from a wet animal: changes with time in the heat balance of a physical model representing a newborn homeotherm. *Journal of Thermal Biology* (in press).

McBride, G.E., Christopherson, R.J. and Sauer, W.C. (1983) Metabolic responses of horses to temperature stress. *Journal of Animal Science* 57 (suppl. 1), 175.

McLean, J.A. (1974) Loss of heat by evaporation. In: Monteith, J.L. and Mount, L.E. (eds), *Heat Loss from Animals and Man.* Butterworths, London, pp. 19–31.

Mangold, D.W., Bundy, D.S. and Hellickson, M.A. (1983) Psychrometrics. In: Hellickson, M.A. and Walker, J.N. (eds), *Ventilation of Agricultural Structures.* ASAE, St Joseph, Michigan, USA, pp. 9–22.

Meyer, A.A. and Webster, A.J.F. (1971) Cold-induced vasodilation in sheep. *Canadian Journal of Physiology and Pharmacology* 49, 901–908.

Mitchell, D. (1974) Convective heat transfer from man and other animals. In:

Monteith, J.L. and Mount, L.E. (eds), *Heat Loss from Animals and Man.* Butterworths, London, pp. 59–76.

Mitchell, M.A. (1985) Measurement of forced convective heat transfer in birds: a wind tunnel calorimeter. *Journal of Thermal Biology* 10, 87–95.

Monteith, J.L. and Mount, L.E. (eds) (1974) *Heat Loss from Animals and Man.* Butterworths, London.

Monteith, J.L. and Unsworth, M.H. (1990) *Principles of Environmental Physics,* 2nd edn. Arnold, London.

Mount, L.E. (1960) The influence of huddling and body size on the metabolic rate of the young pig. *Journal of Agricultural Science, Cambridge* 55, 101–105.

Mount, L.E. (1967) Heat loss from new-born pigs to the floor. *Research in Veterinary Science* 8, 175–186.

Mount, L.E. (1974) The concept of thermal neutrality. In: Monteith, J.L. and Mount, L.E. (eds), *Heat Loss from Animals and Man.* Butterworths, London, pp. 425–439.

Mount, L.E. (1979) *Adaptation to Thermal Environment: Man and His Productive Animals.* Arnold, London.

Ousey, J.C., McArthur, A.J. and Rossdale, P.D. (1991) Metabolic changes in thoroughbred and pony foals during the first 24h *postpartum. Journal of Reproduction and Fertility* (Suppl.) 44, 561–570.

Ousey, J.C., McArthur, A.J., Murgatroyd, P.R., Stewart, J.H. and Rossdale, P.D. (1992) Thermoregulation and total body insulation in the neonatal foal. *Journal of Thermal Biology* 17, 1–10.

Poczopko, P. (1981) The environmental physiology of juvenile animals. In: Clark, J.A. (ed.), *Environmental Aspects of Housing for Animal Production.* Butterworths, London, pp. 109–130.

Tucker, V.A. (1970) Energetic cost of locomotion in animals. *Comparative Biochemistry and Physiology* 34, 841–846.

Van Kampen, M. (1981) Thermal influences on poultry. In: Clark, J.A. (ed.), *Environmental Aspects of Housing for Animal Production.* Butterworths, London, pp. 217–232.

Vansteelant, B., DeShazer, J.A. and Milanuk, M.J. (1988) Computer based humidity temperature controller for a swine farrowing facility. In: *Livestock Environment III.* ASAE, St Joseph, Michigan, pp. 264–271.

Vant'Ooster, A. and Both, A.J. (1988) Towards better understanding of relations between building design and natural ventilation in livestock buildings. In: *Livestock Environment III.* ASAE, St Joseph, Michigan, pp. 8–21.

Wathes, C.M. (1981) Insulation of animal houses. In: Clark, J.A. (ed.), *Environmental Aspects of Housing for Animal Production.* Butterworths, London, pp. 379–412.

Wathes, C.M. and Clark, J.A. (1981) Sensible heat transfer from the fowl: boundary layer resistance of a model fowl. *British Journal of Poultry Science* 22, 161–173.

Webster, A.J.F. (1981) Optimal housing criteria for ruminants. In: Clark, J.A. (ed.), *Environmental Aspects of Housing for Animal Production.* Butterworths, London, pp. 217–232.

Webster, A.J.F. (1987) *Understanding the Dairy Cow.* BSP Professional Books, Oxford.

Webster, A.J.F., Gordon, J.G. and Smith, J.C. (1976) Energy metabolism of veal calves in relation to body weight, food intake and air temperature. *Animal Production* 23, 35–42.

Whittow, G.C. (1962) The significance of the extremities of the ox (*Bos taurus*) in thermoregulation. *Journal of Agricultural Science, Cambridge* 58, 109–120.

Whittow, G.C. and Findlay, J.D. (1968) Oxygen cost of thermal panting. *Journal of Physiology* 214, 94–99.

Wiersma, F. and Nelson, G.L. (1967) Nonevaporative convective heat transfer from the surface of a bovine. *Transactions of the American Society of Agricultural Engineers* 10, 733–737.

Worstell, D.M. and Brody, S. (1953) Environmental physiology and shelter engineering. XX. Comparative physiological reactions of European and Indian cattle to changing temperature. *Missouri Agricultural Experimental Station Research Bulletin* 515.

Yousef, M.K. (1985) Thermoneutral zone. In: Yousef, M.K. (ed.), *Stress Physiology in Livestock, Vol I, Basic Principles.* CRC Press, Inc., Boca Raton, Florida.

Air and Surface Hygiene 6

C.M. WATHES
Animal Science and Engineering Division,
Silsoe Research Institute, UK

Introduction

Hygiene in livestock housing is usually poor by comparison with standards for humans. In particular, hygiene of the air and of building surfaces is often less than satisfactory and is potentially a serious limitation to high efficiencies of production and good health in those intensive systems of animal husbandry which involve housing at some stage of the production cycle. Environmental diseases of livestock, e.g. calf pneumonia, diarrhoea and mastitis, may be controlled as much by improvements in air and surface hygiene as by the development of vaccines or other pharmacological agents.

'Effective' ventilation is one of the principal tenets of intensive animal production and, indeed, is enshrined in the UK Codes of Recommendation for the Welfare of Livestock. However, what is meant by good, effective, sufficient or other adjectives commonly applied to building ventilation is not usually clear (Wathes *et al.*, 1983). What is clear are the objectives of ventilation, i.e. 'an aerial environment in which: (i) the animals' health can be maintained and their productivity sustained; (ii) the stockman can accomplish his tasks in comfort and without risk to his health; and (iii) the building and its equipment are protected from corrosion or physical damage' (Wathes *et al.*, 1983).

Surface hygiene has a similar aura of mystery to aerial hygiene. It can be stated with absolute certainty that all surfaces within livestock buildings may harbour thriving populations of microorganisms. These flourish in the moist, warm microenvironments of beddings and the cracks and crevices of the building's structure and equipment, and find a ready supply of nutrients that is replenished regularly. Complete sterility of surfaces is only feasible under laboratory conditions and it is perhaps astonishing that surface contamination of livestock buildings does not lead to more disease than is apparently the case.

The aims of this chapter are to consider:

1. The roles of air and surface hygiene in the health and performance of housed livestock.
2. The dynamics of aerial pollutants.
3. The microbial ecology of building surfaces.
4. Building designs for improved hygiene.

Attention to air and surface hygiene should be an important part of the design and operation of any building for animals. However, the main thrust of environmental control in livestock buildings over the past decade has been directed towards the performance of predominantly healthy animals, for example via temperature and light control, with little attention given to air and surface hygiene.

Roles of Air and Surface Hygiene in Health and Production

The major roles that air and surface hygiene play in animal health and production are twofold. Firstly, the air and surfaces of buildings may act as reservoirs for primary and opportunistic pathogens of infectious and allergic diseases. Secondly, air- and surface-borne pollutants, including micro-organisms, may contribute to the aetiology of environmental diseases, such as calf pneumonia, by the continuous burden which they impose on non-specific host defence mechanisms. Evidence for these roles has accumulated slowly over recent years from both field and laboratory studies.

Poor air and surface hygiene in livestock buildings is nearly always associated with intensive systems of husbandry and is exacerbated by poor standards of management. Intensive systems usually involve high stocking densities and large flocks or herds, which produce large quantities of wastes on a farm scale. The common aerial pollutants found in livestock buildings are dusts, gases and commensal microorganisms and these are inevitable by-products of the animals' existence. They arise from feed, bedding, excreta and the animals themselves. In winter, ventilation rates are deliberately maintained at slow speeds in intensive pig and poultry houses because of the need to conserve heat and thereby maintain optimum environmental temperatures (see Chapter 1). High concentrations of aerial pollutants are a direct result of this policy. Similarly, poor drainage, infrequent renewal of litter beds or incorrect design of slatted floors can lead to poor surface hygiene. In some cases the remedy is obvious: in others the complexity of the underlying physical, chemical and microbial processes ensures that simple solutions are unlikely to be found. For example, establishment and maintenance of litter quality in a broiler house is essential for satisfactory bird health and performance, but its achievement remains one of the arts of the skilled stockman and has defied exact specification until recently (Tucker and Walker, 1992).

Airborne transmission of disease

The aerial route is the natural pathway for transmission of some pathogenic microorganisms. The hardy spores of fungi and some bacteria, e.g. *Aspergillus fumigatus,* are well adapted to the physiological and physical stresses of aerial transport: in contrast the majority of species of bacteria and viruses are ill-equipped to survive in air. Table 6.1 lists common pathogens of farm animals which are known to be transmitted aerially. However, airborne transmission does not imply that the respiratory tract is the sole or even the major route of inoculation. Dry or wet deposition on vegetative surfaces may lead to ingestion and subsequent infection in grazing animals, as proposed for foot and mouth disease in cattle (Chamberlain, 1970). Furthermore, airborne transmission is not necessarily confined to respiratory pathogens (Table 6.1). For example, inoculation with aerosols of *Salmonella typhimurium* via masks or 'whole body' exposure, led to infection in calves (Wathes *et al.*, 1988). Additional support for this experimental finding comes from epidemiological evidence that contagion only accounts for about 40% of secondary cases of infection with *S. typhimurium* among calves penned individually (Hardman *et al.*, 1991). This observation has clear implications for control of disease spread in intensive calf units and may be of more general application. Similarly, laying hens may be infected by aerosol with *S. enteritidis* (Baskerville *et al.*, 1992) and piglets exposed to aerosols of an enterotoxigenic strain of *Escherichia coli* at weaning may develop severe, sometimes fatal diarrhoea (Wathes *et al.*, 1989).

Foot and mouth disease is the best example of long-range (≈ 10 km) airborne transmission among farm animals. Dispersal of the virus in exhaled breath, faeces, urine and secretions occurs at a rate dependent on the stage of disease (Donaldson *et al.*, 1970). Given the fragility of the virus in aerosol (Donaldson, 1983), it is perhaps surprising that airborne transmission occurs at all. However, a combination of high shedding rates and low infective doses in some farm species, particularly pigs and cattle respectively, ensures the success of this route (Donaldson, 1983). Gloster *et al.* (1981) have devised a numerical model for forecasting the likely airborne spread of foot and mouth disease virus. The model is based on meteorological and geographical information, such as wind vector, humidity and topography and biological data, e.g. virus output. The model predicts spread up to 10 km from the source, has been validated against field outbreaks and is in current operational use by the UK Ministry of Agriculture (Gloster *et al.*, 1981). Extension of the model to other infectious diseases, e.g. Newcastle disease of poultry, is hampered by insufficient biological data (Gloster, 1983). *Ipso facto,* attempts to separate animal houses to prevent airborne transmission

Table 6.1. Common pathogens of pigs and poultry known to be transmitted aerially.

Bacteria	
Bordetella bronchiseptica	*Mycobacterium tuberculosis*
Brucella suis	*Mycoplasma gallisepticum*
Corynebacterium equi	*Mycoplasma hyorhinus*
Erysipelothrix rhusiopathiae	*Mycoplasma suipneumoniae*
Escherichia coli	*Pasteurella multocida*
Haemophilus gallinarus	*Pasteurella pseudotuberculosis*
Haemophilus parasuis	*Salmonella pullorum*
Haemophilus pleuropneumoniae	*Salmonella typhimurium*
Listeria monocytogenes	*Staphylococcus aureus*
Leptospira pomona	*Streptococcus suis* type II
Mycobacterium arium	
Fungi	
Aspergillus flavus	*Coccidioides immitis*
Aspergillus fumigatus	*Cryptococcus neoformans*
Aspergillus nidulans	*Histoplasma farcinorum*
Aspergillus niger	*Rhinosporidium seeberi*
Rickettsia	
Coxiella burnetii	
Protozoa	
Toxoplasma gondii	
Viruses	
African swine fever	Infectious nephrosis of fowls
Avian encephalomyelites	Infectious porcine encephalomyelitis
Avian leukosis	Marek's disease
Foot-and-mouth disease	Newcastle disease
Fowl plague	Ornithosis
Hog cholera	Porcine enterovirus
Inclusion body rhinitis	Swine influenza
Infectious bronchitis of fowls	Transmissible gastroenteritis of swine
Infectious laryngotracheitis of fowls	

Source: After Wathes (1987) with additions.

are likely to be unsuccessful for most infectious diseases of farm animals. The rapid mixing of air within buildings also implies that airborne transmission between stalls, pens or cages, is highly likely, unless 'plug or piston flow' ventilation systems are used. There are several examples of the recovery of primary pathogens from the air of livestock buildings containing infected animals, e.g. foot and mouth disease virus (Donaldson *et al.*, 1970), Newcastle disease virus (Hugh-Jones *et al.*, 1973), mycoplasmas of pigs

(Tamasi, 1973), Marek's disease virus (Carrozza *et al.*, 1973) and Aujeszky's disease virus of pigs (Bourgueil *et al.*, 1992). Other primary pathogens could presumably be isolated from the air given a gentle aerosol sampler and sensitive assay.

Air quality in animal houses

The air of an animal house seethes with a dense miasma of microorganisms, dust particles and gases. There have been innumerable studies of the natural history of air hygiene in livestock buildings (for reviews see Carpenter, 1986; Wathes, 1987; De Boer and Morrison, 1988; Whyte, 1993). As might be expected a priori, the composition and concentration of the miasma vary with husbandry system, season and climate, ventilation system, etc. There are few general conclusions to be drawn except the obvious ones, that air quality in livestock houses is significantly worse than that outdoors; acceptable standards for human occupational exposure are sometimes exceeded (see Table 6.2); and improvements to air quality probably depend on a number of (small) measures taken together.

Nevertheless, a description of typical air quality in animal houses is useful. In addition to the primary pathogens listed above, numerous bacteria and fungal propagules or microbial components, such as endotoxin, will be found in the air at high concentrations, typically $\geq 10^6$ bacteria colony forming particles m^{-3} or $\geq 10^9$ fungal propagules m^{-3}. There are no generally accepted recommendations for tolerable levels of non-pathogenic airborne microorganisms: high concentrations are not necessarily correlated with endemic respiratory disease. Conversely, recovery of primary pathogens from the air is usually associated with the specific disease. Where the skin is the source then commensal bacteria such as *Staphylococcus lentus* and *Staph. xylosus* will be observed (Wathes *et al.*, 1991). Litter provides an attractive medium for the wood-rotting fungus *Paecilomyces* while other common fungi include *Aspergillus* spp., *Penicillium* spp. and *Scopulariopsis* (Madelin and Wathes, 1989). Where hay is fed or straw is used as bedding, then fungal spores will dominate the aerial microflora with over 50 species recorded in hays and beddings typically used in stables (Clarke and Madelin, 1987). Other airborne microorganisms include faecal bacteria such as *E. coli* and *Streptococcus* spp., and actinomycetes. Lengthy catalogues of airborne microbes are given by Clarke and Madelin (1987), Lovett *et al.* (1971), Dennis and Gee (1973), Dutkiewicz (1978), Madelin and Wathes (1989) and Wathes *et al.* (1991). Airborne microbes may be carried aloft either in liquid suspensions, e.g. as from a sneeze, or on rafts of dust particles, dried faeces for example. In either case, aerodynamic size governs substantially their behaviour in the turbulent air streams of an animal house and their site of deposition and subsequent fate in the respiratory tract of animals. Other factors affecting microbial survival in air are considered below.

Table 6.2. Occupational exposure limits of gases and dust in livestock buildings.

	Human occupational exposure limits		Animal exposure limits (Maximum continuous)
	Long term, (8 h time-weighted average)	Short term (10 min)	
Gases (ppm)			
Ammonia, NH_3	25	35	20
Carbon dioxide, CO_2	5,000	15,000	3,000
Carbon monoxide, CO	50	300	10
Formaldehyde, HCHO	20	30	–
Hydrogen sulphide, H_2S	10	15	0.5
Methane, CH_4	Asphyxiant		–
Nitrogen dioxide, NO_2	3	5	–
Dusts (mg m^{-3})			
Grain dust*			
Total inhalable fraction	10	–	–
Non-specific dust			
Total inhalable fraction	10	–	3.4†
Respirable fraction	5	–	1.7†

Source: (For humans) Health and Safety Executive, 1992; (for animals) CIGR, 1992.

* Maximum exposure limit.
† 24h time-weighted average.

Airborne dust particles are the second main pollutant in livestock buildings. The biological origins of most particles ensure that most dust is organic in nature; the major sources are desquamated skin cells, down and feather debris, dried faeces, feed and bedding, and microbial cells or fragments. For example, analysis by scanning electron and light microscopy indicated that most airborne dust in a turkey house was faeces or urates (Feddes *et al.*, 1992). In other building types, feed may be the primary source. Particulate behaviour in air is determined by aerodynamic size. The highest concentrations of airborne dust are found in piggeries and poultry houses; lower levels occur in cattle and sheep sheds. Numerous factors contribute to differences such as these, in particular the rate of ventilation, type and method of feeding, and manure disposal, stocking density, etc. The mean concentrations of airborne dust are usually less than the human occupational exposure standard (8 hour time-weighted average) of 5 mg m^{-3} (respirable fraction) and 10 mg m^{-3} (total inhalable fraction) for nuisance dust (Health and Safety Executive, 1992). However, the range in mean concentration over a 24 h period or at different times of the husbandry cycle can be tenfold (e.g. pigs; Robertson, 1992). These long-term (8h working day) limits apply to non-specific dusts irrespective of any specific allergic or toxic hazards. Animals continuously endure their atmospheres and the CIGR (1992) recommends linear extrapolation over time. In addition, chronic exposure to several pollutants simultaneously may result in synergism in their effects on animal health.

Inhalation of organic dusts elicits specific airborne responses that may induce airway hypersensitivity following repeated exposure (Rylander, 1986). Both organic and inorganic dusts may also simply cause mechanical blockages of macrophages, as shown recently (Gilmour *et al.*, 1989). In addition, dust particles may act as carriers for pathogenic microorganisms, e.g. Marek's disease in poultry (Jurajda and Klimes, 1970).

The most common noxious gas in animal houses is ammonia, though other gases of concern include hydrogen sulfide, carbon dioxide and methane (Table 6.2). Many other compounds are also present at lower concentrations: Hartung (1988) lists 137 trace gases though occupational exposure limits for many of these gases have not been specified for animals. Two distinct problems may arise. Acute exposure to lethal concentrations of manure gases may occur following agitation of slurry in below-ground stores (e.g. Feilden, 1982). However, the effects of chronic exposure are more insidious, especially when they are confounded with those due to dusts or by concurrent respiratory disease. Both ammonia and hydrogen sulfide are irritants; ammonia is highly soluble in water thereby enhancing the potential hazard of exposure on inhalation in the humid environment of the respiratory tract. Early work by Charles and Payne (1966) demonstrated that exposure to 100 ppm ammonia caused keratoconjunctivitis in hens after 6 weeks, while chronic exposure of pigs to ammonia reduced pulmonary clearance of bacteria (Drummond *et al.*, 1978), depressed growth rate (Drummond *et al.*, 1980) and exacerbated turbinate atrophy (Drummond *et al.*, 1981). Mean concentrations of ammonia are usually less than the human or animal exposure standards (Table 6.2) and there are few reports of long-term measurements of other gases in animal houses. Both methane and carbon dioxide are classified as simple asphyxiants and, as such, are unlikely to pose significant hazards to animal health at the levels usually encountered.

Evidence for the harmful effects of poor air quality on animal – and human – health (e.g. Donham, 1987; and Whyte, 1993) has accumulated slowly over the past decade. A recent epidemiological study by Robertson *et al.* (1990) provided strong field evidence for a major effect of poor air quality on the incidence and severity of an endemic respiratory disease in pigs (atrophic rhinitis) and adds good support to the laboratory experiments described above. Tentative guidelines for occupational exposure limits are given in Table 6.2, but these should be kept under continual review pending current research.

Surface hygiene in animal houses

Contamination of surfaces within livestock buildings with pathogenic microorganisms may play a significant role in animal health. Microorganisms are shed continually from animals via numerous routes (Table 6.3) and thereafter may thrive in the warm, moist environment of an animal house in which the rich supply of nutrients from excreta, feed and bedding is replenished regularly. Deep litter bedding and slurry stores are the obvious major reservoirs but any surface may be suitable for colonization including fixed equipment, cracks and crevices in building materials, and ventilation shafts and fan blades. No surface will ever be sterile – even after routine cleaning and disinfection (see also Boon and Wray, 1989). Other sources of contamination include fresh feed and bedding, insects, fomites and the stockman. Subsequent infection of susceptible hosts may occur via the principal routes of inhalation, ingestion, contact and wounds. Nearly all the infectious diseases listed in Table 6.3 are caused by single primary pathogens, though diseases with a complex multifactorial aetiology, e.g. post-weaning diarrhoea in pigs, may also be attributed to poor surface hygiene. Mastitis in dairy cows, joint ill in sheep and salmonellosis in calves are common examples of diseases in which surface hygiene is involved.

Zoonoses form a special class of communicable disease which may infect both animals and man and are of particular importance to public health. Within the context of surface hygiene, zoonoses of interest include orf, salmonellosis, ringworm and various protozoal diseases. Communication of zoonoses from animals to man may be minimized by reduction of contact with infected animals, decontamination of building surfaces, elimination of pests and hygienic disposal of manure, bedding and carcasses. Critical standards of hygiene for zoonoses or other infectious diseases are not available.

Dynamics of Aerial Contaminants

Dynamic model

The concept of a balance sheet can aid understanding of the dynamics of aerial contaminants within livestock buildings. Appreciation of the relative strengths of the various sources and sinks (of contaminants) can help direct efforts to improve air quality by outlining the advantages of different control strategies. Figure 6.1 illustrates this approach. The major sources of air contaminants are the animals themselves by way of their various secretions and excretions, their feed and bedding, and material brought indoors by the incoming airstream. The major sinks are exhaust ventilation (the solution to pollution is dilution – though this practice nowadays is unacceptable

Table 6.3. Examples of routes by which animal pathogens are shed from infected hosts.

Site of exit	Contaminated tissue or fluid	Pathogen	Disease	Host
Body surface	Hair	*Microsporum canis*	Ringworm	Dogs, man, etc.
	Lesion crusts	Poxviruses	Cowpox	Cattle, sheep, etc.
	Exudate (e.g. pus)	*Staphylococcus aureus*	Abscesses	
Nose	Secretions	Paramyxovirus sp.	Distemper	Dog
		Orthomyxovirus sp.	Influenza	Swine, horse, birds
	Exudate (bloodstained)	*Bacillus anthracis*	Anthrax	Cattle, sheep
Mouth	Saliva	Foot-and-mouth virus	Foot-and-mouth	Cattle, sheep
		Lyssavirus sp.	Rabies	Dog
	Sputum	*Mycobacterium tuberculosis*	Tuberculosis (pulmonary)	Cattle, man
	Tonsil	*Erysipelothrix rhusiopathiae*	Erysipelas	Swine
Mammary	Milk	*Streptococcus agalactiae*	Mastitis	Cow
Anus	Faeces	*Mycobacterium johnei*	Johne's disease	Cattle, sheep
		Rotavirus sp.	Enteritis	Swine
		Salmonella dublin	Enteritis, septicaemia	Cattle
Urinogenital tract	Urine, semen	*Leptospira canicola*	Leptospirosis	Dog
		Camphylobacter fetus	Infertility	Cattle
	Eggs	*Salmonella pullorum*	Pullorum disease	Poultry
Eyes	Tears	*Haemophilus influenzae*	Pink eye (New Forest disease)	Cattle
Wound (tick vector)	Blood	*Rickettsia burnetti*	Q-fever	Cattle

Source: Linton, 1987.

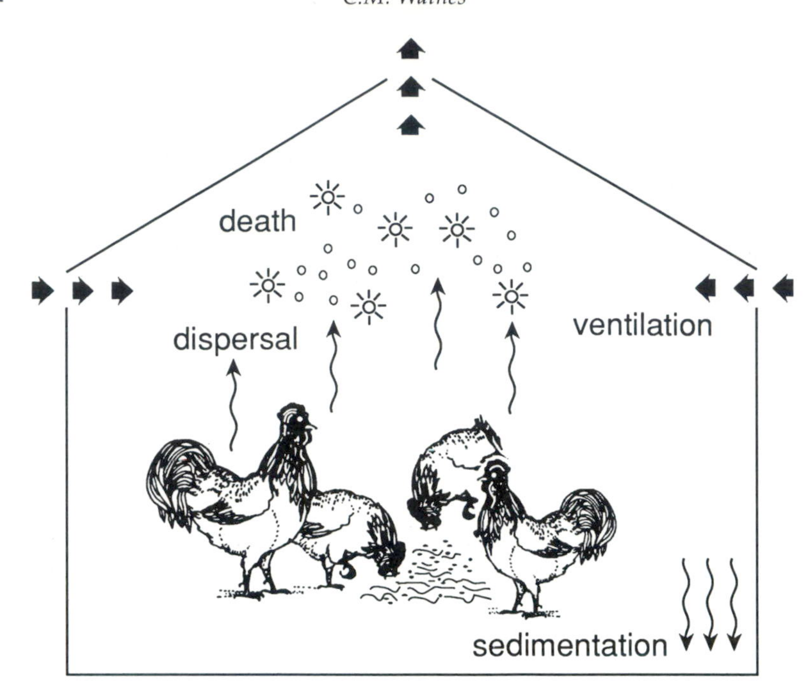

Fig. 6.1. The concentration of aerial contaminants in a livestock building is the net result of a dynamic equilibrium between various sinks and sources.

because of environment pollution from animal agriculture), physical mechanisms such as coagulation, sedimentation and impaction, and, for living microorganisms, death *in situ*.

Within any given volume of air, the concentration of an aerial contaminant represents the instantaneous balance between inflow and outflow fluxes. The volume may be as small as the headspace around a calf in a pen or as large as the entire building. Inhomogeneities in spatial concentration will arise from the corresponding locations of sources and ventilation exhausts. Concentration will also vary over time. This dynamic equilibrium can be modelled mathematically. The mass balance for a contaminant flow into and out of a building is

$$\frac{\mathrm{d}C}{\mathrm{d}t} = \frac{R}{V} - q_e C + q_v (C_a - C) \tag{1}$$

where C is the indoor concentration, t is time, V is the volume of the building, R is the emission rate, C_a is the ambient concentration, q_v is the air change rate, and q_e is the sum of the specific rate constants and represents clearance from the air by mechanisms other than ventilation, e.g. sedimentation, death *in situ*. The solution of Equation (1) is

$$C = C_o e^{-(q_e + q_v)t} + \frac{R + Vq_v C_a}{V(q_e + q_v)} (1 - e^{-(q_e + q_v)t}) \tag{2}$$

where C_o is the initial pollutant concentration at $t = 0$. This solution assumes perfect mixing, constant emission rate and a one-compartment model. Of course, these assumptions are simplistic and deny the complexity of contaminant dynamics in a 'real' building. In most buildings $q_e + q_v$ exceeds $10\,h^{-1}$ and the exponential term becomes negligible after 15 min or so. Hence

$$C = \frac{R + Vq_v C_a}{V(q_e + q_v)} \tag{3}$$

where q_e and q_v are clearance mechanisms that act in series and have the same units (equivalent to air changes per hour, h^{-1}). Ventilation rates in intensive livestock buildings may be as slow as $2\,h^{-1}$ during winter when heat must be conserved, rising to $20–30\,h^{-1}$ during summer while q_e represents a 'catch all' for other clearance mechanisms, e.g. the physical processes of coagulation, sedimentation and impaction and the biological process of death *in situ* for microbial aerosols. Typical values of q_e for unit density particles dispersed at 1 m height into still air and settling on to a horizontal surface are $0.1\,h^{-1}$ and $10\,h^{-1}$ for aerodynamic diameters of 1 and $10\,\mu m$ respectively. Effective rate constants for microbial death can be as rapid as $1000\,h^{-1}$ for fragile bacterial or viral species to less than $0.1\,h^{-1}$ for robust cells.

Figure 6.2 shows graphically the predictions of Equation (3). In this example, air quality in a calf house is estimated from a simple steady-state model, assuming perfect mixing from a uniform source in a constant climate. The concentration of aerial contaminants, e.g. gases, respirable dusts and viable microbes, is expressed in arbitrary units. Gas concentration well illustrates the law of diminishing returns with faster air change rates. In addition to dilution by ventilation, particles are cleared by the physical mechanisms described above, typically at $q_e = 5\,h^{-1}$ for a particle of $6\,\mu m$ aerodynamic diameter. Furthermore, inactivation of microbes reduces concentration even more, by $q_e = 10\,h^{-1}$ in this example. Perhaps the most interesting conclusion to be drawn from this analysis concerns the relative benefits of doubling airspace from 6 to $12\,m^3$ per calf. For viable microbes, the reduction in concentration achieved by doubling cubic capacity can only be reproduced by raising ventilation rates from 6 to $30\,h^{-1}$. Such a rapid rate could only be realized in practice by creating large openings in the building or by using fans of larger capacity than would normally be necessary: both practices would undoubtedly make the building undesirably draughty. Satisfactory air quality can therefore be promoted not only by minimum ventilation rates, but also by generous stocking densities.

Recently, attention has turned to more complex theoretical models of

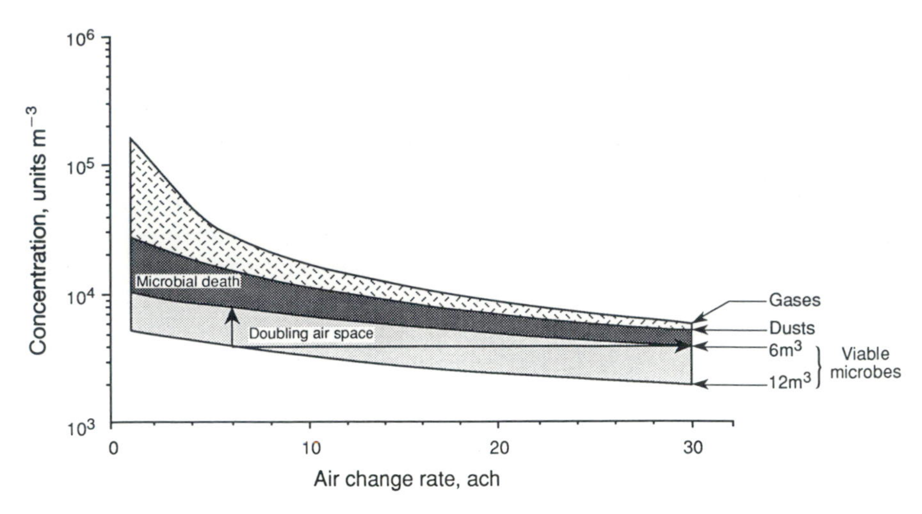

Fig. 6.2. Model relationship between air change rate and aerial concentration of gases, respirable dusts and viable microbes in a calf house stocked at either 6 m^3 or 12 m^3 per calf (after Wathes *et al.*, 1988).

temporal and spatial distribution of aerial pollutants in livestock buildings (e.g. Liao and Feddes, 1989; Maghirang *et al.*, 1990). Pollutant dynamics can be modelled numerically by solving the equations governing the transport of momentum and energy of the airflow and the mass transport of the pollutant. Scales ranging from the microscopic to the macroscopic can be employed and the effects of turbulence considered. This adoption of techniques of computational fluid dynamics for air hygiene studies is most welcome and timely. While verification of model predictions has yet to be undertaken under full-scale conditions, this approach allows rapid identification of the benefits of various control strategies, e.g. location of air inlets, and of the existence of stagnant zones, while providing a fundamental insight into the physical behaviour of aerial pollutants in ventilated airspaces.

Emission rates

The sources of aerial pollutants are manifold but yet data on their rates of emission are sparse. Knowledge of the primary and net emission rates from the various sources would aid in the appraisal of different control strategies: at present, relative source strengths can only be inferred from studies of the natural history of aerial pollutants that report concentration and composition as a function of system of husbandry or management practices. In principle, the method of measuring overall emission rate from all sources within a livestock building is simple, though separation into the various sources is most difficult. Simultaneous measurements of C, C_a, q_e and q_v can yield R (Equation 3), provided that the assumptions of a well-mixed distribution of pollutants in a steady state are satisfied.

This approach was first used by Feddes *et al.* (1982) to estimate emission rates of ammonia, carbon dioxide and moisture from broilers kept on deep litter. More recently Qi *et al.* (1992) observed net generation rates of respirable and total dust of 1.32 and 1.84 $mg\,h^{-1}$ per bird for caged layers. Generation rates were faster at rapid ventilation rates, probably due to turbulent air currents suspending dust from cage surfaces, etc. Similar approaches have been used for emission rates of gaseous pollutants, e.g. dairy cows (Clark and McQuitty, 1987) and farrowing sows (Clark and McQuitty, 1986). Litter beddings are clearly a major source of dust and bioaerosols but the animals themselves are a second source. In a study with veal calves kept in crates on slats (now outlawed in the UK), Wathes *et al.* (1984) measured the rate of release of aerobic bacteria from the animal's body surface using a ventilated cup technique. Release rates were rapid, typically 2×10^6 colony forming particles $h^{-1}m^{-2}$ (calf surface area), and were similar to rates recorded for man. Skin squames are shed during normal replacement of the epidermis and a proportion carry aloft single cells or microcolonies of both aerobic and anaerobic bacteria (Noble, 1975).

Ventilation

Dilution by ventilation is clearly one of the most effective means by which aerial pollutants are cleared from the air of livestock buildings. The principles and practice of building ventilation are well understood in terms of thermal environments (this volume, Chapter 7), but it is only recently that the role of ventilation in determining acceptable air quality has been researched. Some widespread beliefs are now being challenged. For example, Maghirang *et al.* (1991) have observed that concentrations of aerial dust *rise* with building ventilation rate. This surprising result may be explained by increased animal activity leading to faster generation rates. Alternatively, fast turbulent air currents may suspend or resuspend settled surface layers of dust. Confirmation of this and other novel findings is required before long established concepts can be refuted.

Local ventilation

Unless fresh air entering a livestock building is perfectly mixed with existing air, then some zones will be ventilated at faster rates than others. Ventilation rates are widely quoted for livestock buildings (see this volume, Chapters 1 and 7) but normally refer to an overall rate specified at the buildings' exhaust. Observation of the movement of smoke tracers within the large air spaces of animal houses readily reveals the existence of stagnant zones, e.g. in the lee of pen divisions, that expose the fallacy of uniform ventilation. Spatial inhomogeneities of pollutant concentration, humidity or air temperature will result (Conceição *et al.*, 1989; Barber *et al.*, 1991; Maghirang *et al.*, 1991), though these may also arise from location of sources.

Theoretical studies of air flow and pollutant distribution demonstrate significant spatial gradients in pollutant concentration, though validation of their predictions is confined to scale models and full-scale measurements are desirable (Barber and Ogilvie, 1982; Liao and Feddes, 1989; Maghirang *et al.*, 1990). The movement of air through buildings is determined by airflow patterns, which can be characterized in terms of air velocity and turbulence intensity and are determined by air temperature and building characteristics, e.g. location of ventilation openings, pen divisions and stock. Incomplete mixing of air may arise from short circuiting of air between inlets and exhaust or the establishment of stagnant zones by virtue of design of the ventilation system or the buildings' construction. For crossflow exhaust ventilation, Maghirang *et al.* (1990) predicted a maximum concentration of a gaseous pollutant (at animal level) of 2.5 times that at the exhaust: fine, respirable aerosols that follow the microscopic air flows would be expected to have a similar range in concentration. Perfect mixing of air within a livestock building is not particularly desirable because of the possible spread of airborne pathogens. Contrariwise, thorough mixing is most desirable where animals are kept for breeding. For example, olfactory stimulation by sex pheromones helps induce oestrus in pre-pubertal gilts, encourages sexual development in immature boars and increases copulatory performance in mature boars (Baxter, 1984).

Alternative criteria for ventilation rates

The criteria against which a ventilation rate can be set quantitatively are thermal environment, concentration of aerial pollutants and humidity. Control of these variables within a livestock building via the ventilation system requires an accurate and reliable sensor capable of withstanding harsh operating conditions. Various types of thermostats are widely available but it is only recently that sensors for ammonia and humidity have been developed for agricultural applications. Sensors for aerial dust are not yet available commercially but could be adapted from those used in laboratories. Thermal environments, specified principally in terms of air speed and temperature (this volume, Chapter 5), are widely used in temperate climates to set ventilation rates within pig and poultry buildings. Optimum temperatures are well known for all classes of livestock (this volume, Chapter 1). Table 6.2 gives tentative values for acceptable limits of aerial pollutants while relative humidities in the range 30–90% have been recommended and the exact value is probably not critical (Wathes *et al.*, 1983).

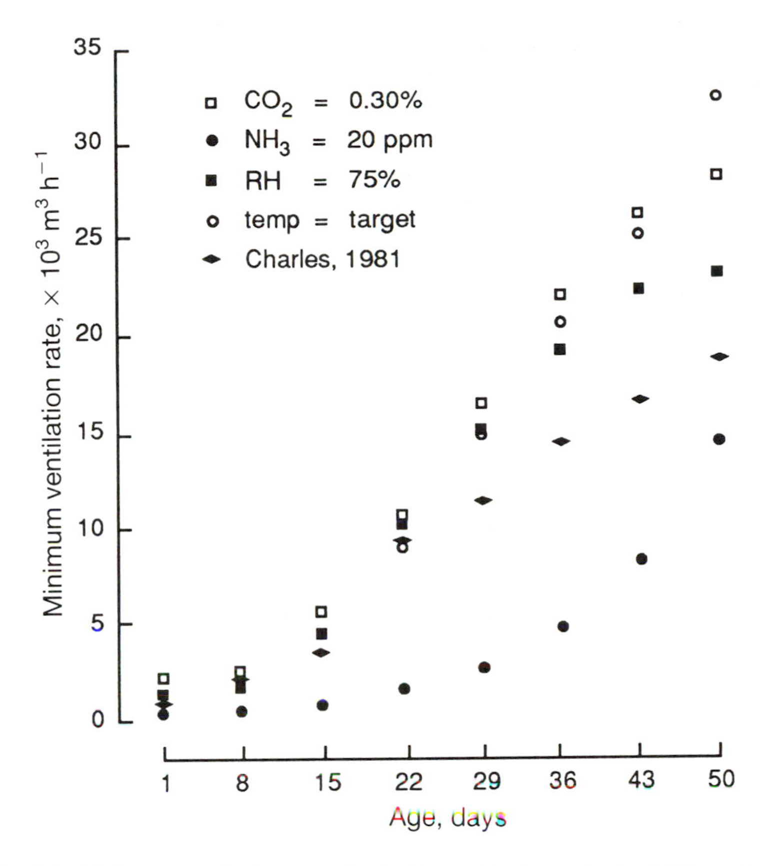

Fig. 6.3. Minimum ventilation rates for broilers using four criteria. Building details: volume = 4000 m^3; floor area = 1440 m^2; ridge height = 6 m; eaves height = 2 m; overall *U* value = 0.5 W m^{2}°C^{-1}; temperature = 31.5°C at 1 day reducing by 0.5°C day^{-1} to 21°C at 22 days. Ambient conditions: CO_2 = 0.034%; NH_3 = 0 ppm: moisture content = 4.85 g m^{-3}, 100% RH at 0°C; temperature = 0°C. Rates for heat balance (temp. = target) only shown after 22 days and are calculated without allowance for supplementary heating (from Wathes *et al.*, 1983).

Figure 6.3, from Wathes *et al.* (1983), shows the consequences of employing four alternative criteria to set the minimum ventilation rate in a broiler house for a flock of 20,000 birds housed on litter at 20 birds m^{-2}. Production or emission rates of heat, carbon dioxide, ammonia and moisture from the birds and the litter were taken from Feddes *et al.* (1982). Recommendations by Charles (1981) for ventilation rates, which are still equally valid a decade later, were based on bird production responses to minimum ventilation rates established experimentally. The alternative criteria only produce different recommendations for minimum ventilation rates after two weeks of age. Thereafter adoption of different criteria means that some optimum limits are unsatisfied. For example, use of ammonia as the criterion produces carbon dioxide levels that greatly exceed the limit of 0.30%. The practical recommendations of Charles (1981) are a little slow to maintain carbon dioxide and relative humidity at optimum levels but ensure that air temperature and ammonia concentration are maintained at acceptable levels. There is, however, insufficient knowledge to apply cost–benefit analysis to the alternative criteria. Should a fattening piggery be kept cool to lower the burden of aerial pollutants but thereby increase maintenance energy intake, or kept warm with a correspondingly poor air quality?

Microbial survival in air

The most important climatic determinants of the survival of airborne microorganisms in animal houses are air temperature and relative humidity (RH). In general, the rate of inactivation of airborne microorganisms increases with temperature (see reviews by Strange and Cox, 1976; Sattar and Ijaz, 1987). Viruses with structural liquids, i.e. equine herpes virus, are not stable at low RH while those lacking a lipoprotein envelope, e.g. foot-and-mouth disease virus, survive best in high RH. However, subtle exceptions to this rule may arise from differences between microbial strains or composition of the suspension fluid (e.g. Donaldson, 1972; Barlow and Donaldson, 1973). The response of airborne bacteria to atmospheric humidity is also species dependent. For example, the death rate of *E. coli* in air is fastest at low RH, though a more fundamental study of death mechanisms revealed that oxygen toxicity rather than desiccation damage *per se* was the true cause of viability loss (Cox, 1989). Furthermore, the relationship between survival and RH may not be smooth: narrow zones of instability have been reported for aerosolized *E. coli* (Cox, 1989).

The numerous reports from 1960s onwards of the airborne survival of bacteria and viruses employed simple regression models to describe the loss of viability of the microbe over time. Such models were limited in their predictive ability outwith the range of experimental conditions and provided little insight into biophysical and biochemical mechanisms of death. An important contribution was made by Cox (1989), who proposed mathematical models of microbial survival based upon either probability or catastrophe theory and first- and second-order denaturation kinetics. He postulates that changes in temperature and humidity of the air induce phase transitions in the microbe's membranes which lead to structural reorganization and hence loss of viability. Some of these transitions may be reversible given appropriate conditions, such as occur in the moist, warm microenvironment of the respiratory tract, and thereby enable microbes to repair the damage arising from aerosolization.

Given that numerous, important diseases are transmissible by the aerial route and that other non-pathogenic microorganisms are present at high concentrations in the air of livestock buildings, could climate be used to control airborne microbes? The feasibility of this method depends on the desirability and ease of modification of the building's climate and knowledge of the climatic optima for the microbes of interest. For livestock buildings in temperate climates, control of air temperature is directed towards thermoregulation (see this volume, Chapters 1 and 5) while control of humidity is practised rarely owing to the high costs of air conditioning plant for the rapid ventilation rates in use. Manipulation of air temperature and humidity could be employed to lower burdens of airborne microorganisms, though the critical values for each species, if known, are unlikely to be similar and a general specification could not be given. Pending better evidence of the costs and benefits, then control of airborne microbes by climate modification is not a sensible stratagem.

Microbial Ecology of Building Surfaces

An animal house is an attractive environment for surface-borne microorganisms. The atmosphere is warm and moist, the supply of nutrients in the form of animal feed, bedding, excreta and detritus is rich, colonization sites are plentiful and are disturbed only irregularly, and natural disinfectants, particulary UV radiation, are absent (see also Wray, 1975). Two 'surfaces' are of interest, e.g. those of the building's internal structures and bedding where present.

Interest in the hygiene of building surfaces arises from their role as a reservoir for potential pathogens, for example *Salmonella typhimurium* infection in calves. Surface hygiene may be promoted in building design by common-sense details, e.g. the elimination of unnecessary horizontal surfaces such as window ledges, avoidance of condensation on cold surfaces, e.g. water pipes, through lagging, and closely-fitting joints between wall and ceiling panels (Morgan-Jones, 1987). Regular cleaning is a tiresome chore that could benefit from some mechanization but is usually accorded a low priority in the stockman's diary. However, higher standards of surface hygiene in poultry houses are being demanded increasingly by food retailers. Furthermore, the inaccessibility of some surfaces like fan ducts ensures that residual colonies of microbes can remain to reinfect cleaned surfaces. Choice of building material may have some bearing on surface hygiene. Sundahl (1975) assessed the ease with which typical building materials could be cleaned by power hosing. Plywood coated with either phenolic resin or bitumen solution was easiest to clean while bare wood, asbestos cement and galvanized steel were the most difficult. More recently, Richie *et al.* (1989) reported that cleaning times, without presoaking, were shortest for vinyl and PVC dropping boards (for caged poultry) compared with plywood, glass, stainless steel and aluminium. Pre-soaking for 10 min prior to pressure washing reduced cleaning times by at least one quarter.

The survival times of surface-borne microorganisms under the favourable conditions found in most animal houses can be surprisingly long. For example, some serotypes of salmonella survive several months in moist faeces, and much longer in dried faeces (Wray, 1975). Wray's extensive review demonstrated similar persistence for other pathogens, particularly brucella, leptospira, listeria and coliforms while the spores of fungi and some bacteria are particularly well adapted to resist environmental stresses.

Methods of cleaning and disinfecting livestock buildings are well established in theory, though practical implementation may be tiresome and not all the recommendations are followed in practice. Morgan-Jones (1987) presents hygiene programmes for all classes of farm livestock for both routine and terminal treatments. The main elements of a terminal cleaning and disinfection routine are removal of gross dirt, especially organic matter, further reduction of microbes by disinfection, a minimum period of rest of the building of at least several weeks, and fumigation if the building can be sealed. The UK Ministry of Agriculture, Fisheries and Food also produces excellent leaflets describing practical aspects of cleaning and disinfection. However, the most meticulous care is needed to render all surfaces sterile – though they quickly become recontaminated – and reservoirs of some microorganisms are almost inevitable (e.g. Wray *et al.*, 1987).

Management of litter beddings is more an art than a science and a proper understanding of the physical, chemical and microbiological processes in litter is not yet available. Litter in a broiler house can be maintained in a 'working', friable state by a skilled poultryman through attention to house humidity by control of ventilation rate, artificial heating in the first few weeks of the crop, prevention of water spills and condensation and renewal of patches of poor litter. Quality and quantity of dietary fat and protein are also important (Tucker and Walker, 1992). Failure to follow these precautions can lead to greasy or capped litters, causing breast blisters, hock burns and dirty birds.

Bedding management is important for other housed species, not only to provide a warm, comfortable mattress and firm platform for movement but also a hygienic surface for disease control (see also Chapter 3). An obvious example is the bed of a cubicle house (Chapter 11). Certain forms of mastitis, e.g. coliform, result from environmental contamination of the bedding by the pathogen. Growth and persistence of the microbe is better in some bedding materials than in others. For example, the hollow scrape formed in deep cubicle beds of sawdust promotes wet conditions that favour the survival of species of klebsiella and coliform. While several means of reducing coliform contamination by heat or chemical sterilization are available, re-establishment of the microbial reservoir occurs usually within a week or so (Eberhart *et al.*, 1979). Regular removal of manure pats and urine-soaked bedding and replenishment with fresh litter is the solution.

Hygiene Blueprints for Livestock Housing

Control strategies

Seekers of a universal solution to poor hygiene in livestock buildings will search in vain. A successful control strategy requires an understanding of the primary sources, reservoirs and sinks of air- and surface-borne contaminants. The stratagem of first choice must be based on control or elimination of the contaminant at source. Once contaminants have become dispersed throughout a large building, then the large area and volume ensures that subsequent control becomes less feasible or more expensive. While most contaminants are amenable to this approach, the component of dust arising from desquamated skin cells and detritus of fur and feather can only be controlled after dispersal. Determination of the relative strengths of the various sinks for aerial pollutants is also necessary if initial controls prove ineffective.

The roles that air and surface hygiene play in animal disease demand an economic analysis of the cost–benefit relationships for different control strategies and diseases. McInerney *et al.* (1992) have devised recently a framework for such an analysis which describes economic costs as the sum of losses (a benefit figure such as reduced growth rate) and expenditure (additional treatments necessary to control or prevent disease, e.g. higher heating costs resulting from faster ventilation rates). Given the technical limitations on disease control imposed by current management skills and scientific knowledge, they demonstrate convincingly that the avoidable – as distinct from the total – costs of disease are minimized at a level of disease above the minimum obtainable with maximum control expenditure. Using subclinical mastitis as an example, they show that the economic cost could be reduced from £172.7 million to £159.6 million (UK annual costs at 1988 prices) by adoption of the optimal control strategy. This reduction of £13.1 million is achievable with current knowledge: further research would be necessary to reduce the baseline figure. Clearly, an economic analysis of control strategies for air and surface hygiene would be most valuable, though the added complexity of environmental disease may make the task harder. Turner *et al.* (1993) have used this approach to investigate environmental influences on the incidence and severity of atrophic rhinitis in pigs. This initial work appears to demonstrate the validity of economic modelling in determining control strategies but needs refinement and further validation before it can be put to general use.

Control techniques

Control techniques for air- and surface-borne contaminants fall into two categories: reduction or elimination of sources and decontamination following dispersal. Clearly, feed and bedding materials should be of high quality without obvious signs of microbial or other contamination. In stables the potential hazards from 'mouldy' hay may be ameliorated – but not eliminated – by thorough soaking overnight though putative toxins and allergens will not be removed. While some bedding materials are intrinsically less dusty (see Chapter 14), air hygiene will depend subsequently on bedding management.

The system of feeding would appear to be a major determinant of dust burdens, though conclusive evidence is hampered by the lack of standard techniques of assessment. Mechanical systems of delivery from the bulk bin to the food trough may create fine dust particles through grinding or crushing, even though the original pellets or crumbs are comparatively dust free. One recent study of feeding systems for pigs showed that the burden of total airborne dust under restricted feeding was twice that for *ad libitum* feeding (Robertson, 1992). Part of the explanation for this perhaps surprising finding is the intense activity of restricted-fed pigs at feeding time, which may then disturb settled dust. Animal activity is a major contribution to high dust burdens. Robertson's study was confounded by differences in the delivery system – feed was usually delivered to the floor in the restricted system and to hoppers and troughs for the *ad libitum* group. Comparisons of dry and wet feeding systems for pigs also show conflicting results (see Dawson, 1990). Wet systems may cause higher dust levels after spilt feed has deposited and dried on body and building surfaces, thereby acting as a secondary source.

An alternative approach that seems particularly promising is modification of the feed itself by addition of fats or oils. Reductions of around 50% in dust mass concentration (total fraction) can be achieved by supplementation of pig feed with 5% tallow (Chiba *et al.*, 1985, 1987), though not all reports show a benefit (Welford *et al.*, 1992). Similar reductions in the amount of settled dust have been reported when 5% soyabean oil is added to weaner diets for pigs (Gore *et al.*, 1986). Comparable studies with poultry may prove of similar value. If feed is modified or supplemented for the control of airborne dusts then the consequences for animal nutrition and product quality must also be considered.

Atmospheric ammonia is released from slurry stores and litter beddings during microbial breakdown of urea or uric acid. Inhibition of some of the chemical pathways in the formation of ammonia has been assisted by addition of novel dietary binders, usually derived from extracts of the yucca plant. Some success has been reported, though there is not yet a widespread consensus for these claims (Whyte, 1993). The main sources of methane and carbon dioxide are the animals themselves, though microbial processes within litter can generate small quantities of carbon dioxide. It is possible to minimize nitrogen excretion through dietary modification and precision feeding. Carbon monoxide is produced by propane gas heaters that are improperly adjusted. Other gases, such as nitrogen dioxide and hydrogen sulfide, may be liberated at high rates during emptying of slurry pits and rapidly reach lethal concentrations (McLoughlin *et al.*, 1985): the obvious precaution is to remove all animals, including man, from the confines of the building during this operation.

Various end-of-pipe methods were devised in the 1980s to remove aerial contaminants from the air of livestock buildings. These techniques were based on air cleaners using a variety of principles, such as dry filtration, wet scrubbing or electrostatic precipitation, ionization, etc. (see Pearson, 1988). They were only successful in those few cases where the cleaned air could be returned to the vicinity of all livestock without significant interference with the existing ventilation system, e.g. flat decks for weaner pigs (Carpenter *et al.*, 1986a,b; van't Klooster *et al.*, 1993). While these air cleaners may be efficient on a small scale, the large volumes of most livestock buildings coupled with technical difficulties in maintenance and high installation and/ or running costs, suggest that this control technique is unlikely to be of commercial benefit.

Overall, a control strategy for promoting an acceptable quality of air and surface hygiene in livestock houses should be based on several techniques operating in parallel. Attention to litter or slurry management, assured supplies of high quality feed and bedding, a well-designed system of ventilation, calm animals kept at a low stocking rate and the judicious use of feed additives will all aid this goal.

Conclusions

Knowledge of and interest in hygiene in livestock buildings has grown significantly in the 1980s. While optimum thermal environments can now be specified and have been adopted widely on farms, several complementary issues must be resolved before similar attention can be given to air and surface hygiene. Definitive statements of tolerable levels of aerial contaminants are needed, together with a detailed understanding of the physical, chemical and microbiological processes governing contaminant dynamics. A proper appraisal of control techniques based upon a sound strategy is required, supported by an economic analysis of costs and benefits. Parallel studies of surface hygiene may finally convert the art of litter management into a science. Such challenges are amenable to both laboratory experiments and farm trials, and should be in the interests of both farmers and animals alike.

References

Barber, E.M. and Ogilvie, J.R. (1982) Incomplete mixing in ventilated airspaces. Part 1 – Theoretical considerations. *Canadian Agricultural Engineering* 24, 25–29.

Barber, E.M., Dawson, J.R., Battams, V.A. and Nicol, R.A.C. (1991) Spatial variability of airborne and settled dust in a piggery. *Journal of Agricultural Engineering Research* 50, 107–127.

Barlow, D.F. and Donaldson, A.I. (1973) Comparison of the aerosol stabilities of foot-and-mouth disease virus suspended in cell culture fluid or natural fluids. *Journal of General Virology* 20, 311–318.

Baskerville, A., Humphrey, T.J., Fitzgeorge, R.B., Cook, R.W., Chart, H., Rowe, B. and Whitehead, A. (1992) Airborne infection of laying hens with *Salmonella enteritidis* phage type 4. *Veterinary Record* 130, 395–398.

Baxter, S. (1984) *Intensive Pig Production.* Granada, London.

Boon, C.R. and Wray, C. (1989) Building design in relation to the control of diseases of intensively housed livestock. *Journal of Agricultural Engineering Research* 43, 149–161.

Bourgueil, E., Hutet, E., Cariolet, R. and Vannier, P. (1992) Air sampling procedure for evaluation of viral excretion level by vaccinated pigs infected with Aujeszky's disease (pseudorabies) virus. *Research in Veterinary Science* 52, 182–186.

Carpenter, G.A. (1986) Dust in livestock buildings – review of some aspects. *Journal of Agricultural Engineering Research* 33, 227–241.

Carpenter, G.A., Cooper, A.W. and Wheeler, G.E. (1986a) The effect of air filtration on air hygiene and pig performance in early-weaner accommodation. *Animal Production* 43, 505–515.

Carpenter, G.A., Smith, W.K., Maclaren, A.P.C. and Spackman, D. (1986b) Effect of internal air filtration on the performance of broilers and the aerial concentrations of dust and bacteria. *British Poultry Science* 27, 471–480.

Carrozza, J.H., Fredrickson, T.N., Prince, R.P. and Luginbuhl, R.E. (1973) Role of desquamated epithelial cells in transmission of Marek's disease. *Avian Diseases* 17, 767–781.

Chamberlain, A.C. (1970) Deposition and uptake by cattle of airborne particles. *Nature* 255, 99–100.

Charles, D.R. (1981) Practical ventilation and temperature control for poultry. In: Clark, J.A. (ed.), *Environmental Aspects of Housing for Animal Production.* Butterworths, London, pp. 183–195.

Charles, D.R. and Payne, C.G. (1966) The influence of graded levels of atmospheric ammonia on chickens. II Effects on the performance of laying hens. *British Poultry Science* 7, 189–198.

Chiba, L.I., Peo, E.R., Lewis, A.J., Brumm, M.C., Fritschen, R.D. and Crenshaw, J.D. (1985) Effect of dietary fat on pig performance and dust levels in modified-open-front and environmentally regulated confinement buildings. *Journal of Animal Science* 61, 763–781.

Chiba, L.I., Peo, E.R. and Lewis, A.J. (1987) Use of dietary fat to reduce dust, aerial ammonia and bacterial colony forming particle concentrations in swine confinement buildings. *Transactions of the American Society of Agricultural Engineers* 30, 464–468.

Clark, P.C. and McQuitty, J.B. (1986) Air quality in commercial farrowing barns. Paper No. PNR 86-302. American Society of Agricultural Engineers, St Joseph, Michigan.

Clark, P.C. and McQuitty, J.B. (1987) Air quality in six Alberta commercial free-stall dairy barns. *Canadian Agricultural Engineering* 29, 77–80.

Clarke, A.F. and Madelin, T. (1987) Technique for assessing respiratory health hazards from hay and other source materials. *Equine Veterinary Journal* 19, 442–447.

Commission International du Génie Rural (1992) *Climatization of Animal Houses.* Second Report of a Working Group. Publ. Centre for Climatization of Animal Houses – Advisory Services, State University of Ghent, Belgium, 147pp.

Conceição, M.A.P., Johnson, H.E. and Wathes, G.M. (1989) Air hygiene in a pullet house: spatial homogeneity of aerial pollutants. *British Poultry Science* 30, 765–776.

Cox, C.S. (1989) Airborne bacteria and viruses. *Science Progress* 73, 469–500.

Dawson, J.R. (1990) Minimising dust in livestock buildings: possible alternatives to mechanical separation. *Journal of Agricultural Engineering Research* 47, 235–248.

De Boer, S. and Morrison, W.D. (1988) *The Effects of the Quality of the Environment in Livestock Buildings on the Productivity of Swine and Safety of Humans.* University of Guelph, Ontario, 121pp.

Dennis, C. and Gee, J.M. (1973) The microbial flora of broiler-house litter and dust. *Journal of General Microbiology* 78, 101–107.

Donaldson, A.I. (1972) The influence of relative humidity on the aerosol stability of different strains of foot-and-mouth disease virus suspended in saliva. *Journal of General Virology* 15, 25–33.

Donaldson, A.I. (1983) Quantitative data on airborne foot-and-mouth disease virus: its production, carriage and deposition. *Philosophical Transactions of the Royal Society, London* B 302, 529–534.

Donaldson, A.I., Herniman, K.A.J., Parker, J. and Sellers, R.F. (1970) Further investigations on the airborne excretion of foot-and-mouth disease virus. *Journal of Hygiene* 68, 557–564.

Donham, K.J. (1987) Human health and safety for workers in livestock housing. In: *Latest developments in livestock housing.* Proceedings of Commission Internationale du Génie Rural, Section 2 Seminar. 22–26 June, Illinois, pp. 86–95.

Drummond, J.G., Curtis, S.E. and Simon, J. (1978) Effects of atmospheric ammonia on pulmonary clearance in the young pig. *American Journal of Veterinary Research* 39, 211–212.

Drummond, J.G., Curtis, S.E., Simon, J. and Norton, H.W. (1980) Effects of aerial ammonia on growth and health of young pigs. *Journal of Animal Science* 50, 1085–1091.

Drummond, J.G., Curtis, S.E., Meyer, R.C., Simon, J. and Norton, H.W. (1981) Effects of atmospheric ammonia on young pigs experimentally infected with *Bordetella bronchiseptica. American Journal of Veterinary Research* 42, 963–968.

Dutkiewicz, J. (1978) Exposure to dust-borne bacteria in agriculture. 1. Environmental studies. *Archives of Environmental Health* 33, 250–259.

Eberhart, R.J., Natzke, R.P., Newbould, F.H.S., Nonnecke, B. and Thompson, P. (1979) Coliform mastitis – a review. *Journal of Dairy Science* 62, 1–22.

Feddes, J.J.R., Leonard, J.J. and McQuitty, J.B. (1982) Heat and moisture loads and air quality in commercial broiler barns in Alberta. *University of Alberta Research Bulletin* 82-2, 83pp.

Feddes, J.J.R., Cook, H. and Zuidhof, M.J. (1992) Characterisation of airborne dust particles in turkey housing. *Canadian Agricultural Engineering* 34, 273–280.

Feilden, N.E.H. (1982) Toxic gases from slurry. *Farm Buildings Progress* 68, 7–10.

Gilmour, M.I., Baskerville, A., Taylor, F.G.R. and Wathes, C.M. (1989) The effect of titanium dioxide inhalation on the pulmonary clearance of *Pasteurella haemolytica* in the mouse. *Environmental Research* 50, 157–172.

Gloster, J. (1983) Factors influencing the airborne spread of Newcastle disease. *British Veterinary Journal* 139, 445–451.

Gloster, J., Blackall, R.M., Sellers, R.F. and Donaldson, A.I. (1981) Forecasting the airborne spread of foot-and-mouth disease. *Veterinary Record* 108, 370–374.

Gore, A.M., Korneygay, E.T., Viet, H.P. and Collins, E.R. (1986) Soybean oil effects on nursery air quality and pig performance. *American Society of Agricultural Engineers Paper no:* 86–4040.

Hardman, P.M., Wathes, C.M. and Wray, C. (1991) Salmonella transmission among calves penned individually. *Veterinary Record* 129, 327–329.

Hartung, J. (1988) Zur Einschätzung der biologischen Wirkung von Spurengasen der Stalluft mit Hilfe von zwei bakteriellen Kurzzeittests (On the estimation of the biological effect of trace gases present in animal house air with the aid of two bacterial short-term tests). Fortschritt-Berichte VDI 15, Nr 56, VDI-Verlag, Düsseldorf.

Health and Safety Executive (1992) Occupational exposure limits. *Environmental Hygiene* 40/92, HMSO, London.

Hugh-Jones, M., Allan, W.H., Dark, F.A. and Harper, G.J. (1973) The evidence for the airborne spread of Newcastle disease. *Journal of Hygiene, Cambridge* 71, 325–339.

Jurajda, V. and Klimes, B. (1970) Presence and survival of Marek's disease agent in dust. *Avian Diseases* 14, 188–190.

Liao, C.M. and Feddes, J.J.R. (1989) Modeling and analysis of the dynamic behaviour of airborne dust in a ventilated airspace. ASAE paper No. PNR 89-402, American Society of Agricultural Engineers, Penticton, British Columbia.

Linton, A.H. (1987) Epidemiology of infectious diseases in animals. In: Linton, A.H., Hugo, W.B. and Russell, A.D. (eds), *Disinfection in Veterinary and Farm Animal Practice.* Blackwell Scientific Publications, Oxford, pp. 1–11.

Lovett, J., Messer, J.W. and Read, R.B. (1971) The microflora of Southern Ohio poultry litter. *Poultry Science* 50, 746–751.

McInerney, J.P., Howe, K.S. and Schepers, J.A. (1992) A framework for the economic analysis of disease in farm livestock. *Preventive Veterinary Medicine* 13, 137–154.

McLoughlin, M.F., McMurray, C.H., Dodds, H.M. and Evans, R.T. (1985) Nitrogen dioxide (silo gas) poisoning in pigs. *Veterinary Record* 116, 119–121.

Madelin, T.M. and Wathes, C.M. (1989) Air hygiene in a broiler house: comparison of deep litter with raised netting floors. *British Poultry Science* 30, 23–37.

Maghirang, R.G., Manbeck, H.B. and Puri, V.M. (1990) Numerical study of air contaminant distribution in livestock buildings. ASAE Paper No. 90-4543. American Society of Agricultural Engineers, Chicago, Illinois.

Maghirang, R.G., Manbeck, H.B., Roush, W.B. and Muir, F.V. (1991) Air contaminant distributions in a commercial laying house. *Transactions of the American Society of*

Agricultural Engineers 34, 2171–2180.

Morgan-Jones, S. (1987) Practical aspects of disinfection and infection control. In: Linton, A.H., Hugo, W.B. and Russell, A.D. (eds), *Disinfection in Veterinary and Farm Animal Practice.* Blackwell Scientific Publications, Oxford, pp. 144–167.

Noble, W.C. (1975) Dispersal of skin microorganisms. *British Journal of Dermatology* 93, 477–485.

Pearson, C.C. (1988) Air cleaning for livestock production buildings. *Farm Buildings and Engineering* 5, 13–17.

Qi, R., Manbeck, H.B. and Maghirang, R.G. (1992) Dust net generation rate in a poultry layer house. *Transactions of the American Society of Agricultural Engineers* 35, 1639–1645.

Richie, P.O., Manbeck, H.B. and Graves, R.E. (1989) Cleanability and durability of dropping boards and curtains in cage layer houses. *Transactions of the American Society of Agricultural Engineers* 32, 1069–1074.

Robertson, J.F. (1992) Dust and ammonia in pig buildings. *Farm Building Progress* 110, 19–24.

Robertson, J.F., Wilson, D. and Smith, W.J. (1990) Atrophic rhinitis: the influence of the aerial environment. *Animal Production* 50, 173–182.

Rylander, R. (1986) Lung diseases caused by organic dusts in the farm environment. *American Journal of Industrial Medicine* 10, 221–227.

Sattar, S.A. and Ijaz, M.K. (1987) Spread of viral infections by aerosols. *CRC Critical Reviews in Environmental Control* 17, 89–131.

Strange, R.E. and Cox, C.S. (1976) Survival of dried and airborne bacteria. In: Gray, T.R.G. and Postgate, J.R. (eds), *The Survival of Vegetative Microbes.* 26th Symposium of the Society for General Microbiology, Cambridge University Press, Cambridge, pp. 111–154.

Sundahl, A.M. (1975) Cleanability of building materials. *Farm Buildings Progress* 40, 19–21.

Tamási, G. (1973) Mycoplasma isolation from the air. In: Hers, J.F. Ph. and Winkler, K.C. (eds), *Airborne Transmission and Airborne Infection.* Oosthoek Publishing Company, Utrecht, pp. 68–71.

Tucker, S.A. and Walker, A.W. (1992) Hock burn in broilers. In: Garnsworthy, P.C., Haresign, W. and Cole, D.J.A. (eds), *Recent Advances in Animal Nutrition.* Butterworth, Heinemann, pp. 33–50.

Turner, L.W., Wathes, C.M. and Audsley, E. (1993) Dynamic probabilistic modelling of respiratory disease in swine, including production and economic effects. In: *Proceedings of the IVth International Livestock Environment Symposium.* Warwick, UK, July 1993. American Society of Agricultural Engineers, pp. 89–97.

Van't Klooster, C.E., Roelofs, P.F.M.M. and Den Hartog, L.A. (1993) Effects of filtration, vacuum cleaning and washing in pig houses on aerosol levels and pig performance. *Livestock Production Science* 33, 171–182.

Wathes, C.M. (1987) Airborne microorganisms in pig and poultry houses. In: Bruce, J.M. and Sommer, M. (eds), *The Environmental Aspects of Respiratory Disease in Intensive Pig and Poultry Houses: Including the Implications for Human Health.* Commission of the European Communities, Luxembourg, pp. 57–71.

Wathes, C.M., Jones, C.D.R. and Webster, A.J.F. (1983) Ventilation, air hygiene and animal health. *Veterinary Record* 113, 554–559.

Wathes, C.M., Howard, K., Jones, C.D.R. and Webster, A.J.F. (1984) The balance of airborne bacteria in calf houses. *Journal of Agricultural Engineering Research* 30, 81–90.

Wathes, C.M., Zaidan, W.A.R., Pearson, G.R., Hinton, M. and Todd, J.N. (1988) Aerosol infection of calves and mice with *Salmonella typhimurium. Veterinary Record* 123, 590–594.

Wathes, C.M., Miller, B.G. and Bourne, F.J. (1989) Cold stress and post-weaning diarrhoea in piglets inoculated orally or by aerosol. *Animal Production* 49, 483–496.

Wathes, C.M., Johnson, H.E. and Carpenter, G.A. (1991) Air hygiene in a pullet house: effects of air filtration on aerial pollutants measured *in vivo* and *in vitro. British Poultry Science* 32, 31–46.

Welford, R.A., Feddes, J.J.R. and Barber, E.M. (1992) Pig building dustiness as affected by canola oil in the feed. *Canadian Agricultural Engineering* 34, 365–373.

Whyte, R.T. (1993) Aerial pollutants and the health of poultry farmers. *World's Poultry Science Journal* 49, 139–156.

Wray, C. (1975) Survival and spread of pathogenic bacteria of veterinary importance within the environment. *The Veterinary Bulletin* 45, 543–550.

Wray, C., Todd, J.N. and Hinton, M. (1987) Epidemiology of *Salmonella typhimurium* infection in calves: excretion of *S. typhimurium* in the faeces of calves in different management systems. *Veterinary Record* 121, 293–296.

Ventilation Control and Systems

7

J.M. RANDALL AND C.R. BOON
Animal Science and Engineering Division,
Silsoe Research Institute, UK

Introduction

The functions of a ventilation system are manifold. Yet in most installations only a small subset of those functions is operative. Where they exist at all, control systems are mainly designed to maintain a predetermined temperature in the building with little regard to other conditions. Previous chapters have described the many requirements of livestock, some of which are affected by ventilation, but to design a ventilation system demands a knowledge of their relative importance. The relative penalties of the different interacting factors are needed before an informed decision can be made.

In a fan-ventilated system it is most usual to sense the air temperature inside the building: if it is higher than a pre-set value the air exchange rate is increased thus reducing the inside temperature. Maximum ventilation rates are set by the capacity of the installed fans determined by an appropriate analysis based on parameters such as upper and lower critical temperatures for the animals and internal relative humidity, and the frequency of occurrence of high outside temperatures (Bruce, 1981a). Minimum ventilation rates may be based on balances of sensible heat, water vapour or carbon dioxide (e.g. Bruce, 1981a; Albright, 1990). If criteria for minimum temperature, minimum water vapour removal and maximum carbon dioxide concentration are known, then three estimates of the required minimum ventilation rate may be made. At the minimum ventilation rate contaminants such as dust and gases are at their maximum concentration. Little is known about the relative penalty of allowing the temperature to fall by increasing the ventilation rate above the minimum, yet reducing the contaminant burden. What would then be the relevant benefits of supplying heat to maintain the temperature (this volume, Chapter 1)?

Further to controlling temperature via the ventilation rate it is necessary to obtain control over the distribution of air in the building. Similar conditions for all the stock are usually sought, but for each group or pen of stock variations in space can be used to advantage, e.g. provision of cool dunging areas in a finishing piggery encourages the pigs to keep their lying areas clean (Randall *et al.*, 1983a). Again, in some circumstances partial air mixing can be advantageous, e.g. by providing less contaminated or cooler air over the stock, whereas near-complete mixing can help towards providing large areas of uniform conditions. Perhaps the ideal for most animals is plug or piston flow ventilation providing uncontaminated, fresh air although it is difficult to achieve in practice. Thorough air mixing is required in a service house where good circulation of pheromones is needed. In a building housing broilers which completely cover the floor it is important to supply similar conditions over the floor plane, but in general conditions in the rest of the space are of less significance. However, when the birds are young and heating is employed it is advantageous to get uniform mixing throughout the space in order to prevent excessive heat loss through the roof (Boon and Battams, 1988). Thus there are frequently conflicting requirements of temperature, humidity, dust and gas control for which acceptable strategies of ventilation and heating have to be sought.

The influence of wind on a ventilation system can override the designed control functions, and techniques to overcome such problems must always be incorporated. Backdraught shutters can be used where air leaves a building, but air inlets are less easily wind proofed.

Although the requirements of a ventilation system are complex, interactive and not easily defined it is always essential to lay down a detailed specification of the essential functions before embarking on design. As a result a clear physical basis for design adopting a systems approach is required to ensure the most appropriate system and its control for any particular building. It is not possible in this brief chapter to develop a complete design philosophy, but some of the underlying physical principles are outlined.

Principles of Control of Ventilation Rate

Ventilation, or air exchange, through an opening in a building takes place when a pressure difference is generated across the opening. Thus there are only two strategies for changing a ventilation rate. Either the pressure difference across an opening can be changed or the size of the opening can be adjusted in order to increase or decrease flow. Forced ventilation systems using fans allow the pressure difference to be controlled whereas natural ventilation systems depend on adjustment of openings to control the ventilation rate. In forced ventilation systems the pressure is generated by the use of fans, usually driven by electric motor. If the fan extracts from the building it lowers the internal pressure, causing air to enter through openings elsewhere. In natural ventilation systems the pressure is generated either by an air density difference caused by heaters or animals raising the internal temperature or by wind which generates pressures around the external surfaces of the building which differ from the internal pressure. All of these processes are amenable to description and analysis using the underlying physical principles.

Forced ventilation

There are three criteria which must be satisfied simultaneously in designing a forced ventilation system. These are the Archimedes number and similar parameters which characterize the flow pattern, the system characteristics (i.e. of the building and its vents) and the fan characteristics. The last two are important in controlling ventilation rate. Typical characteristics of buildings and fans are shown in Fig. 7.1 where it may be seen that as air pressure increases, flow through the vents in the building increases, but as pressure against the fan increases it delivers less air.

Propeller fans are usually selected for livestock ventilation systems. This is because they deliver relatively large quantities of air and only a modest static pressure performance is demanded of them. The low pressure requirement arises from the pressure/flow characteristics of air through a typical livestock building.

When control of ventilation rate is affected by varying the voltage to the fan motor and hence the impeller speed, then the different speed characteristics of the fan are required. Figure 7.1 shows typical characteristics at two fan speeds. Where each line meets the air volume axis, the maximum air volume at zero static pressure can be determined. In practice, air inlets and fan boxes cause restriction of air movement and increase the static pressure under which the fan operates. The actual operating point depends on the building characteristic. In Fig. 7.1 three building characteristics are shown. Building ‘A’ develops little static pressure as the fan volume increases because it has many holes and air leaks. It intersects the fan characteristic at ‘a’ very close to the maximum, zero resistance, flow. The static pressure required of the fan can be as low as 10 Pa. The other two building characteristics intersect the fan characteristics at ‘b’ and ‘c’ representing the pressure created in buildings with typical good construction and with the best carefully wind-proofed construction. They intersect at about 25 and 50 Pa respectively. When designing a new building a well-sealed structure is required with air inlets carefully designed to give control of air speeds and air distribution within the building. Although this arrangement causes a reduction in air volume, due to restriction of the air inlets, air distribution and ventilation are more effective. In addition, a building operating at higher pressures is less prone to the effects of wind. Building A

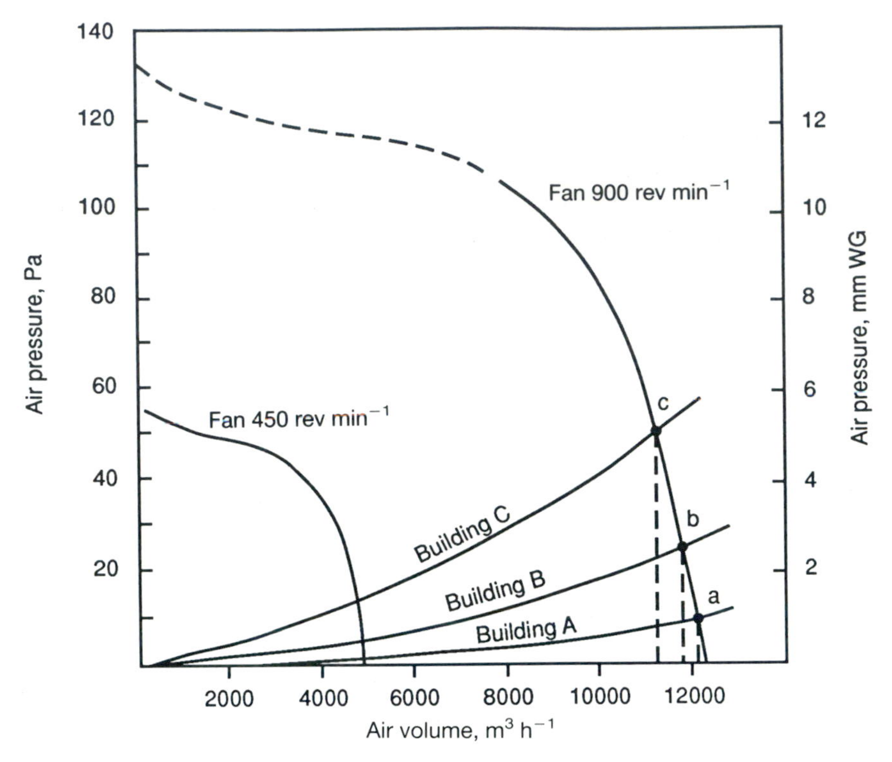

Fig. 7.1. The characteristics of a fan at two speeds and their interaction with three building characteristics. Building 'A' is very leaky, 'B' of typical good construction and 'C' of best carefully wind-proofed construction. WG = water gauge.

will be cold in winter because wind pressures cause uncontrolled ventilation through leaks in the building and it will have poor air distribution. In summer an increased number of openings reduces the static pressure and slightly increases the volume of air passing through the building. This is sometimes desirable in broiler houses to provide additional cooling in very hot weather. Correct air distribution is still important in summer, because increased air speeds can be used to increase heat loss from the animals. Thus some systems, such as 'high speed jets', have adjustable inlets enabling air to be directed over the pigs' lying area and an inlet which can be enlarged as the air volume flow increases (Randall, 1977). A suitable criterion is a static pressure of about 50 Pa within the building and fans should be selected for their air throughput at this pressure.

A number of theories have been proposed to describe the interaction of fan and building characteristics (Albright, 1979; Cole, 1980) and the effects of wind on propeller fan ventilation systems (Bruce, 1981b).

The pressure difference across a simple opening (Bruce, 1981b) may be represented by

$$\Delta P = \tfrac{1}{2} k \rho |V| V = P_e - P_i \qquad (1)$$

where the sign of ΔP is given by the sign of the velocity V, which is a vector and is not affected by the scalar mass velocity $\rho|V|$.

If a fan of diameter D is installed in the opening, the fan total pressure is added to the pressure drop in Equation (1). The fan total pressure is the sum of the fan static pressure and the fan dynamic pressure; the latter being the pressure associated with the quantity of airflow.

$$\Delta P + \frac{D}{|D|} \Delta P_f = \tfrac{1}{2} k \rho |V| V \qquad (2)$$

The algebraic sign of the pressure difference generated by the fan is ascribed to the fan diameter being positive when the fan attempts to move the air from the outside to the inside through the term $D/|D|$. Equation (2) may be solved to give the velocity of the air through the opening, provided a mathematical expression for ΔP_f is used. Within the normal range of operation it is proposed that

$$\Delta P_f = \Delta P_o - aV^2 \qquad (3)$$

where ΔP_o is the notional fan static pressure at zero flow (and coincidentally the total pressure at this point). This equation can be extended outside the normal range of operation, but any results should be used with caution. Accounting for the sign of the flow direction from the fan in relation to the building gives

$$\Delta P_f = \Delta P_o - \frac{D}{|D|} a|V|V \qquad (4)$$

This equation represents the propeller fan characteristics within the normal operating range, and ΔP_o and a are readily found for any fan, from an analysis of the characteristic curves given in manufacturers' catalogues. Typical values for ΔP_o and a are 80–200 and 1.4–0.6 respectively.

Substituting Equation (4) into Equation (2) and solving to give the velocity through the opening.

$$V = \frac{\Delta P + \frac{D}{|D|} \Delta P_o}{\left| \Delta P + \frac{D}{|D|} \Delta P_o \right|^{1/2}} \cdot \frac{1}{(a + \tfrac{1}{2} k \rho)^{1/2}} \qquad (5)$$

If there are n openings in the building then the flow through each

$$Q_n = V_n A_n \qquad (6)$$

and the ventilation rate for the complete building

$$Q = \sum_{(in)} V_n A_n \qquad (7)$$

where the summation is over the openings (in) through which air passes into the building (which is numerically equal to the summation over the openings through which air leaves the building).

The pressure difference across the building is given by Equation (1) where P_e is the external pressure due to wind and P_i is internal pressure. This internal pressure arises from both the fan and the wind and is not necessarily zero when the wind speed is zero. In the absence of wind, P_e equals zero. An iterative computer program is used to solve Equation (5) by making an initial guess for a value of P_i, calculating the velocity at all openings and then checking the deviation from the continuity constraint

$$\sum V_n A_n = 0 \tag{8}$$

If this is not satisfied a new estimate of P_i is made until the continuity condition is adequately satisfied.

Fans should be selected not only on their airflow characteristics as discussed above but also on their cost effectiveness (Moulsley and Randall, 1990; Randall and Moulsley, 1990). The quantity of air delivered per unit of electricity consumed is defined (Albright, 1975) as the ventilation efficiency ratio (V_e) which, over the range of fans generally available in the UK was shown to vary between 5.8 and 4.2 $m^3 kJ^{-1}$ for 630 mm diameter fans and 5.1 and 2.4 $m^3 kJ^{-1}$ for 450 mm diameter fans. Such a variation for a given fan size can affect annual costs by 20% of the initial purchase cost, which could be offset by paying twice the price for the most efficient fan. Annual electricity costs dominate all other annual costs after year 5 and exceed 50% even at year 2.

The annual capital, electricity and maintenance costs all add to the annual cost, whereas the annual contribution of the resale value decreases it. Thus the annual cost

$$A_c = \frac{W_i}{w}\left[c\left(1 + \sum_1^N p_n w^n\right) - Sw^N\right] + \frac{Q_a U}{3600 V_e} \tag{9}$$

where the inflation:interest ratio is defined as

$$w = \frac{100 + q}{100 + r} \tag{10}$$

and we define

$$W_i = \frac{w - 1}{w^N - 1} \tag{11}$$

The first term in Equation (9) represents the annual capital cost. The second term represents the annual maintenance cost given by the summation of separately estimated annual costs, related to the size of the installation and thus to capital cost.

It might be assumed that fans have a repair cost to date as a percentage of the list price proportional to 0.12 $X^{1.5}$ where X is the accumulated hours of use as a percentage of the wear-out life. For a 20 year wear-out life and 60% usage it can be deduced that

$$p_n = 0.624[n^{1.5} - (n-1)^{1.5}] \quad (12)$$

The third term in Equation (9) represents the annual resale value (Audsley and Wheeler, 1978; Randall and Moulsley, 1990) where it might be assumed that

$$S = 56\,(0.885)^N \frac{c}{100} \quad (13)$$

The final term in Equation (9) represents the annual electricity cost where Q_a is the annual air requirement for the installation, U the current electricity price and V_e the ventilation efficiency ratio of the fan.

Methods of detection

In forced ventilation systems it is usual to sense air temperature inside the building and control the ventilation rate to a predetermined value (see above). Different levels of sophistication can be chosen with a thermocouple being the simplest. More frequent are thermistors or platinum resistance thermometers – both of which change resistance in response to changes in air temperature. The sensors' function is to feed back information to the controller so that action may be taken by the ventilation system to ensure that the correct environmental conditions are provided for the housed livestock.

There are many other important factors in the provision of optimum conditions, for example pressure difference across the air inlet, ventilation rate, humidity levels, air speeds over the livestock, level of pollutants such as dust and noxious gases. Many of these can have deleterious effects on the performance of the stock but in commercial situations it is not usually practical to measure their level. While they can all be measured under research conditions, most sensors are usually too delicate to be placed for long periods in the potentially corrosive atmosphere found in many livestock buildings unless suitably protected. In addition, they are too costly to be considered at their present level of development.

While sensors for relative humidity are becoming available for use under commercial conditions, in general only temperature sensors are used for environmental control. High quality devices such as platinum resistance thermometers should be used and more than one position in the building should be monitored. The minimum requirement is for four sensors connected together in an electrical bridge network. These are placed around the building to obtain a representative mean temperature and reduce effects due to variation in livestock size and consequently heat output, though it is probably better to seek to eliminate temperature gradients *a priori*.

Control devices

There are several levels of sophistication for use in control, from simple on/off devices to computer control with complex algorithms. Whichever device is used the objective is to provide optimum conditions for the stock. Over the years many different control strategies have been employed, some more successful in practice than others. As technology has advanced, so the application of modern equipment in livestock buildings has increased but not to the level that might have been anticipated. While this is in part due to the general economics of the livestock industry, a major obstacle is the hostile environment in which the systems are expected to operate. Consequently the housing of the control equipment has become an important aspect of controller design to ensure that the electronics is protected not only from the dust and other aerial pollutants, but also during washing and disinfection.

Many systems employ a simple thermostat to provide an on/off two-stage control function giving a minimum and maximum setting of ventilation rate. An upgrade of this simple system is the mechanical thermostat with up to five switched stages either with a transformer to provide different fan speeds or to switch power to different numbers of fans. In both cases discrete stages of ventilation are achieved.

Variable fan speed control forms one of the most common systems of ventilation. This is achieved by temperature sensors providing information to a solid state controller. This is normally a thyristor device giving a chopped waveform with varying output voltage to drive the fan. Thus a continuously varying ventilation rate is achieved. However, there are many problems associated with such a system and these are highlighted below. A significant improvement is to operate individual fans so that a stepped control is achieved.

The use of microprocessors for control opens up the possibility of using inputs from many different types of sensor but, as discussed above, it is at present only practical to sense air temperature. However, it is possible to have improved control strategies written into the software of the microprocessors to provide not only improved conditions for the stock but also management information on the performance of the controller.

Methods of control

The purpose of control is to provide optimum conditions for the livestock by controlling the thermal environment. In order to achieve this a knowledge of the heat balance for the building is required taking into consideration the heat release from the livestock, supplementary heating if used, and the heat lost through the surfaces and the ventilating air. The equation relating these factors is:

$$q_a + q_h = (C_p\rho Q + \sum_{S=1}^{n} A_s U_s)\,\Delta T \tag{14}$$

From a knowledge of the stocking density and assumed heat release of the stock and also the U value of the building components, a graph may be drawn relating the ventilation rate with the outside temperature which assumes a required inside temperature. This is clearly a non-linear relationship as shown in Fig. 7.2.

There are four basic methods for varying ventilation rate (Randall, 1991):

1. Keeping fan speed constant and recirculating a proportion of the building air.
2. Keeping fan speed constant and restricting the throughput of the fan.
3. Varying the speed of the fans.
4. Altering the number of fans in operation.

The first option, using recirculating systems, is used in many buildings, often in association with ducts, either rigid or flexible, e.g. polythene. The chief characteristic of this system is that the velocities of air discharged into the building are constant which, with good temperature control, give a constant temperature/velocity cooling effect. This may be advantageous for

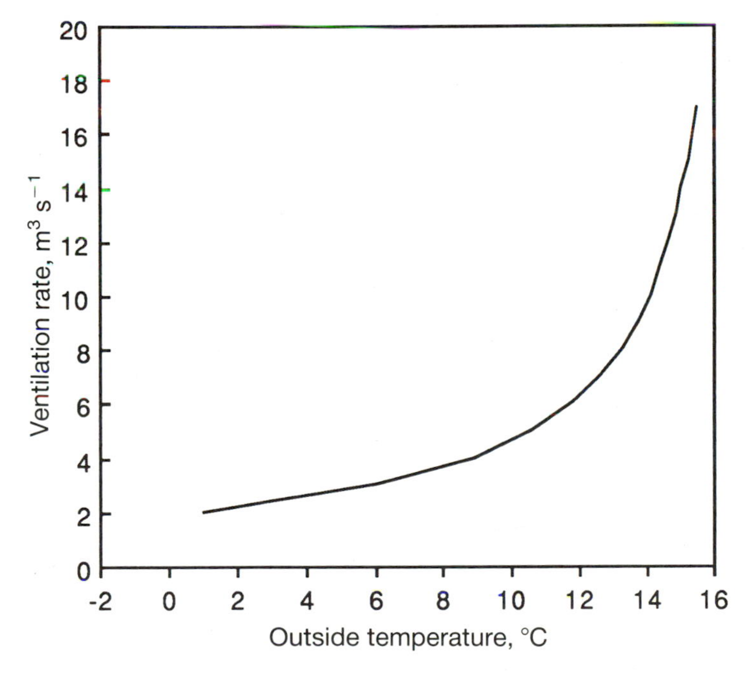

Fig. 7.2. Variation of ventilation rate as a function of outside temperature to obtain an inside temperature of 18°C (500 pigs of average liveweight 64 kg).

some classes of stock but in certain climatic conditions it may be required to increase air speed at higher temperatures to reduce heat stress. A possible disadvantage is that hygiene may be compromised by either increased spread of airborne pathogens or retention of pathogens in the ducting system.

A good method of controlling ventilation rate, particularly for small buildings is to run a fan in combination with a damper mechanism to enable mixing of varying proportions of outside and recirculated air. This system can be controlled automatically by sensing the building temperature and can be made to operate either in a continuous or step mode depending on controller design. The system must be designed so that a minimum proportion of fresh air always enters the building.

The second option entails maintaining the fan speed close to its maximum and controlling the airflow by restriction either at the fan or at the air inlets or outlets. This method is rarely used in practice.

The third option, in varying guises, is used most widely. Control is achieved by variation of fan speed using stepwise or continually variable control. It might be assumed that by continuous variation of the fan speed the control curve (Fig. 7.2) could be achieved. However, a significant disadvantage occurs at low fan speeds when the pressure difference between the inside and the outside of the building is small and quite moderate winds may upset the desired airflow pattern and ventilation rate.

The fourth option, the favoured solution in relatively large buildings, is to apply on/off control to the fans in sequence thus achieving several steps of ventilation rate. Clearly this system is particularly suited to multi-fan ventilation systems where it is relatively straightforward to achieve the minimum required ventilation rate by using one or two fans. To ensure that the required air distribution is achieved, it is essential to link the fan switching control to control of the inlet gap. As discussed on page 172 an inlet air speed of $5\,m\,s^{-1}$ is the optimum design criterion. The design of such a system (Randall, 1977) has been fully tested (Randall and Armsby, 1983; Randall *et al.*, 1983a, b). It is suitable for all classes of livestock.

With fewer than ten fans installed it is necessary to consider the option of time switching of the fan to produce a mean low ventilation rate. By switching off a single fan for periods of time it is possible to reduce the ingress of cold air but, during the off period, there is no control of the air pattern. It has been suggested that a cycle of 10 min should be used, i.e. for 50% of one fan it is on for 5 min and off for 5 min. However, if the time constant of the buildings for a step change in ventilation rate is about 10 min then the switching period should be approximately an order of magnitude lower than this, i.e. 1 min. By using a 100 second period it is possible to extend the jet ventilation system to smaller buildings. This has consequences in buildings adopting an all-in all-out routine which calls for smaller rooms for housing the stock, particularly for pigs. Poultry are raised using all-in all-out as standard practice.

With the advent of relatively cheap microprocessor technology it is now possible to extend the control algorithm from a purely climatic orientated system to one that takes into account the thermal requirements of the stock themselves. For pigs it is possible to employ the concept of lower critical temperature (LCT) which has been developed by Bruce and Clark (1979) and Bruce (1981a). They developed a model based on the heat balance between the pig and its surroundings taking into account the radiative and convective heat transfer, the sensible heat transfer to the air and the minimum latent heat loss. The model gives

$$\mathrm{LCT} = T_{\mathrm{b}} - \frac{q_n(r_{\mathrm{a}} + r_{\mathrm{t}}) - q_{\mathrm{e}} r_{\mathrm{a}}}{A_{\mathrm{p}}[1 + (A_{\mathrm{f}}/A_{\mathrm{p}})\,((r_{\mathrm{a}} - r_{\mathrm{t}})/(r_{\mathrm{t}} + r_{\mathrm{f}})) - A_{\mathrm{g}}/A_{\mathrm{p}}]} \qquad (15)$$

The equation parameters can be written in terms of five practical variables, liveweight, group size, feeding level in relation to maintenance, air speed at pig level and the floor thermal resistance. With a typical floor thermal resistance of 0.065 °C m^2 W^{-1}, a group size of 12 and a feeding level of 2.7 times maintenance, the equation for LCT is reduced to a function of liveweight and air speed. Figure 7.3 shows this relationship for a range of air speeds normally encountered in a well controlled fan ventilation system.

A practical control system based on these criteria was developed (Boon and Lowe, 1987) and successfully implemented in a commercial building. By maintaining the climatic environment at 2°C above LCT, as opposed to a fixed value, it was shown that financial savings could be obtained (Boon, 1984).

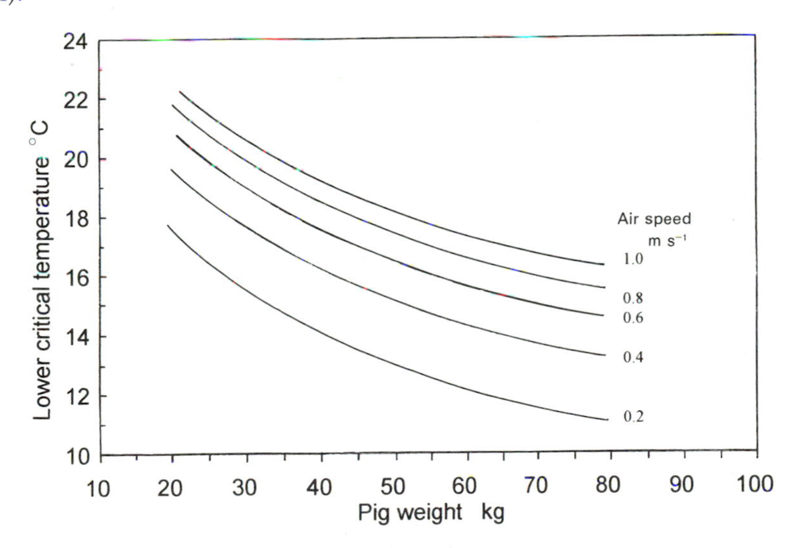

Fig. 7.3. Lower critical temperature as a function of pig liveweight for various air speeds.

Natural ventilation

Natural ventilation operates by pressure difference across an opening and arises from two sources. In the first, heat generated inside the building raises the temperature of the air, lowers its density in relation to the outside air and consequently generates a pressure difference causing flow. In the second, wind generates a range of pressure differences around the outside and within the building causing an inflow where the outside pressure is the higher and vice versa. Theories for both these modes of natural ventilation have been well developed.

In practical applications of natural ventilation it is wise to design the openings based on thermal effects alone unless a certain wind speed can be guaranteed. This is rarely so. For systems using non-adjustable vents a check should be made that over-ventilation will not occur in the presence of a strong wind.

Thermally induced ventilation

Many theories have been published for thermally induced ventilation, some of them have been shown by Foster and Down (1987) to be either incorrect or of very limited applications. A generalized analysis of natural convection in buildings has been developed and verified by Bruce (1978, 1982) using independent data and by Down *et al.* (1990). The exact expressions for some vent openings are given below, based on the theory of Bruce (1978).

When the air densities (caused by temperature differences) between the inside and outside of a building are different, then ventilation arises through any openings due to the pressure difference (Fig. 7.4). Air enters through the lower parts of the opening and leaves through the upper parts. Between the two is a plane at which no flow occurs, which is defined as the neutral plane (Bruce, 1978). In order to calculate the ventilation rate it is necessary to establish the position ($\bar{h}$) of this neutral plane.

It may be shown that

$$\tfrac{1}{2}\rho V^2 = g\Delta\rho(\bar{h} - h) \tag{16}$$

where it may be assumed that air is a perfect gas at constant pressure and consequently

$$\frac{\Delta\rho}{\rho} \approx \frac{\Delta T}{T} \tag{17}$$

Here ΔT is the difference in temperature between inside and outside.

The values of ΔT and T can be established from a heat balance on the building based on heat supplied by the stock and that lost through ventilation and through the structure.

Hence the velocity of flow at any height in the opening, where the

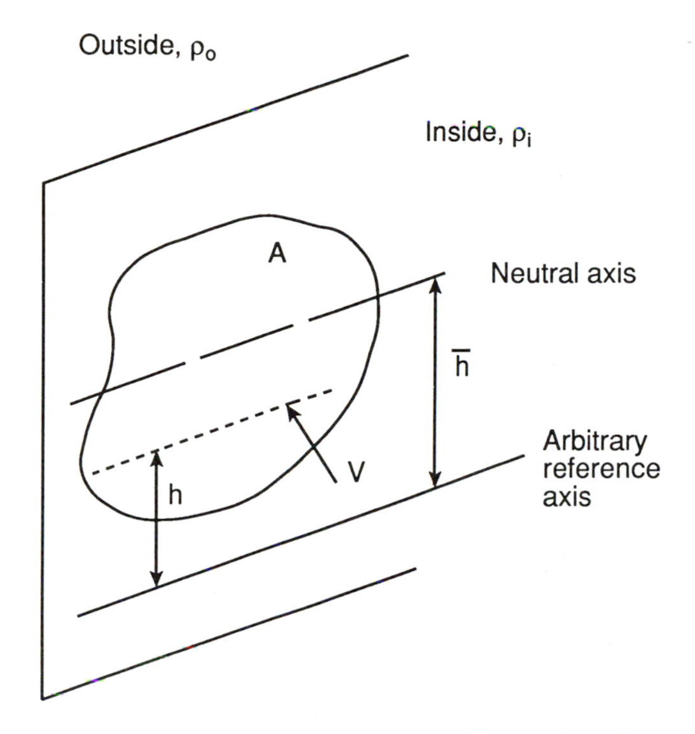

Fig. 7.4. Natural ventilation generated by a pressure difference through an opening of area *A*.

direction of flow from inside to outside is positive above the neutral axis and negative below it

$$V = \frac{|\bar{h} - h|}{\bar{h} - h}\left[2g\,\frac{\Delta\rho}{\rho}\,|\bar{h} - h|\right]^{1/2} \tag{18}$$

When there is no net flow across the opening, the position of the neutral axis is given by solving

$$C\int_A V\mathrm{d}A = 0 \tag{19}$$

which becomes

$$\int_A \frac{|\bar{h} - h|^{3/2}}{\bar{h} - h}\,\mathrm{d}A = 0 \tag{20}$$

The rate of ventilation

$$Q = C\left(\frac{2g\Delta\rho}{\rho}\right)^{1/2}\int_A \frac{|\bar{h} - h|^{3/2}}{\bar{h} - h}\,\mathrm{d}A \tag{21}$$

where the integration is over the area either below or above the neutral axis.

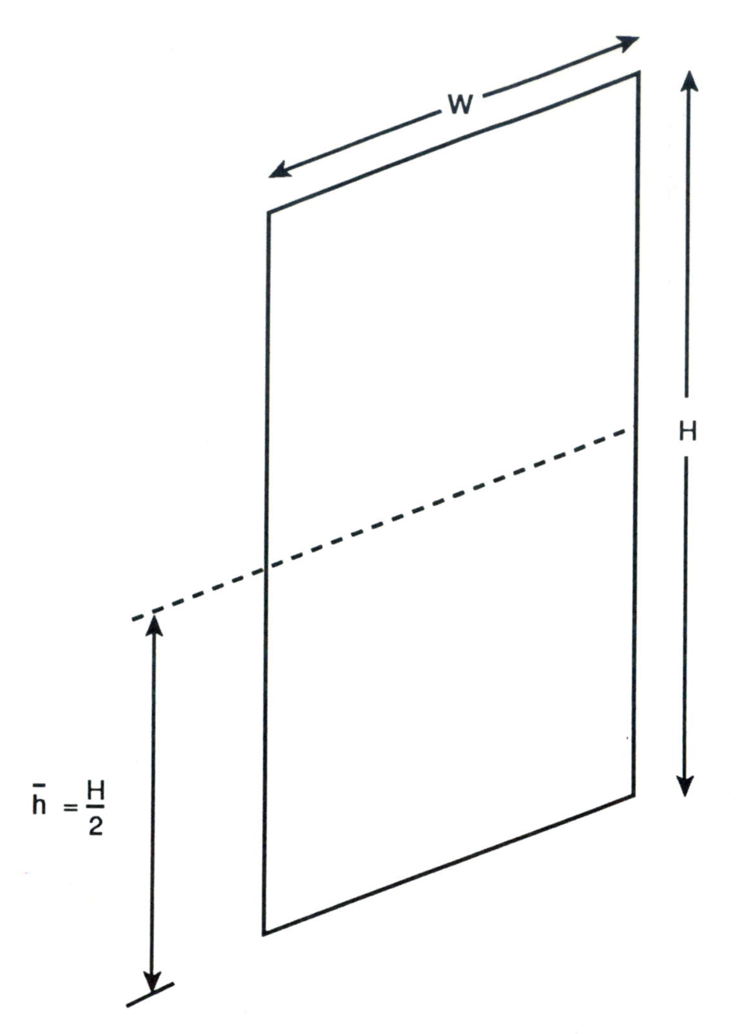

Fig. 7.5. Natural ventilation through a single rectangular opening of width *W* and height *H*.

The value of *C* may be taken as 0.65 for most bluff openings as commonly used to ventilate livestock buildings.

These equations are general and are not restricted by shape, position or orientation of the opening or openings.

For a building with a single rectangular opening, for example a door of horizontal length *W* and height *H* (Fig. 7.5) the neutral axis is at a height *H*/2 and the ventilation rate,

$$Q = \frac{AC}{3}\left(g\,\frac{\Delta\rho}{\rho}\,H\right)^{1/2} \tag{22}$$

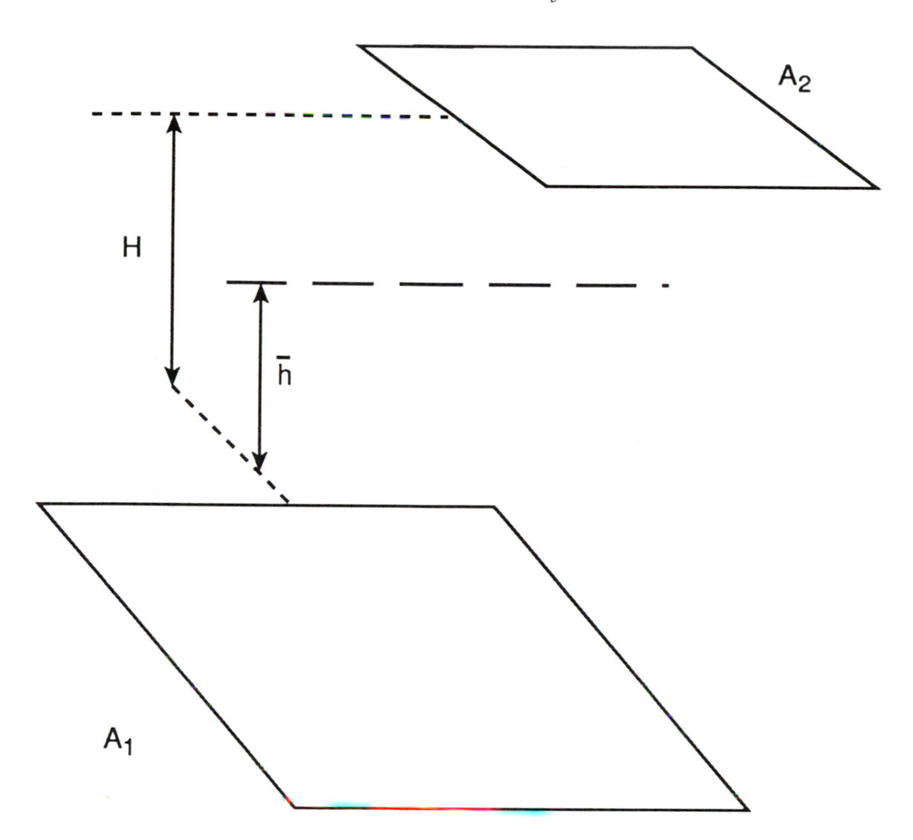

Fig. 7.6. Natural ventilation through two horizontal openings of areas A_1 and A_2, separated by a distance H.

This depends on both the area and height of the opening and can be readily determined.

Although a perforated floor combined with a ridge opening may be used occasionally, the solution for two horizontal openings has little direct application. However, its advantage of having an analytical solution allows certain analyses to be carried out and these can be relevant to arrangements with two vertical openings, the heights of which are small in comparison to their vertical separation. With similar constraints the analysis may be applied to the combination of a vertical wall vent and a horizontal ridge vent. If the two horizontal openings (Fig. 7.6) have areas of A_1 and A_2, the neutral axis is at

$$\bar{h} = H/\left\{1 + \left(\frac{A_1}{A_2}\right)^2\right\} \tag{23}$$

The resulting ventilation rate is

$$Q = CA_1 \left\{ 2g \frac{\Delta\rho}{\rho} \frac{H}{\left[1 + \left(\frac{A_1}{A_2}\right)^2\right]} \right\}^{1/2} \tag{24}$$

Ventilation systems using one vertical and one horizontal opening are commonly found in cattle buildings (Bruce, 1978). The height of the neutral axis (Fig. 7.7) is computed (Foster and Down, 1987) from

$$\left|\bar{h} - \frac{d}{2}\right|^{3/2} - \left|\bar{h} + \frac{d}{2}\right|^{3/2} - \frac{3W}{2} \frac{|\bar{h} - H|^{3/2}}{\bar{h} - H} = 0 \tag{25}$$

where W is the width of the ridge opening and d the height of the wall opening.

The neutral axis may fall in one of two regions, giving the following expressions for the corresponding ventilation rates. For the neutral plane

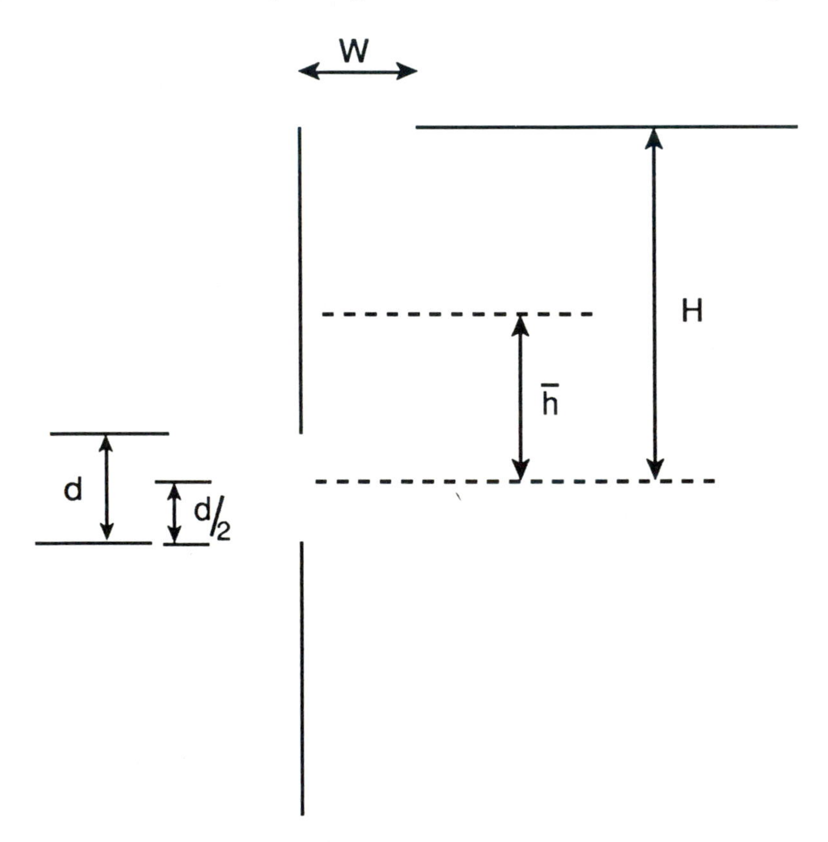

Fig. 7.7. Natural ventilation through one horizontal and one vertical opening separated by a height *H*.

above the side opening, $\bar{h} \geq d/2$ and by integrating above the neutral plane

$$Q = C\left(2g\,\frac{\Delta\rho}{\rho}\right)^{1/2} [WL(H - \bar{h})^{1/2}] \tag{26}$$

or similarly when integrating below the neutral axis

$$Q = C\left(2g\,\frac{\Delta\rho}{\rho}\right)^{1/2} \frac{2L}{3}\left(\left|\bar{h} + \frac{d}{2}\right|^{3/2} - \left|\bar{h} - \frac{d}{2}\right|^{3/2}\right) \tag{27}$$

Either Equation (26) or (27) may be used to determine the ventilation rate.

When the neutral plane intersects the side opening $\bar{h} < d/2$ and integrating above the neutral plane

$$Q = C\left(2g\,\frac{\Delta\rho}{\rho}\right)^{1/2} \left[WL(H - \bar{h})^{1/2} + \frac{2L}{3}\left(\frac{d}{2} - \bar{h}\right)^{3/2}\right] \tag{28}$$

or integrating below the neutral plane

$$Q = C\left(2g\,\frac{\Delta\rho}{\rho}\right)^{1/2} \frac{2L}{3}\left[\left|\bar{h} + \frac{d}{2}\right|^{3/2} + 2\left|\frac{d}{2} - \bar{h}\right|^{3/2}\right] \tag{29}$$

This last equation may be used when substituting only the dimensions of the opening in the vertical plane.

Since these equations do not have analytical solutions, more generalized simplified forms cannot be derived. However, Bruce (1975a, 1977, 1978) has taken Equations (23) and (24) to provide generalized solutions provided the neutral plane lies above the upper edge of the vertical opening (Down *et al.*, 1990). If it intersects the opening then exact solutions derived from Equations (25) and (28) should be applied. The theory is general and may also be applied to the ventilation of slotted roofs in cattle buildings (Bruce, 1978).

Size of openings

For a cattle building with open ridge and eaves ventilation, the ventilation rate due to buoyancy is given by Equation (24). To enable this equation to be used for design it is assumed that air is a perfect gas so that Equation (17) holds and thus

$$\frac{1}{A_i^2} + \frac{1}{A_0^2} = \frac{2\,C^2\,g\,H\,\Delta\,T}{TQ^2} \tag{30}$$

Assuming that the heat output of the animals is proportional to the 0.67 power of their mass (Bruce, 1978) and the building heat balance is given by Equation (14), a relationship may be derived between outlet area per animal, liveweight over the range 10 to 600 kg, and floor area per animal as shown in Figure 7.8. This applies for a total inlet area twice that of the total outlet area and a separation between them of 1 m. For separations other than 1 m

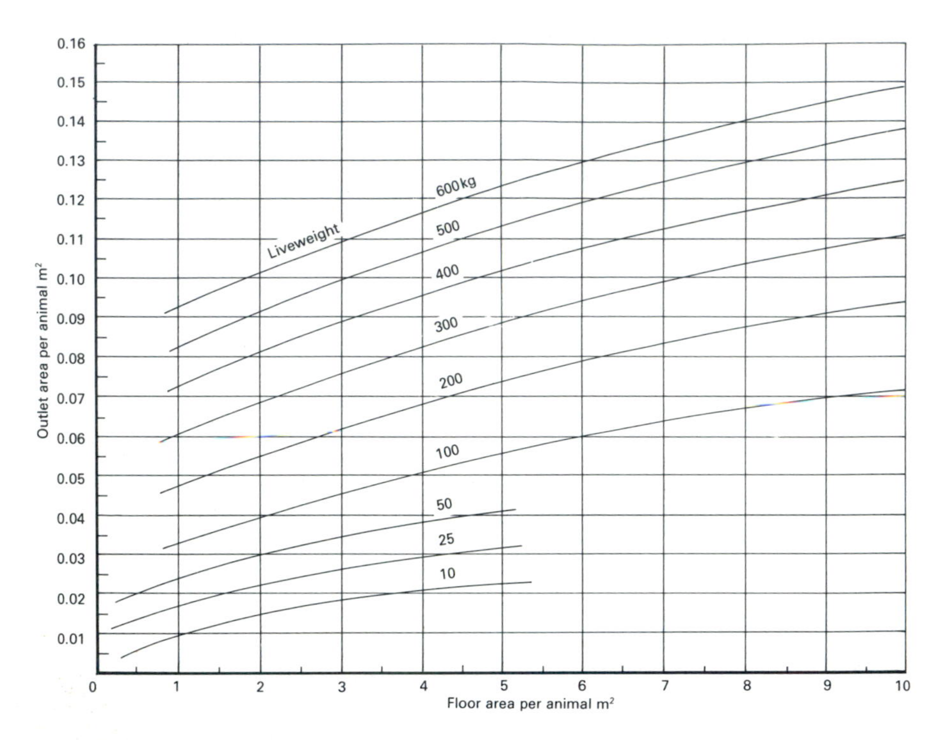

Fig. 7.8. Outlet area as a function of floor area per animal for various liveweights.

in height a correction factor of $H^{-0.5}$ should be used as a multiplier of the outlet area per animal.

Combined thermal buoyancy and wind

Analysis of the combined effects of wind and thermal buoyancy have been made by Bruce (1975b), Brockett and Albright (1987) and Zhang *et al.* (1989).

The aerodynamic pressure across an opening in a building is

$$\Delta P = \frac{1}{2}\rho V^2(C_{pe} - C_{pi}) \tag{31}$$

The external pressure coefficient at the position of a vent is the ratio of the external pressure to the kinetic pressure of the free wind, usually taken at a height of 10 m.

The internal pressure coefficient is defined similarly, but is usually considered to be constant throughout the volume of the building.

The pressure coefficients need to be measured on full-sized buildings (e.g. Hoxey, 1984), on a model in a wind tunnel (e.g. Bruce, 1975b, 1977, 1986; Shrestha *et al.*, 1990) or determined by computational fluid dynamics.

As the internal pressure varies, the air velocity through any opening, n, is

$$V_n = V_{10} C \frac{|C_{pen} - C_{pi}|^{3/2}}{C_{pen} - C_{pi}} \tag{32}$$

Thus the total volume flow rate may be derived from the continuity

$$\Sigma A_n V_n = 0 \tag{33}$$

and

$$\Sigma A_n \frac{|C_{pen} - C_{pi}|^{3/2}}{C_{pen} - C_{pi}} = 0 \tag{34}$$

This equation is first solved iteratively to find the internal pressure coefficient which gives values of V_n satisfying Equation (33). The result is then used in Equation (32) to calculate the air velocity through each of the openings. Consequently the overall volume flow or ventilation rate is calculated from

$$Q = \Sigma A_n V_n \tag{35}$$

where only the negative or positive values of V_n are used.

By studying a model based on these equations, Zhang *et al.* (1989) have concluded that as wind speed increases, the ventilation rate induced by wind increases linearly, and that induced by thermal buoyancy decreases slowly. The net result is that the total ventilation rate increases slowly with wind speed when the effect of thermal convection predominates; and is similar to that of the wind increasing linearly with wind speed when the effect of wind predominates.

As the direction of the wind moves away from being perpendicular to the side-wall, the ventilation rate due to wind decreases and that due to thermal buoyancy increases. The total ventilation rate decreases. The total ventilation rate increases almost directly with an increase in the size of the openings.

Methods of control

Manual control of natural ventilation can be achieved by opening or closing vents and adjustment of side curtains. These methods are labour intensive and require good management to achieve optimum conditions. The more the short-term variability in the climate the more difficult it becomes to achieve good control, and adjustments are extremely unlikely to be made at night. With several buildings on a site it becomes more efficient to automate the process.

This logical extension of natural ventilation has been researched by the Centre for Rural Building in Scotland (Robertson, 1984). As with the temperature control systems described above, ACNV (automatically controlled natural ventilation) adjusts ventilation rate in the standard manner by checking the internal air temperature at regular intervals and adjusting the inlet vents to control the air exchange. The flaps are operated mechanically either by a motor, wire and pulley or by linear actuators. Performance in cold weather has been reported by Burnett and MacDonald (1987) who showed that, with different designs of pig housing, air temperature could be kept above the lower critical temperature of the pigs for more than 90% of the time.

The system described above was designed taking into account the effect of wind. However, the design of ACNV systems can be based on thermal buoyancy alone. Strom and Morsing (1984) have shown that such a system may be improved by automatically controlling both inlet and outlet areas.

Failsafe systems

A well-designed forced ventilation livestock building is almost free from the influence of wind and thus a power failure can result in a slow ventilation rate, depending on the size of the inlet. The result is obviously an increase in air temperature and a possible significant change in relative humidity, as well as noxious gases, inside the building. These effects are clearly shown by Boon *et al.* (1983) where temperatures in an experimental building rose within two hours from 18 to 26°C and humidity increased from 11.5 to 88%. It is thus necessary to incorporate a failsafe system to cope with power failure, overheating or overcooling.

Many pigs, calves and poultry are housed in buildings that are ventilated either by fans or by automatically controlled natural ventilation. Faults in these systems can put the livestock at risk and cause severe stress and eventually death. For poultry, for instance, failure of ventilation can cause deaths in 20 min in hot weather.

Although a failsafe system can be automatic, it is mandatory in the UK and some other countries that an alarm be incorporated in the system. This can be visual, audible or telephone linked and should be able to detect not only power failure, but high and low temperatures. Normally the sensory device for the latter two conditions will be a temperature sensor. The correct limits (either high or low) will depend on the many factors associated with the husbandry of the stock, e.g. class and age of stock, stocking density, group size, etc. It is also important that each livestock building be fitted with a mains power failure detector. This should incorporate a delay of approximately 5–10 min so that short-term interruptions to the electricity supply are ignored. The delay time again is dependent on the susceptibility of the stock to temperature changes.

Figure 7.9 shows how an alarm system could be incorporated into a central system. An installed ventilation system, whether powered or ACNV

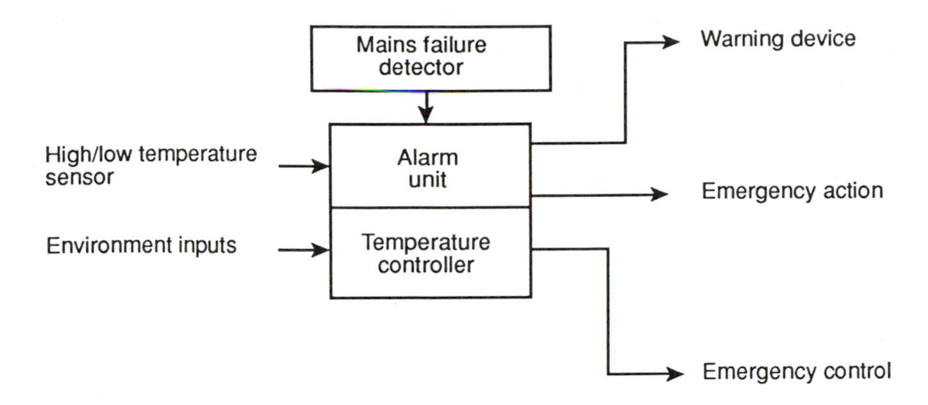

Fig. 7.9. Block diagrams of alarm system integrated with a control system.

should be adequate for the stock in the building but provision should be made to ensure that the animals receive sufficient fresh air in an emergency. Apart from using a back-up generator when mains power has failed, provision can only be by using natural ventilation and this requires openings at both high and low levels in the building. The number and size of the emergency openings depend on the total area required and the existing layout of fan and vents. The total area required depends on the number and type of stock housed as described above.

For a building with open ridge or side wall ventilation Equation (31) relates the total area of the inlet and outlet. The corresponding air exchange rate is given by Equation (14).

To determine A_i and A_o from these two equations two decisions are required. Firstly, the ratio of inlet to outlet areas is often recommended to be 1.5 to 2. However, in practice this is usually difficult to achieve and there is very small benefit from having the inlet area larger than the outlet. The inlet area should never be smaller than the outlet area and, where the building design is not limiting, the factor should approach 1.5.

Secondly, the value of ΔT adopted determines the risk taken in the design of the emergency ventilation system by the choice of an acceptable rise in internal air temperature. The value should be based on an appraisal of local climatic conditions throughout the year and the tolerance of the housed animals to significant departures of temperature from the normal condition. A general recommendation is that ΔT should not be greater than 5 K.

ACNV systems are normally designed with an assumed wind speed of $1\,m\,s^{-1}$. Provision must be made to operate existing vents in the event of excessive temperature rise or power failure, for example by a low voltage actuator.

Principles of Air Distribution

Air distribution within a building is important in order to achieve the required conditions for the stock. In some husbandry systems the aim is to achieve uniformity of environment throughout the entire space, in others it may be adequate to achieve uniformity or alternatively a range of environmental conditions over the floor.

There is often debate over the use of pressurized and exhaust systems. In order to control ventilation rate it matters little which one is used, and in principle the method also has little consequence on air distribution apart from the influence of adventitious leaks. If the building is pressurized, then all the air enters through the inlet vents and the air distribution is controlled. When the building is exhausted, air enters not only through the designed inlet vents, but also through cracks around doors and between cladding panels. This air leakage creates localized air jets which are likely to be colder than the internal conditions and which may impinge directly on the stock.

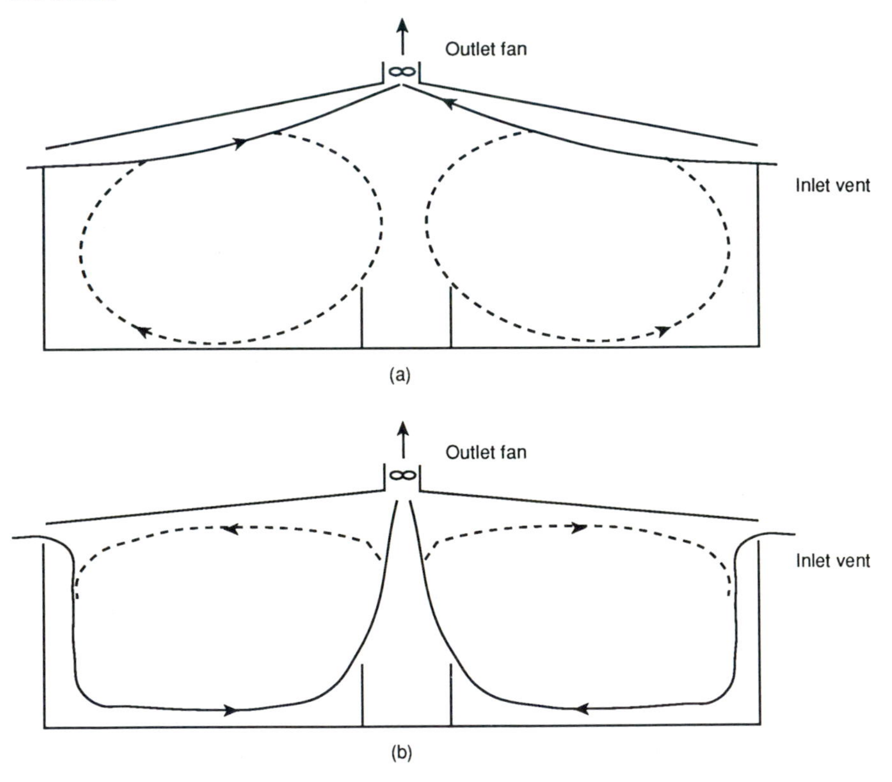

Fig. 7.10. Airflow patterns with primary flow paths (——) and secondary flow paths (----) for $Ar_c < 30$ (a) and $Ar_c > 75$ (b).

Air leakage through small cracks around closed doors can be expressed in the form

$$Q = LK(\Delta P)^m \tag{36}$$

where L is the length of the crack and K takes a value of about $0.2 \times 10^{-3} m^3 s^{-1}$ per metre of crack length at a pressure difference of 1 Pa. A typical value for m is about 0.65.

In general air distribution can be controlled by forced ventilated systems but only under special circumstances (e.g. Hoff *et al.*, 1992) with natural ventilation.

Physics of internal air movement

The pattern of air movement in a livestock building forms the link between the ventilation system and the microclimate around the animals. General rules have been derived to predict the form of the air pattern in typical livestock buildings (Fig. 7.10) with forced ventilation (Randall, 1975).

1. Air moves in a series of rotary motions.
2. A primary airflow path can be defined from the inlet to the outlet vent along the direction of flow.
3. Secondary paths are induced by the primary paths to complete one or more rotary motions.
4. Even small obstacles in the path of an air stream cause substantial changes of direction and pattern.
5. At high ventilation rates the rotary pattern is established initially by the design of the air inlet and subsequently by the internal obstructions in the building.
6. At low ventilation rates thermal buoyancy causes the incoming air jets to fall, and thereby modifies patterns established at high ventilation rates.

The direction of flow of the incoming air jet may be characterized by the Archimedes number (Müllejans, 1966) which represents the ratio of the buoyancy and dynamic pressures in the jet.

$$Ar = \frac{gD_h}{V^2}\left(\frac{\Delta\rho}{\rho}\right) \tag{37}$$

where D_h is the hydraulic diameter of the room

$$D_h = \frac{2BH}{B + H} \tag{38}$$

The air speed in the room, V, is represented by the hypothetical mean air speed

$$V = \frac{Q}{BH} \tag{39}$$

where Q is the volume flow of air through the room.

To account for the effects of different vent geometries (Müllejans, 1966) and for bluff vents (Van Gunst *et al.*, 1967) the Archimedes number may be expressed in the form

$$Ar_c = Ar\,C\frac{Ld}{D_h^{\,2}} \tag{40}$$

Using this definition Randall and Battams (1979) have shown that for a limited range of building geometries, the path of the air entering a rectangular room through an inlet just beneath the ceiling remains horizontal if $Ar_c < 30$ and will fall if $Ar_c > 75$ (see Fig. 7.10). Between these values unstable intermediate patterns exist. An inlet air speed of $5\,\mathrm{m\,s^{-1}}$ is likely to give a value of $Ar_c < 30$ and a stable airflow pattern in most well-built commercial livestock buildings for external temperatures down to 0°C. In these circumstances the incoming air travels for some distance beneath the roof enhancing entrainment causing the temperature to be increased before it enters the space occupied by the livestock (see Fig. 7.10).

Further evaluation of these criteria by Leonard and McQuitty (1986a) for external temperatures down to −10°C shows them to be somewhat conservative. They propose $Ar_c < 50$ for all ceiling or full width inlets and $Ar_c < 40$ for part width inlets set well below the ceiling to ensure that the incoming air jet does not fall on entry.

All of the above criteria assume that the relationship

$$\frac{\Delta\rho}{\rho} \approx \frac{\Delta T}{T} \tag{41}$$

is a good approximation where ΔT is the difference between the temperature of a heated surface inside the building (e.g. animal surface temperature) and the temperature of the air entering the building. Because of the difficulties of measuring surface temperatures and the variety of surface temperatures in a building the temperature difference between the exhaust air and incoming air has been proposed (Leonard and McQuitty, 1986a) as being more practical. Using this temperature difference values of $Ar_d < 27$ and $Ar_d < 21$ for full-width or part-width vents give equally good criteria.

The criterion of an inlet air speed of $5\,\mathrm{m\,s^{-1}}$ is adequate for external temperatures down to about 0°C, but is unsuitable for colder conditions (Barber *et al.*, 1982). Other criteria of adequate air circulation and acceptable air speeds near to the stock are also important (Barber *et al.*, 1982; Albright, 1989; Ogilvie *et al.*, 1990; Jin and Ogilvie, 1992).

A jet momentum function (Kaul *et al.*, 1975) defined as

$$J_i = QV\rho/R \tag{42}$$

was proposed to have a functional relationship with air circulation patterns for stable circulation under isothermal conditions when $J_i > 0.01\,\mathrm{kg\,m^{-2}s^{-2}}$.

A dimensionless jet momentum number (Barber *et al.*, 1982) of

$$J = \frac{QV}{gR} \tag{43}$$

modifies the stability criteria of Kaul to $J > 7.5 \times 10^{-4}$. Using both the Archimedes and Jet momentum numbers Barber *et al.* (1982) conclude that for a jet velocity of $5\,m\,s^{-1}$, stable air circulation can be expected only for temperatures greater than −10°C. Below this, airflow rates are too low to give good air circulation unless the jet velocity is increased to $10\,m\,s^{-1}$. However, because of building and fan characteristics it is rarely possible to achieve this condition in practice (Leonard and McQuitty, 1986b) (see page 151).

The volume airflow:floor area factor (Q/A) used as an index of air energy input into a room (in addition to the non-dimensional jet momentum number) has been investigated to predict air speeds over the floor or near to the stock (Ogilvie *et al.*, 1990). It was shown to correlate well with floor air speed for some building configurations. However, it is not possible to specify a single value of J which applies to all configurations; J is specific to the building layout. Since Q/A is mathematically related to J for a fixed building size and inlet jet velocity, similar correlations are obtained.

In recirculating ventilation systems a range of jet momentum numbers can be achieved for a fixed internal recirculation rate. Thus the jet velocity and recirculation rate can be varied independently to obtain a desired jet momentum number and floor air speed. Q/A is not very useful in practice because it characterizes only the recirculation rate and not the jet velocity.

Air inlets and outlets

When the ventilating air enters an enclosure in the form of a jet, the design of the air inlet is the dominant factor controlling the airflow pattern, as discussed in the previous section. The positions of the air outlets have little effect on the overall pattern (Turnbull and Coates, 1971; Kaul *et al.*, 1975; Randall, 1975). However, the position of the air outlet can affect other aspects of ventilation performance. Short-circuiting of air may occur if the inlet jet is directed towards and is close to the air outlet (Randall, 1973; Kaul *et al.*, 1975).

In a well-designed ventilation system, the air outlets do not affect the distribution of the fresh incoming air and thus the major airflow pattern. However they do affect the distribution of the air leaving the building. Thereby outlet position can affect the uniformity of steady-state thermodynamic and contaminant balances (e.g. Barber and Ogilvie, 1982; Krause and Janssen, 1990). This occurs particularly in airspaces where there are two major rotary flow regions and fresh air is directed into only one of these.

Although it is generally accepted that the position of the outlet does not

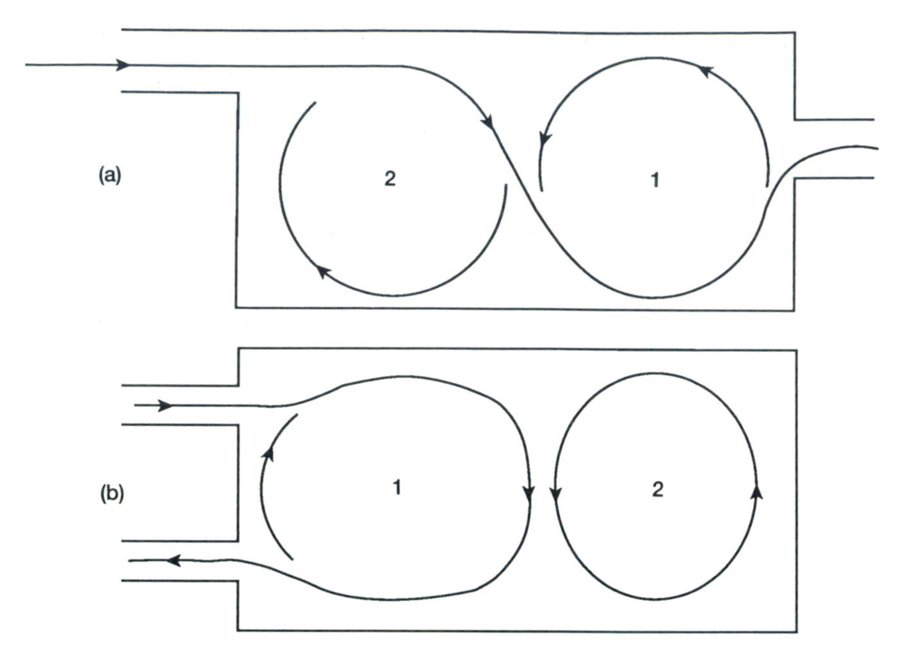

Fig. 7.11. Effect of outlet position on air mixing: (a) tanks in series; (b) secondary zone.

affect the pattern of airflow (Randall, 1975), it can be argued that the location of the outlet may affect the degree of air mixing in the ventilated space. Figure 7.11 shows the same airspace with similar flow patterns, but with the outlets in different positions. With the width of the building more than two or three times the height, two rotary flow regimes are likely to exist (e.g. Kaul *et al.*, 1975; Randall, 1975). Where the inlet is on the opposite side of the room to the outlet, there are two airflow regions connected in series. The zone (2) nearest the inlet is relatively better ventilated than the zone (1) nearest the outlet (Barber and Ogilvie, 1982). With the inlet and outlet in the same wall, the zone (2) furthest from the inlet is relatively less well ventilated than the zone (1) next to the outlet. Hence for the same ventilation rate the *steady state* thermal properties of the *exhaust air* are the same in each system. However, the mean temperature and humidity in the airspace of the first system (a) are less than the corresponding conditions in the second (b). The position of the air outlet affects the steady-state thermodynamic properties in the airspace for a given ventilation rate without affecting the airflow pattern.

The zone remote from the outlet is either under- or over-ventilated. In tracer gas experiments using scaled models Barber and Ogilvie (1982) showed that by changing the outlet location a 30% difference of effective ventilation rate occurred in a slot-ventilated enclosure. A second consequence is that these effects are localized within the building and are not evident in the overall contaminant concentration in the exhaust air.

In some specialized circumstances outlets may be positioned to minimize adverse conditions. For example, in piggeries with slurry pits beneath a perforated floor, it may be advantageous to have the air outlets rather than the air inlets beneath the floor in order to minimize the transfer of contaminants into the occupied space. However, it is essential in either case that the free area of the floor when fully occupied by recumbent pigs is large enough (e.g. twice the normal air vent area) to permit the total required airflow without restricting it. It may also be possible to site outlets in positions where they are least likely to be influenced by wind.

Air inlets may be fixed in size, adjustable or in the form of a diffusing surface. Fixed sized vents are adequate where it is not necessary to maintain temperature in cold weather (e.g. naturally ventilated cattle buildings) or to control the airflow pattern (e.g. dry sow housing). For control of both of these features it is generally advisable to use adjustable vents. Some small benefit can sometimes accrue from manually adjusted vents, but in most circumstances for a worthwhile benefit, fully automatic vent control is required to be sufficiently responsive to diurnal temperature variations (Randall, 1975).

With large areas of diffusing inlets such as glass fibre ceilings used in poultry houses, the incoming air enters at very low speeds, well below those of the stock convection currents. Thus the latter dominate the airflow pattern. With tiers of poultry cages air tends to rise over the birds and fall between each row of cages to set up a series of rotary flows (Randall, 1975).

Incoming air entering through a duct can usually be directed as required (Carpenter, 1972). If ducts are made of a perforated material with many holes, their surface becomes equivalent to a diffusing inlet. In these circumstances no strong directional current arises but if the incoming air is somewhat cooler than the internal air, the inlet air tends to fall slowly beneath the duct.

Internal mixing

Heat balance equations for the ventilated building assume the hypothesis of complete mixing within the airspace. Thus the thermodynamic properties of the exhaust air are equal to the average properties in the airspace. In practice there is departure from complete mixing due to short-circuiting between inlet and outlet, the presence of stagnant zones or the existence of a multiple airflow region (Barber and Ogilvie, 1982). Incomplete mixing also causes variation in the concentration of gases and particulate aerosols within the airspace.

Ventilation systems such as the high speed jet system (Randall, 1977) go some way to improving mixing but, even with this system problems are still evident at low ventilation rates, especially where supplementary heating is used. The air movement in the building airspace is defined by the imposed airflow pattern caused by the main ventilation system, to which is added the convection from both heaters and the stock. At minimum ventilation rates convection currents dominate, the more so when heaters are in use, and the resultant effect is a stratification of the temperature. Temperatures in the roof space may exceed temperatures at floor level by at least 10 K. Figure 7.12 shows the result of efficient destratification (Boon and Battams, 1988).

Three relatively simple ways of mixing air in open plan livestock buildings such as broiler rearing units can be considered. Firstly, air can be mixed by using a standard propeller fan blowing down each side of the building to set up a horizontal rotating pattern normal to the convection pattern. This is an efficient method of destroying the stratification but perhaps should only be employed in severe conditions of stress as the air speeds at stock level of about 3 to 4 $\mathrm{m\,s^{-1}}$ are too high for the stock, especially young animals. For older stock the method is often employed in hot climates to reduce heat stress.

Secondly, air can be discharged through the holes of a pressurized perforated duct constructed of either tubular polyethylene film or a rigid

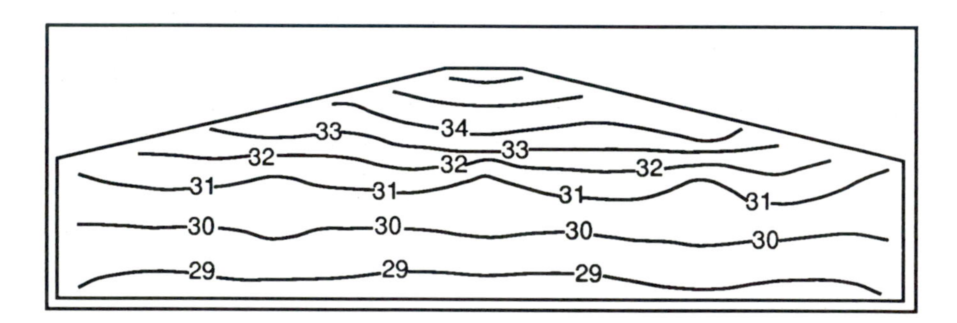

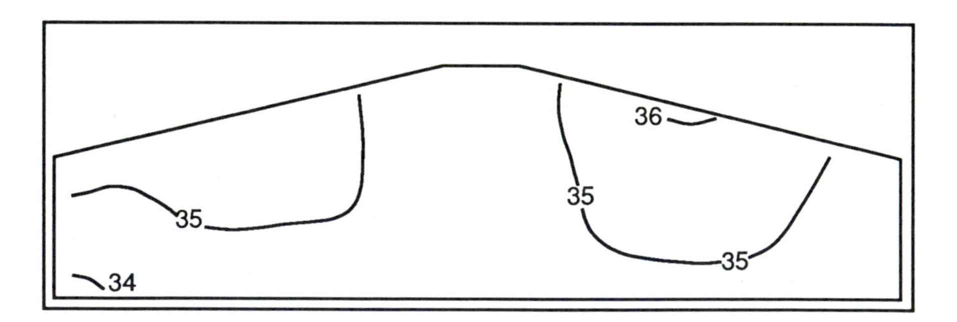

Fig. 7.12. Upper: stratification of temperatures due to heaters in a broiler building. Lower: destratification effected by the use of ceiling fans.

material. This is an efficient way of distributing the air and, indeed, can be part of the main circulating system using damper proportioning of the incoming and house air. Design of the duct is important (Carpenter, 1972) to achieve uniform discharge of air along the length of the duct. The total area of hole should be 1.5 to 2 times the duct cross-sectional area and their spacing along the duct depends on whether the duct is parallel sided or tapered. To facilitate manufacture, a tapered duct allows uniform hole spacing. Small improvements in design, such as D-shaped holes with a flap formed by the 'D', ensure that the air is discharged normal to the duct. This relatively cheap solution to mixing suffers from the problem of build-up of dust within the duct.

The last method uses a ceiling fan of either the paddle type that produces vertical motion of the air or the radial (centrifugal) type that produces horizontal radial motion. The former is the simplest to install and remove and has low power consumption. Ceiling fans are efficient at eliminating stratification of temperatures (see Fig. 7.12) but care must be taken in their use. The normal mode of operation is to blow the air downwards towards the floor but this produces air speeds in excess of $1\,m\,s^{-1}$ which are too high for young stock, e.g. day-old chicks. By reversing the fan motor electrically, and also reversing the blades for higher efficiency, the air is blown upwards to create an acceptable airflow pattern with low air speeds at floor level. Boon and Battams (1988) have shown that for buildings 12–15 m wide a single 1.5 m diameter fan per 12 m length of building, blowing upwards and rotating at full speed gave efficient mixing. For buildings 15–24 m wide, two such units per 12 m length would be required. Such an arrangement not only provides a good environment for the stock but reduces fuel energy costs by at least 20%.

The Future

An important aspect of the design of systems for controlling the environment in livestock buildings has always been production efficiency but, in the future, more account will be taken of the problems associated with the welfare of the confined livestock. This inevitable change is due to consumer pressures followed by government legislation.

Studying animal behaviour will allow the conditioned responses of animals to be used to advantage in control system design. Baldwin and Ingram (1968) and Curtis and Morris (1982) have already shown that in a cold environment pigs can be taught to operate a switch to obtain a reward in the form of heat. It is likely that similar behaviour could be exploited to improve air quality, for example by reducing ammonia concentration.

The increase in the use of microprocessors and computers as standard components in ventilation control systems allows the design of total farm systems for a multi-building site. Distributed processor technology has been used for some years in the glasshouse industry and, with suitable modifications, is suitable for livestock enterprises. Each building will require unique conditions depending upon age and class of stock thus requiring its own local controller which is monitored and set by a central processor.

Improvements in ventilation system design will continue and are likely to incorporate the ideas and technology outlined above. However, their uptake will depend upon the state of the economics of the livestock industry.

Symbols

a	empirical constant, kg m^{-3}
A	area, m^2
A_c	annual cost of a fan installation, £ a^{-1}
A_f	surface area in contact with floor, m^2
A_g	surface area in contact with other animals, m^2
A_i	inlet area of vents, m^2
A_n	area of the nth opening, m^2
A_o	outlet area of vents, m^2
A_p	surface area of pigs, m^2
A_s	surface area of building elements, m^2
Ar	Archimedes number
Ar_c	corrected Archimedes number
Ar_d	corrected Archimedes number (based on air temperature difference after Leonard and McQuitty)
B	length of a building supplied by a vent of length L, m
c	initial capital cost of the fan installation, £
C	discharge coefficient for an opening
C_p	specific heat of air, 1010 J kg^{-1} K^{-1}
C_{pe}	external pressure coefficient
C_{pen}	external pressure coefficient in nth opening
C_{pi}	internal pressure coefficient
d	vertical dimension of an opening, m
D	fan diameter, m
D_h	hydraulic diameter, m
g	acceleration due to gravity, m s^{-2}
h	variable height, m
$\bar{h}$	height of neutral axis, m
H	fixed height, m
J	jet momentum number
J_i	jet momentum function, kg m^{-2} s^{-2}
k	resistance coefficient
K	air leakage factor, m^3 s^{-1} per metre length
L	length of an opening, m
m	empirical exponent

n	year of ownership of a fan installation
N	term of loan or ownership of the fan installation, a
p_n	factor in nth year, related to annual value
ΔP	pressure difference, $N m^{-2}$
P_e	external pressure, $N m^{-2}$
P_f	fan total pressure, $N m^{-2}$
P_i	internal pressure, $N m^{-2}$
ΔP_o	fan static pressure at zero flow, $N m^{-2}$
q	inflation rate, %
q_a	heat output of animals, W
q_e	evaporative heat loss, W
q_h	heat output of heaters, W
q_n	thermoneutral heat production, W
Q	rate of air flow, $m^3 s^{-1}$
Q_a	annual air requirement for a fan installation, $m^3 a^{-1}$
Q_n	volume flow rate through the nth opening, $m^3 s^{-1}$
r	interest rate receivable on bank account, %
r_a	thermal resistance of skin–air interface, °C $m^2 W^{-1}$
r_f	effective thermal resistance of floor, °C $m^2 W^{-1}$
r_t	thermal resistance of pig tissue, °C $m^2 W^{-1}$
R	volume of a room, m^3
S	current resale value of fans when N years old, £
T	absolute temperature, K
T_b	deep body temperature, °C
U	current electricity price, £ $kW^{-1}h^{-1}$
U_s	thermal transmittance of building elements s, $W m^{-2} K^{-1}$
V	air velocity, $m s^{-1}$
V_e	ventilation efficiency ratio, $m^3 kJ^{-1}$
V_n	air velocity in the nth opening, $m s^{-1}$
V_{10}	wind speed at a height of 10 m, $m s^{-1}$
w	inflation/interest ratio
W	horizontal distance, m
W_i	inflation/interest factor
X	accumulated hours of use of a fan as a percentage of the wear-out life, %
ρ	density, kg m^{-3}

References

Albright, L.D. (1975) *Air Moving Efficiencies of Ventilating Fans.* Paper number NA75-304. American Society of Agricultural Engineers, St Joseph, Michigan, pp. 1–18.

Albright, L.D. (1979) Designing slotted inlet ventilation by the system characteristic technique. *Transactions of the American Society of Agricultural Engineers* 22, 158–161.

Albright, L.D. (1989) Slotted inlet baffle control based on inlet jet momentum numbers. *Transactions of the American Society of Agricultural Engineers* 32, 1764–1768.

Albright, L.D. (1990) *Environment Control for Animals and Plants.* ASAE Textbook Number 4. The American Society of Agricultural Engineers, St Joseph, Michigan, USA, 453pp.

Audsley, E. and Wheeler, J.A. (1978) The annual cost of machinery calculated using actual cash flows. *Journal of Agricultural Engineering Research* 23, 189–201.

Baldwin, B.A. and Ingram, D.L. (1968) Factors influencing behavioural thermo-regulation in pigs. *Physiology and Behaviour* 3, 409–415.

Barber, E.M. and Ogilvie, J.R. (1982) Incomplete mixing in ventilated air spaces. Part 1: Theoretical considerations. *Canadian Agricultural Engineering* 24, 25–29.

Barber, E.M., Sokhansanj, S., Lampman, W.P. and Ogilvie, J.R. (1982) *Stability of Airflow Patterns in Ventilated Air Spaces.* Paper Number 82-4551. American Society of Agricultural Engineers, St Joseph, Michigan, pp. 1–10.

Boon, C.R. (1984) The control of climatic environment for finishing pigs using lower critical temperature. *Journal of Agricultural Engineering Research* 29, 295–303.

Boon, C.R. and Battams, V.A. (1988) Air mixing fans in a broiler building – their use and efficiency. *Journal of Agricultural Engineering Research* 39, 137–147.

Boon, C.R. and Lowe, J.C. (1987) Microprocessor control of the environment for finishing pigs, using lower critical temperature. In: Clark, J.A., Gregson, K. and Saffell, R.A. (eds), *Computer Applications in Agricultural Environments.* Butterworths, London, pp. 251–264.

Boon, C.R., Hague, P. and Shillito Walser, E. (1983) Effects of temporary power failure on temperature, humidity and the activity of pigs in an experimental piggery. *Applied Animal Ethology* 10, 219–232.

Brockett, B.L. and Albright, L.D. (1987) Natural ventilation in single airspace buildings. *Journal of Agricultural Engineering Research* 37, 141–154.

Bruce, J.M. (1975a) Natural ventilation of cattle buildings by thermal buoyancy. *Farm Building Progress* 42, 17–20.

Bruce, J.M. (1975b) A computer program for the calculation of natural ventilation due to wind. *Farm Building R&D Studies* 7, 1–7.

Bruce, J.M. (1977) Natural ventilation. Its role and application in the bioclimatic system. *Farm Building R&D Studies* 8, 1–8.

Bruce, J.M. (1978) Natural convection through openings and its application to cattle building ventilation. *Journal of Agricultural Engineering Research* 23, 151–167.

Bruce, J.M. (1981a) Ventilation and temperature control criteria for pigs. In: Clark, J.A. (ed.), *Environmental Aspects of Housing for Animal Production.* Butterworths, London, pp. 197–216.

Bruce, J.M. (1981b) Modelling the effect of wind on propeller-fan ventilation systems. In: *Modelling, Design and Evaluation of Agricultural Buildings* (Supplementary papers). CIGR Section II Seminar, Aberdeen, 31 Aug–4 Sept 1981. Scottish Farm Buildings Investigation Unit, Craibstone, Aberdeen, pp. 3–11.

Bruce, J.M. (1982) Ventilation of a model livestock building by thermal buoyancy. *Transactions of the American Society of Agricultural Engineers* 25, 1724–1726.

Bruce, J.M. (1986) Theory of natural ventilation due to thermal buoyancy and wind. *Proceedings of CIGR Seminar on Pig Housing.* Rennes, France, 8–11 September, CIGR, pp. 1–9.

Bruce, J.M. and Clark, J.J. (1979) Models of heat production and critical temperature for growing pigs. *Animal Production* 28, 353–369.

Burnett, G.A. and MacDonald, J.A. (1987) ACNV in pig finishing houses:

temperature control in winter. *Farm Building Progress* 87, 27–31.

Carpenter, G.A. (1972) The design of permeable ducts and their application to the ventilation of livestock buildings. *Journal of Agricultural Engineering Research* 17, 219–230.

Cole, G.W. (1980) The derivation and analysis of the differential equations for the air temperature of the confined animal housing system. *Transactions of the American Society of Agricultural Engineers* 23, 712–720.

Curtis, S.E. and Morris, G.L. (1982) Operant supplemental heat in swine nurseries. In: *Livestock Environment II. Proceedings of the 2nd International Livestock Environment Symposium.* ASAE, St Joseph, Michigan, pp. 295–297.

Down, M.J., Foster, M.P. and McMahon, T.A. (1990) Experimental verification of a theory for ventilation of livestock buildings by natural convection. *Journal of Agricultural Engineering Research* 45, 269–279.

Foster, M.P. and Down, M.J. (1987) Ventilation of livestock buildings by natural convection. *Journal of Agricultural Engineering Research* 37, 1–13.

Hoff, S.J., Janni, K.A. and Jacobson, L.D. (1992) Three-dimensional buoyant turbulent flows in a scaled model, slot-ventilated, livestock confinement facility. *Transactions of the American Society of Agricultural Engineers* 35(2), 671–686.

Hoxey, R.P. (1984) Design wind loads for closed farm buildings. *Journal of Agricultural Engineering Research* 29(4), 305–311.

Jin, Y. and Ogilvie, J.R. (1992) Airflow characteristics in the floor region of a slot ventilated room (isothermal). *Transactions of the American Society of Agricultural Engineers* 35(2), 695–702.

Kaul, P., Maltry, W., Müller, H.J. and Winter, V. (1975) *Scientific–Technical Principles for the Control of Environment in Livestock Houses and Stores.* Translation Number 430. National Institute of Agricultural Engineering, Silsoe, 47pp.

Krause, K.-H. and Janssen, J. (1990) Measuring and simulation of the distribution of ammonia in animal houses. *Proceedings of the Second International Conference,* Roomvent 90, 13–15 June 1990, Oslo, Norway, pp. 1–12.

Leonard, J.J. and McQuitty, J.B. (1986a) The use of Archimedes Number in the design of ventilation systems for animal housing. *Conference on Agricultural Engineering,* Adelaide, 24–28 August 1986, pp. 1–6.

Leonard, J.J. and McQuitty, J.B. (1986b) Archimedes Number criteria for the control of cold ventilation air jets. *Canadian Agricultural Engineering* 28, 117–123.

Moulsley, L.J. and Randall, J.M. (1990) Propeller fans for ventilating livestock buildings. 2. Performance criteria. *Journal of Agricultural Engineering Research* 47, 101–113.

Müllejans, H. (1966) The similarity between non-isothermal flow and heat transfer in mechanically ventilated rooms. Translation 202, Heating and Ventilating Research Association, Bracknell.

Ogilvie, J.R., Barber, E.M. and Randall, J.M. (1990) Floor air speeds and inlet design in swine ventilation systems. *Transactions of the American Society of Agricultural Engineers* 33, 255–259.

Randall, J.M. (1973) Air distribution in a full scale section of a livestock building – Part I Unpublished Departmental Note DN/FB/319/3020 National Institute of Agricultural Engineering, Silsoe, 107pp.

Randall, J.M. (1975) The prediction of airflow patterns in livestock buildings. *Journal of Agricultural Engineering Research* 20, 199–215.

Randall, J.M. (1977) *A Handbook on the Design of a Ventilation System for Livestock Buildings Using Step Control and Automatic Vents.* NIAE Report No. 28. National Institute of Agricultural Engineering, Wrest Park, Silsoe, Bedford, 47pp.

Randall, J.M. (1991) Ventilation and temperature control in pig production. *Proceedings of the Congresso Internacional de Zootécnia,* Universidade de Évora, 3–6 April 1991. University of Évora, Portugal, pp. 1–12.

Randall, J.M. and Armsby, A.W. (1983) Cooling gradients across pens in a finishing piggery. I. Measured cooling gradients. *Journal of Agricultural Engineering Research* 28, 235–245.

Randall, J.M. and Battams, V.A. (1979) Stability criteria for airflow patterns in livestock buildings. *Journal of Agricultural Engineering Research* 24, 361–374.

Randall, J.M. and Moulsley, L.J. (1990) Propeller fans for ventilating livestock buildings. 3. Selection for least cost. *Journal of Agricultural Engineering Research* 47, 115–122.

Randall, J.M., Armsby, A.W. and Sharp, J.R. (1983a) Cooling gradients across pens in a finishing piggery. II. Effects on excretory behaviour. *Journal of Agricultural Engineering Research* 28, 247–259.

Randall, J.M., Sharp, J.R. and Armsby, A.W. (1983b) Cooling gradients across pens in a finishing piggery. III. Effects on performance and health. *Journal of Agricultural Engineering Research* 28, 261–268.

Robertson, K. (1984) *ACNV Automatically Controlled Natural Ventilation for Pig Housing.* Scottish Farm Buildings Investigation Unit, Aberdeen, 13pp.

Shrestha, G., Cramer, C. and Holmes, B.J. (1990) Wind induced natural ventilation of an enclosed building. Paper Number 904001. American Society of Agricultural Engineers, St Joseph, Michigan, pp. 1–26.

Strom, J.S. and Morsing, S. (1984) Automatically controlled natural ventilation in a growing and finishing pig house. *Journal of Agricultural Engineering Research* 30, 353–359.

Turnbull, J.E. and Coates, J.A. (1971) Temperatures and air flow patterns in a controlled environment, cage poultry building. *Transactions of the American Society of Agricultural Engineers* 14, 109–113, 120.

Van Gunst, E., Erkelens, P.J. and Coenders, W.P.J. (1967) Some results of investigations regarding the supply of cooled air in a test room. *4th Congress International du Chauffage et de la Climatization.* Paris, May 1967, pp. 1–45. Paris, May 1967.

Zhang, J.S., Janni, K.A. and Jacobson, L.D. (1989) Modelling natural ventilation induced by combined thermal buoyancy and wind. *Transactions of the American Society of Agricultural Engineers* 32, 2165–2174.

Structures and Materials 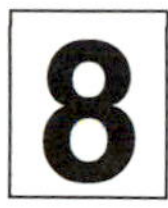

J.E. OWEN
Farm Building Research Team, ADAS Bridgets, UK

Introduction

Livestock housing, whether it is simple or sophisticated, must perform the required function. Firstly, it must be appropriate to the needs of the particular species being farmed, with ruminants generally requiring far simpler housing than monogastric animals. Secondly, it must be designed to meet the particular climatic conditions. Thirdly, construction methods and materials must be appropriate for the working conditions bearing in mind the availability and cost of materials and local construction workers' skills. If these requirements are to be met, careful consideration must be given to animal, climatic, materials and construction, workmanship, management and costs factors at the design and construction stages.

There are many aspects to the design, selection and use of structures, and to the selection and use of materials. Many of these relate to buildings of all types, e.g. strength, stability, durability, and costs, and not to livestock buildings alone. British and other standards cover a wide range of aspects of structure, materials and design for agricultural, including livestock, buildings and other structures. Costs of materials and rates of building work are listed in various cost guides. This chapter concentrates mainly on those aspects of structure and materials which are considered of importance to the environmental and climatic aspects of livestock housing.

Climatic Indices and Outside Design Conditions

Any structure and its associated environmental control systems must be designed to meet the particular climatic conditions that prevail in the locality. Various indices have been developed which describe climate in terms of 'design conditions' rather than extremes, and are usually derived from meteorological records. They are often described in relation to their frequency of occurrence, e.g. the percentage of time such values can be expected to be exceeded, or coincidence with some other climatic variable, e.g. the coincidence of wind speed and low temperature.

Two sources of such climatic data are the American Society of Heating, Refrigeration and Air-Conditioning Engineers (ASHRAE, 1967) and the Chartered Institution of Building Services (CIBS, 1982) guide books. These provide information on most of the parameters discussed below, for a number of countries in the world. These publications also discuss the derivation of data presented and offer guidance on their use.

Outside air dry-bulb design temperature, T_{ao}

Minimum design temperatures

These are the lowest values of outside air temperature that normally need to be considered for the determination of insulation and heating needs in buildings.

Maximum design temperatures

These are the highest values of outside air temperature that normally need to be considered when considering the insulation or cooling needs in buildings.

Outside air wet-bulb temperature, T_{aow}

Wet bulb temperatures are generally of greatest interest in hot conditions and are usually quoted alongside dry bulb temperatures for warm weather. They are used for the design of air conditioning systems.

Solar data

Direct and diffuse solar radiation

Solar radiation on the perpendicular to the sun's rays at the top of the earth's atmosphere has an annual mean irradiance of approximately $1370\,W\,m^{-2}$. In passing through the earth's atmosphere this energy either is absorbed, scattered (with the fraction eventually reaching the earth's surface termed 'diffuse sky' radiation) or passed directly to the earth. By applying relationships based on solar geometry, the direct solar irradiance on specific surfaces at particular latitudes can be predicted. Other empirical relationships can be used to predict diffuse sky irradiation on horizontal surfaces.

Design radiation data

Basic irradiances for a particular locality must be corrected to give design irradiances appropriate to the prevailing radiation climate. Normally height, k_a, direct, k_D, and diffuse, k_d, radiation factors need to be applied to achieve such corrections. Height correction factors depend on solar altitude and height of a locality above sea level. Direct and diffuse radiation factors depend on sky clarity and cloud cover in the locality. Design direct irradiance, I_{Dd}, on vertical and horizontal surfaces and design diffuse sky irradiance, I_{dd}, for horizontal surfaces can be calculated from the following equations.

$$I_{Dd} = k_a k_D I_D$$

and

$$I_{dd} = k_a k_d I_d$$

The two radiation factors, k_D and k_d, both require radiation to be measured at a locality, generally total horizontal surface radiation being measured. The *CIBS Guide* (CIBS, 1982) suggests values of k_D and k_d that can be used for evaluating overheating design in both temperate and tropical localities.

Design monthly 'maximum' irradiance

For some design purposes it is required to know the near maxima, hourly and daily mean irradiances which might occur each month. Such values of design 'maxima' of irradiances (e.g. likely to be exceeded on 2.5% of occasions) are sometimes calculated for different locations and radiation climates.

Design total irradiance

Horizontal surfaces receive both direct irradiance and diffuse irradiance. Vertical surfaces receive direct irradiance, diffuse irradiance and that component of both direct and diffuse irradiance that is reflected from the ground. The total design irradiance on such surfaces is calculated as follows.

$$I_{THd} = I_{DHd} + I_{dHd}$$

where I_{THd} = design total irradiance on a horizontal surface, $W m^{-2}$, I_{DHd} = design direct irradiance on a horizontal surface, $W m^{-2}$, I_{dHd} = design diffuse irradiance on a horizontal surface, $W m^{-2}$ and

$$I_{TVd} = I_{DVd} + 0.5 I_{dHd} + 0.5 k_r I_{THd}$$

where I_{TVd} = design total irradiance on a vertical surface, $W m^{-2}$, I_{DVd} = design direct irradiance on a vertical surface, $W m^{-2}$, k_r = ground reflectance factor (0.2 for temperate and humid tropical regions; 0.5 for arid tropical regions).

The direct irradiance on sloping surfaces depends on the position of the sun relative to the surface. The diffuse irradiance on a roof is partly from the sky and partly from reflection from the ground. The analysis is complex and is usually simplified for design purposes. For sloping roofs the direct components are calculated by dividing the roof into three sectors of the wall–solar azimuth and using sloping roof factors to compensate for roof–solar azimuth. These factors are applied to direct values of design vertical and horizontal radiation. The diffuse irradiance on the sloping roof is assumed to be the same as for a horizontal surface. Even in its simplified form (CIBS, 1982) the analysis is tedious.

Sol-air temperature, T_{eo}

To make the estimation of solar gain to buildings easier the concept of sol-air temperature has been developed. Sol-air temperature is defined as *the outside air temperature which, in the absence of solar radiation, would give the same temperature distribution and rate of energy transfer through a wall or roof as exists with the actual outside air temperature and incident solar radiation.* It is described by the following equation

$$T_{eo} = (\alpha I_t - \varepsilon I_1)R_{so} + T_{ao} \qquad (1)$$

where T_{eo} = sol-air temperature, °C, T_{ao} = outdoor air temperature, °C, α = absorption coefficient of outer surface of building element, I_t = intensity of direct plus diffuse solar radiation on surface, $W m^{-2}$, ε = emissivity of outer surface to longwave radiation, I_1 = longwave radiation from a black surface, $W m^{-2}$, R_{so} = external surface resistance of element, $m^{2}°C W^{-1}$.

Values of T_{eo} have been calculated for different building elements with differing surface orientations and absorption coefficients, for various times of day and months of the year. Figures for UK conditions are published in the *CIBS Guide* and for US conditions in the *ASHRAE Guide.* Such figures may be selectively determined for design purposes, e.g. only values corresponding to irradiances exceeded for 2.5% of the time may be calculated.

Sol-air temperatures can be used directly with '*U*' values and surface areas (see page 190) to evaluate heat gains through various structural elements.

Exposure

The exposure of a building to wind of different speeds and driven rain can affect its heat loss and energy use. Often the exposure of a building needs to be known when estimating its thermal properties or energy use.

Wind speed

Information on wind speed is produced in a variety of forms. For structural design purposes the maximum gust wind speeds that occur and their incidence might be of most interest. For the design of natural ventilation systems it might be the occurrence of minimum wind speeds that is more important. A variety of such information is available.

Driven rain exposure index

In the UK a general exposure rating of sheltered, moderate or severe exposure has long been adopted (Lacy, 1971). This driven rain index is given in units of $m^2 s^{-1}$, i.e. the product of annual total rainfall (m) and annual mean wind speed ($m s^{-1}$). The various ratings were originally specified as follows:

1. *Sheltered.* Driven rain index = $< 3 m^2 s^{-1}$ but excluding areas within 8 km of the sea or large estuaries, within which exposure should be regarded as moderate.
2. *Moderate.* Driven rain index between 3 and $7 m^2 s^{-1}$, except in areas with an index of 5 or more within 8 km of the sea or large estuary, within which exposure should be regarded as severe.
3. *Severe.* Driven rain index = $> 7 m^2 s^{-1}$.

Such exposure ratings have been indicated as maps with guidance provided on how to interpret the effects of height and other site factors when rating buildings for exposure (Prior, 1985).

Temperature and Comfort

Most people think of thermal comfort in terms of air temperature. However, earlier chapters (e.g. Chapter 5) clearly indicate that other climatic parameters (e.g. air speed and solar radiation), housing parameters (e.g. floor thermal characteristics, radiant temperatures of surfaces) and animal behavioural responses (e.g. huddling, postural changes) are involved in heat transfer between an animal and its surroundings.

Comfort indices

For design purposes in human habitation a number of different definitions and indices have been developed to ensure that such variables can be accommodated. Fanger (1972) has developed the concept of the 'comfort equation' for humans, to incorporate activity, clothing, air temperature, mean radiant temperature, air velocity and humidity. ASHRAE (1967) has postulated the use of 'effective temperature' as an index which accommodates as air temperature, air movement and humidity. McArthur (1990) has proposed a 'standard environmental temperature' for livestock exposed to sunlight, wind and different humidities.

Dry resultant temperature

CIBS (1978) has recommended the use of *dry resultant temperature,* which involves inside air and mean radiant temperatures and the assumption that indoor air speed is $0.1\,m\,s^{-1}$, as a measure of the comfort of room occupants. Dry resultant temperature, T_c is calculated from

$$T_c = 0.5\ T_{ai} + 0.5\ T_m \tag{2}$$

where T_{ai} = inside air temperature, °C and T_m = mean surface temperature, °C.

Differing values of dry resultant temperature are recommended for different types of buildings in which different activities take place.

Building 'design' temperatures

For heat transfer calculations and for the design of air conditioning systems, CIBS illustrates the use of another index, *environmental temperature,* T_{ei}, (CIBS, 1979a,b). Again this involves both air and mean surface temperatures, and is evaluated as shown in Equation (3).

$$T_{ei} = T_{ai}/3 + 2T_m/3 \tag{3}$$

The mean surface temperature, T_m, described above is itself determined as the product of the areas and temperatures of the surrounding surfaces divided by the sum of the areas.

Such indices have rarely been adopted for the design of livestock buildings, where reliance is largely placed upon designing on an air temperature basis. This does, however, raise problems in particular circumstances. For example, when radiant heating is used its use should allow a reduction in air temperature; however, the reduction that might be anticipated cannot be quantified by any well-established methods.

Steady State Heat Transfer in Buildings

Designing a building to modify climate requires a knowledge of the fundamentals of heat and moisture transfer and of the principles of ventilation. Thermal considerations involved in the design of livestock buildings are generally based on the assumption of steady state heat transfer between the animal and its enclosure and between the enclosure and the

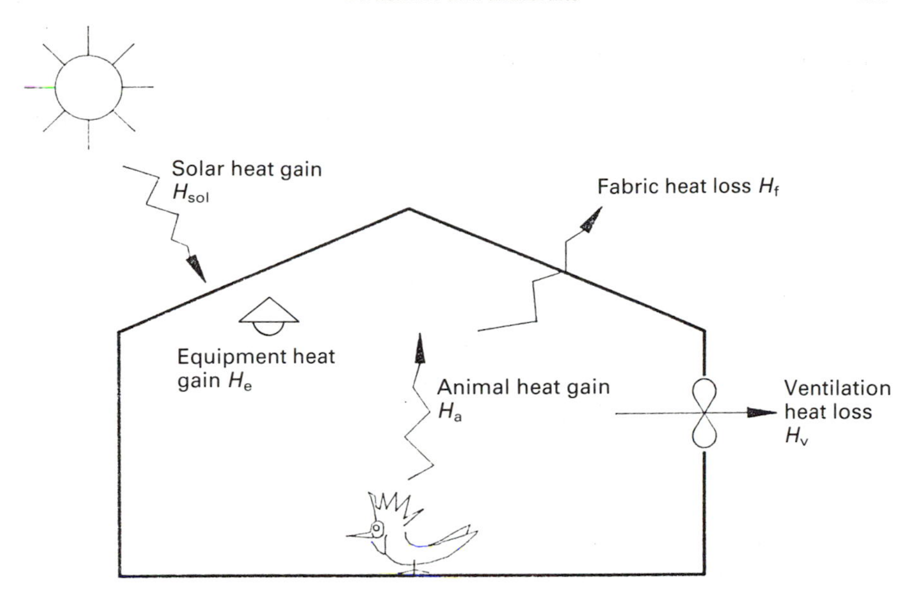

Fig. 8.1. Typical heat gains and losses associated with livestock buildings.

external environment. Typically, the 'heat balance' (see below) of a building is considered under two design conditions, i.e. cold and hot conditions, which determine the required thermal insulation of the building, and the capacity of the heating, cooling and ventilation system.

Heat balances

Figure 8.1 illustrates the typical heat gains and losses associated with a livestock building. To maintain a constant internal air temperature in a building these gains and losses must be balanced. If the heat balance is not maintained then the internal air temperature will rise or fall. Changes in outside conditions, e.g. air temperature, solar radiation, wind speed, etc., will affect the heat gains and losses and consequently the heat balance. Therefore, to achieve temperature control, one must continuously manipulate the controllable gains or losses, e.g. heating or cooling, to maintain the heat balance.

While all these gains and losses need to be quantified for design purposes, the materials and construction of the building will mainly affect the fabric and radiation heat losses and the solar heat gain. These will be dealt with here, while other losses and gains are dealt with elsewhere (see Chapters 1 and 7).

Table 8.1. Thermal conductivities of some typical building materials.

Material	Thermal conductivity ($Wm^{-1}K^{-1}$)
Walls	
Fibre cement sheet	0.36
Brick (outer leaf)	0.84
Brick (inner leaf)	0.62
Concrete block (heavyweight)	1.63
Concrete block (medium weight)	0.51
Concrete block (lightweight)	0.19
Roofs	
Fibre cement sheet	0.36
Steel sheet	50.00
Tile	0.84
Wood wool slab	0.10
Floors	
Cast concrete	1.13
Metal tray	50.00
Screed	0.41
Timber	0.14
Insulation	
Expanded polystyrene slab (EPS)	0.035
Glass fibre quilt	0.040
Glass fibre slab	0.035
Mineral fibre slab	0.035
Phenolic foam	0.040
Polyurethane board	0.025
Urea formaldehyde foam	0.040

Source: Data reproduced from *CIBS Guide*, Volume A, by permission of the Chartered Institution of Building Services Engineers.

Fabric heat losses, H_f

There are well-established methods for determining the thermal properties of structures (CIBS, 1980) and for calculating fabric heat losses. These are widely documented and therefore will only be briefly dealt with here.

Thermal conductivity, k, *and resistivity,* r

Any individual material will have some thermal conductivity, normally known as its '*k* value' which is related to the thermal characteristics of the material, its area, its thickness and the temperature difference across the material. The reciprocal of thermal conductivity is thermal resistivity, r. Table 8.1 shows some typical k values for building materials.

Thermal resistance, R, *and transmittance,* U

Most building elements such as roofs, walls, windows and floors are not made of single materials, but are of composite construction, made up of layers of materials, often separated by air spaces. Figure 8.2, shows a typical wall construction with its various components.

Each individual component of the wall shown will have a resistance to heat flow, the individual components being subscripted, R_1, R_2, etc.

These resistances can be calculated from Equation (4) below.

$$R = l/k \tag{4}$$

where R = resistance of structural component, m^2KW^{-1}, l = thickness of structural component, m and k = thermal conductivity of material, $Wm^{-1}K^{-1}$.

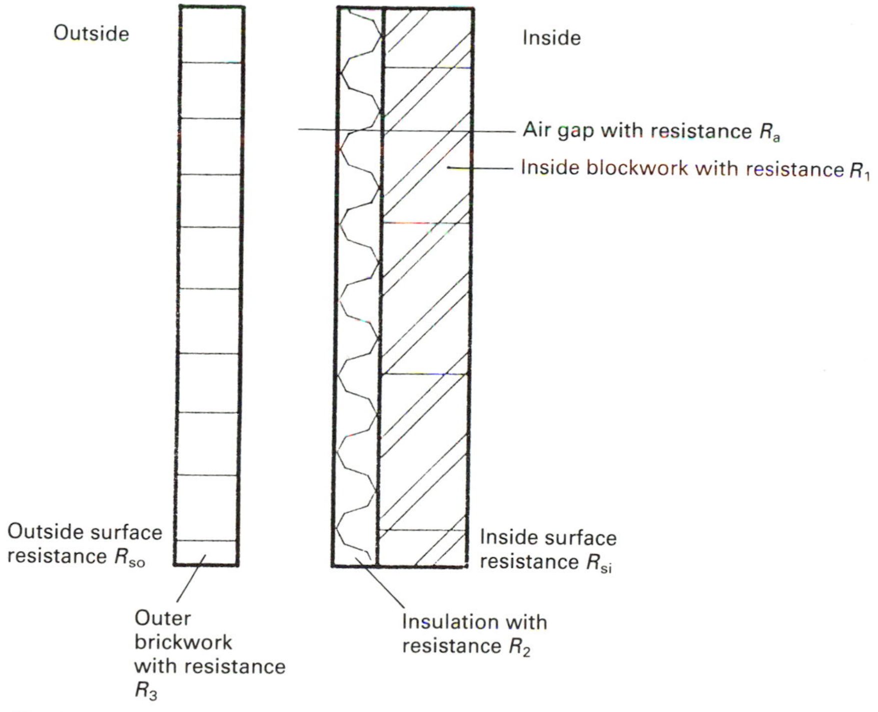

Fig. 8.2. Typical wall construction and its thermal resistances.

Table 8.2. Standard thermal resistance of ventilated airspaces.

Type of airspace (thickness 25 mm minimum)	Thermal resistances ($m^2K^{-1}W^{-1}$)
Airspace between asbestos cement or black metal cladding with unsealed joints, and high emissivity lining	0.16
Airspace between asbestos cement or black metal cladding with unsealed joints, and low emissivity surface facing airspace	0.30
Loft space between flat ceiling and unsealed asbestos cement sheets or black metal cladding pitched roof	0.14
Loft space between flat ceiling and pitched roof with aluminium cladding instead of black metal or low emissivity upper surface on ceiling	0.25
Loft space between flat ceiling and pitched roof lined with felt or building paper	0.18
Airspace between tiles and roofing felt or building paper	0.12
Airspace behind tiles on tile-hung wall*	0.12
Airspace in cavity wall construction	0.18

Source: Data reproduced from *CIBS Guide*, Volume A, by permission of the Chartered Institution of Building Services Engineers.

*For tile hung wall or roof, the value includes the resistance of the tile.

Table 8.3. Internal surface resistances, R_{si}.

		Surface resistance ($m^2K^{-1}W^{-1}$)	
Building element	Heat flow	High emissivity	Low emissivity
Walls	Horizontal	0.12	0.30
Ceilings or roofs, flat or pitched, floors	Upward	0.10	0.22
Ceilings and floors	Downward	0.14	0.55

Source: Data reproduced from *CIBS Guide*, Volume A, by permission of the Chartered Institution of Building Services Engineers.

Notes:
1. See original for exact calculation
2. Surface temperature is assumed to be 20°C
3. Air speed at the surface is assumed to be not greater than 0.1 m s^{-1}.

Table 8.4. External surface resistances, R_{so}.

Building element	Emissivity of surface	Surface resistance for stated exposure ($m^2K^{-1}W^{-1}$)		
		Sheltered	Normal	Severe
Wall	High	0.08	0.06	0.03
	Low	0.11	0.07	0.03
Roof	High	0.07	0.04	0.02
	Low	0.09	0.05	0.02

Source: Data reproduced from *CIBS Guide*, Volume A, by permission of the Chartered Institution of Building Services Engineers.

In addition there will be resistance to heat flow associated with the air space, R_a, due to the cavity in the construction, and with internal and external surfaces boundary layers of air, i.e. R_{si} and R_{so}. The surface resistances are influenced by the direction of heat flow, the emissivity of the surface and, in the case of external surface resistance, the exposure of the surface. The values associated with these particular air spaces and surfaces are not normally calculated but can be found from Tables 8.2, 8.3 and 8.4 (CIBS, 1980). All the resistances involved can be added together to give the total thermal resistance, R_t, of the particular structural element being considered. Thus the R_t value of the wall shown in Fig. 8.2 is given by

$$R_t = R_{si} + R_1 + R_2 + R_3 + R_{so} \text{ m}^2\text{KW}^{-1} \quad (5)$$

The reciprocal of this thermal resistance is thermal transmittance, U, thus

$$U = 1/R_t \text{ Wm}^{-2}\text{K}^{-1} \quad (6)$$

Both of the above terms are used to describe the heat transfer characteristics of building structural elements. In Europe, U value is commonly used while in other parts of the world R value may be preferred.

Special building elements

PITCHED ROOFS

For simple pitched roofs the U value is calculated normal to the slope of the roof. However, when there is a flat ceiling below the pitched roof then the U value must be determined with respect to the plane of the ceiling. This can be done as follows:

$$U_r = 1/[R_a \cos S + R_v + R_b] \quad (7)$$

where U_r = U value of roof, $W m^{-2} K^{-1}$, R_a = combined resistance of materials in the pitched part of the roof, including outside surface resistance, $m^2 K W^{-1}$, S = pitch angle of roof, degrees, R_v = resistance of roof void, $m^2 K W^{-1}$, R_b = combined resistance of materials in ceiling including inside surface resistance, $m^2 K W^{-1}$.

BRIDGED WALLS

The U value of some building elements cannot be calculated using the simple methods shown above. Walls may be built with mortar which has a different thermal conductivity to the walling unit (brick or block). Walls might have thermal bridges, such as steel lintels, columns or beams in their construction. In such cases, proportional area or combined methods are advocated (CIBS, 1980). These are too involved to describe here and are unlikely to be of great significance in livestock buildings.

GLAZING

Windows and other glazed elements may be single, double or triple glazed and may have different exposures. These factors affect their U value. In addition, the frame supporting such glazing can be of differing materials which will usually have different thermal properties to the glazing material. The frame might also comprise differing proportions of the glazed element. To simplify the determination of the U value of such differing window combinations, tables of U values for typical windows are often provided (CIBS, 1980).

FLOORS

The *CIBS Guide* (CIBS, 1980) sets out a procedure for calculating the U values of floors and it covers solid and insulated ground floors and suspended floors. It deals with floors with four or fewer exposed edges and gives tables of calculated U values and predicted reductions in floor heat losses due to the use of edge insulation.

More recently a procedure has been developed (Anderson, 1990) which simplifies these calculations, yet still gives good agreement with the *CIBS Guide* solutions for floors with areas in excess of $25 m^2$. This simplified procedure is outlined below.

1. Uninsulated ground floors

The heat loss from on-ground floor slabs, concrete raft, suspended timber and suspended beam and block floors can all be predicted by considering their area and perimeter length. The U value of the floor can be found from

$$U_f = 0.05 + 1.65(P/A) - 0.6(P/A)^2 \quad (8)$$

where U_f = U value of floor, $W m^{-2} K^{-1}$, P = perimeter length of floor measured inside boundary walls, m, A = area of floor measured inside the boundary walls, m^2, and it is assumed that: (i) the value of earth conductivity is $1.4 W m^{-1} K^{-1}$; (ii) the floor slab has the same conductivity; and (iii) the floor is surrounded by a 0.3m thick wall. These are also the normal assumptions in the *CIBS Guide* calculations.

Equation 8 can be applied without modification to floors with fewer than four exposed edges, the perimeter length, P, however, must only include exposed edges. It can also be applied to floors of irregular shapes.

2. Insulated ground floors
If floors are insulated by means of an insulating surface finish or a screed, then the U value can be determined by adding the thermal resistance of the insulating component, R_{ins}, to that of the floor, R_f (the reciprocal of the U_f value as determined in Equation (8) above) and taking their reciprocal. Thus

$$U_{inf} = 1/[1/R_f + R_{ins}] \qquad (9)$$

where U_{inf} = U value of insulated floor, $W m^{-2} K^{-1}$.

If the floor is insulated at the edge only (usually the most cost-effective method), then the U value can be determined by correcting the U_f value appropriately. Table 8.5 (CIBS, 1980) sets out the percentage reductions of U value that might be anticipated with various depths of edge insulation.

Total fabric loss, H_f

The total fabric loss from the building is determined from the individual U values and areas of the various building components. This is best done by

Table 8.5. Reduction in U_f of solid ground floors with edge insulation.

Floor dimension (m)	Percentage reduction in U_f for edge insulation extending to indicated depth	
	(0.5 m)	(1.0 m)
Very long × 40	7	11
Very long × 20	8	11
Very long × 10	9	14
60 × 60	11	17
40 × 40	12	18
20 × 20	13	19
10 × 10	14	22

Source: Data reproduced from *CIBS Guide*, Volume A, by permission of the Chartered Institution of Building Services Engineers.

Table 8.6. Building heat loss computation.

Building component	Area (m^2)	U Value ($Wm^{-2}K^{-1}$)	Component heat loss (WK^{-1})
Roof	650	0.35	227.5
Walls	300	0.45	135.0
Floor	600	0.3	180.0
Windows	10	5.0	50.0
Doors	15	1.2	18.0
Fabric heat loss factor, h_f			610.5

drawing up a simple table of components, their areas, U values and the component heat loss per unit temperature difference, i.e. the product of the component area and U value. A simple table to illustrate this is shown (Table 8.6) for a building with five components.

The advantage of such a table is that the heat loss through the various building components can be compared and judgements made about reducing the fabric heat loss. In the above example the roof obviously loses most heat: halving its heat loss would be much more beneficial than, say, halving the window heat loss.

The building heat loss factor, h_f, represents the total fabric loss per K temperature difference

$$h_f = \Sigma A_c U_c \tag{10}$$

where h_f = heat loss factor, WK^{-1}, A_c = area of building component, m^2, U_c = U value of building component, $Wm^{-2}K^{-1}$.

The total fabric heat loss, H_f, at any particular inside temperature will obviously vary with outside temperature. Thus

$$H_f = h_f(T_{ei} - T_{ao}) \tag{11}$$

where T_{ei} = inside environmental temperature, °C, T_{ao} = outdoor air temperature, °C.

The use of inside 'air' rather than 'environmental' temperature

In determining H_f, inside and outside air temperatures, T_{ai} and T_{ao}, are commonly used. However the *CIBS Guide* (CIBS, 1979b) recommends the use of T_{ei} not T_{ai}, to describe inside conditions, which in turn requires the determination of T_m and hence knowledge of the surface temperatures of the surrounding surface. Surface temperatures of the ceiling, walls, floor and other surfaces are usually unknown and the *CIBS Guide* (CIBS, 1979b) therefore recommends the use of temperature ratios. Two such ratios are used

$$F_1 = (T_{ei} - T_{ao})/(T_c - T_{ao})$$

and

$$F_2 = (T_{ai} - T_{ao})/(T_c - T_{ao})$$

where T_c is the dry resultant temperature (see below).

Values for F_1 and F_2 are tabulated for different types of heating systems, i.e. from fully convective systems, through various part convective/part radiant systems to effectively full radiant systems. The values of F_1 and F_2 vary with the mean U value of the building (the building fabric heat loss factor, h_f, divided by the total surface area) and the ventilation heat loss factor for the building expressed per unit area of the building surfaces. These factors are intended to compensate for the relationship between inside air and mean surface temperatures. This should ensure comfort at the centre of a space whatever heating system is used.

The value of T_{ei} required to provide comfort for humans, i.e. in terms of the dry resultant temperature, T_c, is defined as follows:

$$T_{ei} = F_1(T_c - T_{ao}) + T_{ao}$$

The methodology, while it has been severely criticized, notably by Davies (1986, 1988a, b), has been widely adopted for design purposes. The first question that arises from the above discussion is, 'Can the concept of comfort as described by T_c be used for animals as well as humans?' This is unlikely, since no values of T_c have been postulated for farm animals in livestock buildings. While Monteith and Unsworth (1990) have described the concept of 'apparent equivalent temperature' for animals, it is different from dry resultant temperature and they have not suggested how values can be determined for differing species and circumstances. Therefore, comfort needs for animals are likely to be described in terms of air temperature for some time to come. Such air temperatures may well be evaluated on the basis of the animal's metabolic rate, air speed over the animal, floor type, group size and other such factors.

The second question that arises is, 'How appropriate are the methods described above if T_{ai} is used instead of T_{ei}?' The probability is that the methods will be appropriate in some circumstances and much less appropriate in others. For well-insulated, windowless, lightweight structures, with low internal air speeds, with relative humidities in the range 40–70% humidity and no use of radiant heating then the use of T_{ai} to describe internal requirements is probably satisfactory. However, for poorly insulated, heavyweight structures, with windows, high air speeds and radiant heating, then the use of T_{ai} may be totally inappropriate. These questions still need to be resolved for livestock buildings. In the meantime most people will continue to determine the total fabric heat loss, H_f, from a building by using Equation (12).

$$H_f = h_f[T_{ai} - T_{ao}] \qquad (12)$$

Holmes (1988) in a comparison of the various inside temperatures to calculate steady state heat losses concluded that the use of dry resultant temperature, T_{ei}, would give similar results to using air temperature, T_{ai}.

Longwave radiation heat loss, H_{rad}

Buildings can lose heat by longwave radiation from external surfaces of buildings to the sky, ground and other buildings. This loss depends on cloud cover, dry bulb temperature, orientation of the surface and the nature of the external environment.

In the derivation of sol-air temperature (see above), this longwave radiation component from roofs is determined by taking the radiation loss from a horizontal black surface to a cloudless sky ($100\,W\,m^{-2}$ for UK conditions), and multiplying it by the emissivity of the outer surface (0.9 for most surfaces) and the external surface resistance of the roof. For vertical walls the longwave radiation loss is taken as being equal to that received from the ground and other buildings, thus the net effect is zero loss. Therefore, using sol-air temperatures to evaluate building fabric heat exchange will inherently estimate longwave radiation losses, since sol-air temperatures lower than outside air temperature will result at night on horizontal surfaces. Alternatively the *CIBS Guide* (CIBS, 1982, Section A2, p. 69) suggests the longwave radiation loss, I_l can be determined by the following simplified relationships

For a horizontal surface $I_l = 93 - 79\,C$

For a vertical surface $I_l = 21 - 17\,C$

where C = cloudiness factor (varies monthly – see Table 8.7).

Table 8.7. Cloudiness factor for UK conditions.

Month	Cloudiness
June	0.14
July & May	0.18
August & April	0.23
September & March	0.27
October & February	0.31
November & January	0.35
December	0.40

Ventilation heat loss

When outside air is used to ventilate livestock buildings, it is generally at a lower temperature than the inside air. Consequently, such ventilation removes heat from the building as cold air comes in, while warm air goes out. This ventilation heat loss can represent a major part of the heat loss from buildings, particularly if the buildings are leaky or ventilation rate is poorly controlled. The heat loss due to ventilation can be determined as follows

$$H_v = M_v\, C_p(T_{ai} - T_{ao})$$

where H_v = ventilation heat loss, W (J s^{-1}), M_v = ventilation rate in kg s^{-1}, C_p = specific heat of air J kg^{-1} K^{-1}. For normal design purposes, by incorporating typical values for the density and specific heat of air and describing ventilation rate in m^{3}h^{-1} rather than kg s^{-1}, the following simplified form of the above equation is used.

$$H_v = 1/3\ V(T_{ai} - T_{ao}) \tag{13}$$

where H_v = ventilation heat loss, W, V = ventilation rate, m^{3}h^{-1}.

Solar heat gain, H_{sol}

The heat gain to buildings due to solar radiation is mainly of concern in the summer when the temperature rise must be limited. Solar gain will occur either via the glazing (uncommon in animal houses), H_w, or via the fabric, H_f, and both need to be considered. In buildings occupied by people there might be large window areas and the heat gain through these can be greatly in excess of that through the fabric. Therefore, traditional methods evaluate window gain and fabric gain separately when assessing cooling loads (CIBS, 1979b). These losses are then added together to give the total solar heat gain. Thus

$$H_{sol} = H_w + H_f \tag{14}$$

Heat gain through windows, H_w

A simple methodology is outlined in the *CIBS Guide* for evaluating H_w, based on tables which have been prepared for direct use. These refer to buildings having single clear glass with and without white, internal, venetian blinds. Tables are given for specified conditions in the UK (51.7°N) and other latitudes. The conditions are as follows:

(a) *Building* – lightweight construction, with de-mountable partitions, suspended ceilings, solid carpeted or wood block floors or suspended floors.
(b) *Plant Operation* – 10 hours per day, i.e 0800 to 1800 hours sun time.

Table 8.8. Cooling load due to solar gain through vertical glazing, $W m^{-2}$ (10 hour plant operation).

Date	Climatic constants	Orientation	Sun time						Orientation
			0800	1000	1200	1400	1600	1800	
June 21	$I = 0.66$	N	81	114	138	137	111	122	N
	$k_c = 1.96$	E	328	254	88	151	125	89	E
	$k_r = 0.20$	S	102	179	238	197	89	61	S
	$C = 0.14$	W	78	114	139	227	314	274	W
July 23 and May 22	$I = 0.89$	N	85	128	157	156	125	86	N
	$k_c = 1.33$	E	306	250	90	167	136	93	E
	$k_r = 0.20$	S	75	194	252	212	59	68	S
	$C = 0.18$	W	80	123	152	222	293	239	W
August 24 and April 22	$I = 0.93$	N	59	102	131	129	100	58	N
	$k_c = 1.34$	E	277	229	71	138	108	65	E
	$k_r = 0.20$	S	118	212	272	231	111	52	S
	$C = 0.23$	W	59	102	130	207	273	177	W
September 22 and March 21	$I = 0.97$	N	32	76	104	102	73	29	N
	$k_c = 1.61$	E	427	220	52	104	75	31	E
	$k_r = 0.20$	S	137	262	333	285	137	48	S
	$C = 0.27$	W	31	75	103	201	258	43	W
October 23 and February 21	$I = 1.18$	N	10	53	81	80	50	8	N
	$k_c = 1.31$	E	136	170	37	80	49	7	E
	$k_r = 0.20$	S	78	241	313	264	108	10	S
	$C = 0.31$	W	9	52	81	159	158	21	W

November 21 and January 21	$I = 1.29$	N	4	28	55	54	25	4	N
	$k_c = 1.34$	E	7	120	103	55	26	5	E
	$k_r = 0.20$	S	6	198	284	226	30	5	S
	$C = 0.35$	W	5	29	56	192	28	5	W
December 21	$I = 1.18$	N	3	16	40	39	14	3	N
	$k_c = 1.70$	E	5	177	85	41	16	5	E
	$k_r = 0.20$	S	5	267	273	206	26	5	S
	$C = 0.40$	W	3	17	41	160	20	3	W

Correction factors for tabulated values

Type of glass (outside pane for double glazing)	Building weight	Single glazing			Double glazing, internal shade			Double glazing, mid-pane shade		
		Light slatted blind		Linen roller blind	Light slatted blind		Linen roller blind	Light slatted blind		Linen roller blind
		Open	Closed		Open	Closed		Open	Closed	
Clear 6 mm	Light	1.00	0.77	0.66	0.95	0.74	0.65	0.58	0.39	0.42
	Heavy	0.97	0.77	0.63	0.94	0.76	0.64	0.56	0.40	0.40
Additional factor for air point control	Light	0.91	0.91	0.91	0.91	0.91	0.91	0.80	0.80	0.80
	Heavy	0.83	0.83	0.83	0.90	0.90	0.90	0.78	0.78	0.78

Source: Data reproduced from *CIBS Guide*, Volume A, by permission of the Chartered Institution of Building Services Engineers.

(c) *Sunshine* – four to five days sunny spell.
(d) *Climate Factors* – direct and diffuse radiation, ground reflectance and cloudiness factors are assumed for the UK and other latitudes.

The tables show the calculated cooling load through vertical glazing for various orientations at different sun times for different months. Correction factors are included in the tables to allow for other types of glazing, building weight and various types of blinds. An additional factor is also shown for use if internal air temperature is used, rather than internal environmental temperature in any assessment of cooling load. Table 8.8 is a partial example of the tables.

Using Table 8.8, the solar gain at mid-day (1200 hours) in a lightweight building in late August through a south facing, 5 m² window with clear 6 mm, double glazing, with closed, internal, light slatted blinds, is calculated as follows:

$$H_w = 272 \times 0.74 \times 5 = 1006.4\,\mathrm{W}$$

This solar gain will impinge on the comfort of a human occupant both as radiation from the blinds and as increased air temperature, due to convective transfer to the room air. If expressed in terms of convective transfer to the air then the amount of heat transferred to the air would now be reduced to 1033.6 × the additional factor for 'air point' control, i.e. 0.90. Obviously the total heat gain through glazing would be the sum of that through all glazing. The heat gain via unglazed walls or roofs elements is determined in exactly the same way as fabric losses. However, to determine solar gain, instead of using T_{ao} in Equation (11), the sol-air temperature, T_{eo}, is used instead. However since T_{eo} will have different values for surfaces with different orientations then:

$$H_f = \Sigma A_c U_c (T_{ei} - T_{eoc}) \tag{15}$$

where T_{eoc} = sol-air temperature pertaining to component, °C. Consequently in summer conditions, surfaces with high values of T_{eoc} will have a negative heat loss, i.e. a heat gain.

Dynamic Heat Transfer

Since outside climate is changing all the time, both seasonally and diurnally, steady state conditions are rarely a true description of the performance of a building. In the lightweight structures often used for housing livestock, variations in outside conditions can elicit a very rapid change in internal conditions. For example, changes in outside temperature will cause a rapid change in inside temperature when high ventilation rates are used.

While the assumption of steady state conditions is normally acceptable for determining plant size, i.e. maximum heating or cooling requirements, such an assumption does not suffice when considering the extremes of temperature that might occur in a building. As well as climate, the intermittent operation of plant and intermittent occupancy of buildings will contribute to the dynamic nature of a building's performance. In hot conditions particular problems can arise if there is a failure of mechanical ventilation systems or when calm conditions occur, when wind driven natural ventilation systems are being used. If ventilation is reduced it can lead to a rapid rise in internal temperatures. To predict the response of buildings to such circumstances requires an analysis of the dynamic response of the building. Such analyses are feasible, but are beyond the scope of this chapter. Those interested in pursuing this topic are referred to Milbank and Harrington-Lynn (1974) and the *CIBS Guide* (CIBS, 1979a).

Moisture Transfer

Moisture in livestock buildings is important for a number of reasons (see Chapter 1). In respect of structures and materials the main importance is related to the condensation of moisture on surfaces (surface condensation) or within the structure (interstitial condensation). Such condensation can lead to deterioration of the structure due to corrosion, rotting, swelling, warping and other such effects. It can also cause problems by dripping on to animals, their bedding or lying area.

Air moisture indices

Air which is said to be *dry* contains no moisture at all, conversely air which is said to be *saturated* cannot hold any more moisture. Since the amount of moisture air can hold depends upon its temperature, then air will have some *saturation temperature* at which it is completely saturated. As the temperature of air rises then it can hold more moisture and as it cools it can hold less. When air is cooled there comes a point when it can no longer hold moisture and the moisture will start to appear as dew, or perhaps, more familiarly as condensation on some cold surface. The temperature at which this occurs is known as the *dew point temperature,* at which the air is saturated.

The amount of moisture in air can be described in a variety of ways, the most obvious being *moisture content* in kg moisture per kg of dry air; this is also known as 'absolute humidity' or 'humidity ratio'. The term *percentage saturation* can also be used to describe the moisture content of air, this being the mass of moisture in air expressed as a percentage of its moisture content (by mass) when saturated and at the same temperature. Associated with the increasing moisture content of air there will be an increasing *water vapour pressure,* i.e. that part of atmospheric pressure due to the vapour component in the air. This is sometimes known as partial water vapour pressure. The use of water vapour pressure to describe the amount of moisture in air leads to the most common term used to describe the moisture condition of air, i.e. *relative humidity*. Relative humidity is given by

$$RH = 100\ p_v/p_s$$

where RH = relative humidity of air, %, p_v = vapour pressure of air at temperature t, Pa, p_s = saturated vapour pressure of air at temperature t, Pa. Relative humidity and percentage saturation are often confused, having very similar numerical values.

Table 8.9. Vapour resistivities of common building materials.

Material	Typical vapour resistivity ($MNs\,g^{-1}m^{-1}$)
Airgap	5
Blockwork:	
lightweight	30
medium weight	50
heavyweight	100
Brickwork: common/facing	50
Cast concrete:	
lightweight	40
dense	200
no fines	20
Chipboard	500
Fibre board	40
Fibre cement: sheet	300
Fibre: glass or mineral	7
Hardboard	600
Phenolic foam: closed cell	300
Plaster	60
Plasterboard	60
Polystyrene:	
expanded bead	300
expanded extruded	1000
Polyurethane: foam – closed cell	600
Plywood:	
sheathing	450
decking	2000
Timber	60
Urea formaldehyde	15
Wood wool slab	20

Source: Adapted from BSI, 1989.

Moisture movement

Moisture movement is driven by vapour pressure and moisture will move from high to low vapour pressure regions. Resistance to vapour movement will be caused by any boundaries through which vapour must move. In buildings such boundaries are the walls, roofs, floors, etc. Their resistance to vapour movement will be largely dictated by the materials used in their construction. Some materials will be quite specifically selected to prevent water and vapour movement, i.e. damp proof courses and damp proof membranes.

Vapour permeability and resistivity

The mass of water vapour moving through a material is described by a material's *vapour permeability, d,* with units kg m$N^{-1}s^{-1}$. Vapour resistivity is simply the reciprocal of vapour permeability. Table 8.9 lists the vapour resistivity for common building materials and components.

Vapour transmittance and resistance

There is a direct analogy between vapour and thermal resistances and transmittances. For any single material in a construction the vapour resistance is given by:

$$G_v = l/d \tag{16}$$

where G_v = vapour resistance, Nskg^{-1}, l = thickness of material, m, d = vapour permeability of material, kgm$N^{-1}.s^{-1}$. The total vapour resistance, G_t, of a composite structure made of n different materials is given by

$$G_t = G_{v1} + G_{v2} + G_{v3} \ldots + G_{vn} \tag{17}$$

The rate of vapour movement, Q_v, through area, A, of such a composite structure with an internal vapour pressure p_{vi} and an external vapour pressure p_{vo} is given by:

$$Q_v = A(p_{vi} - p_{vo})/G_t \tag{18}$$

where Q_v = rate of vapour transmission, kgs^{-1}, A = area of construction, m^2. Table 8.10 gives vapour resistances of some typical vapour barriers.

Temperature and vapour pressure gradients in structures

Temperature gradients

In the wall structure illustrated in Fig. 8.3, there is a temperature drop from the air inside the building to the outside air. There will also be a temperature

Table 8.10. Vapour resistances of typical vapour barriers.

Material	Typical vapour resistance ($MNs\,g^{-1}$)
Aluminium foil	1,000
Asphalt	10,000
Building paper, bituminized	10
Glass	10,000
Metal claddings	10,000
Polyester film	250
Polyethylene	
500 gauge	250
1,000 gauge	500
Roofing felt in bitumen	1,000
Vapour resistant paint	250

Source: Adapted from BSI, 1989.

drop from the inside air to the inside wall surface, from the inside wall surface to the inner surface of the cavity, from the inner to the outer surface of the cavity, and so on. These various temperature drops are in proportion to the thermal resistance of the elements across which they are measured and the rate of heat loss through the wall H_l.

From Fig. 8.3, since the heat loss H_l flows through all components of the structure, it can be seen that the following set of equations all equate to H_l.

$$\begin{aligned} H_l &= (T_{ai} - T_{ao}) \times U \\ &= (T_{ai} - T_{ao}) \times 1/(R_{si} + R_1 + R_a + R_2 + R_{so}) \\ &= (T_{si} - T_{ao}) \times 1/(R_1 + R_a + R_2 + R_{so}) \\ &= (T_1 - T_{ao}) \times 1/(R_a + R_2 + R_{so}) \\ &= (T_2 - T_{ao}) \times 1/(R_2 + R_{so}) \\ &= (T_{so} - T_{ao}) \times 1/(R_{so}) \end{aligned}$$

Thus knowing U and the various resistances from which it is made up, then any of the surface interface temperatures can be predicted for different inside and outside conditions. For example if one wishes to find T_1 then from:

$$[(T_1 - T_{ao}) \times 1/(R_a + R_2 + R_{so})] = H_1 = [(T_{ai} - T_{ao}) \times U]$$
$$T_1 = [(T_{ai} - T_{ao})(R_a + R_2 + R_{so})U] + T_{ao}$$

Vapour pressure gradients

Referring to Fig. 8.3, just like temperature gradients in structures there will

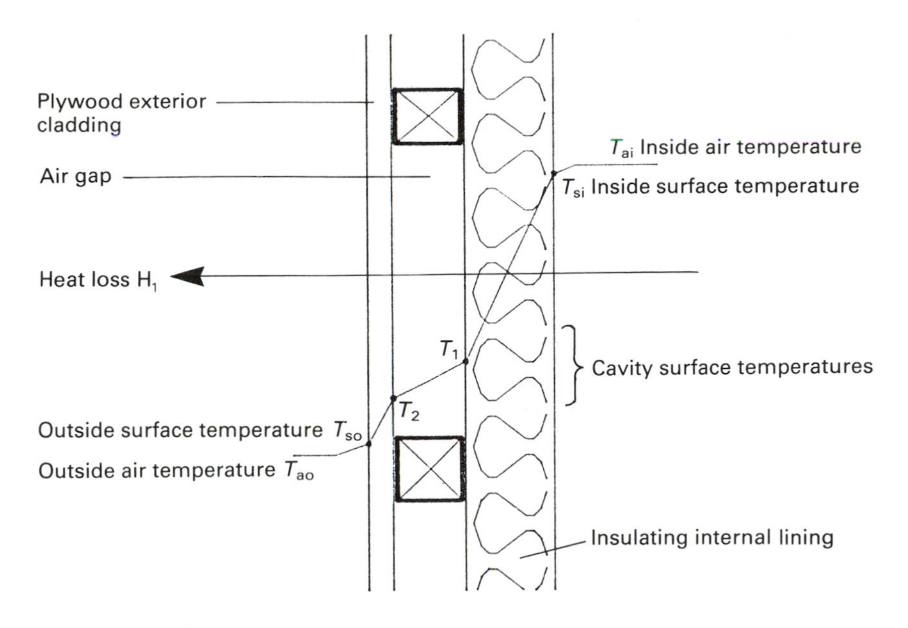

Fig. 8.3. Temperature gradient across a wall construction.

also be vapour pressure gradients. These will be dictated by the vapour pressure across the structure and the vapour resistances of the constructional elements. Thus for the wall shown in Fig. 8.3, with a vapour resistance G_1 for the inner leaf and G_2 for the outer leaf, the rate of vapour transmission, Q_v, is given by:

$$Q_v = A(p_{vi} - p_{vo})/(G_1 + G_2)$$
$$= A(p_{v1} - p_{vo})/G_2$$

where p_{v1} = vapour pressure in cavity of wall, Pa. The analysis is similar to that for predicting temperature gradients; however, it should be noted that the vapour resistances of air boundaries and gaps are negligible, unlike their thermal resistances.

Assessment of condensation risk

It is most important to be able to predict condensation problems before they arise, so that preventive measures can be taken at an early stage. Solving condensation problems after moulds, rots, deterioration and damage have occurred is often fraught with difficulties. Too little attention has been given to condensation in the past, as is evidenced by the high incidence of condensation problems found in all sorts of buildings. Despite the widespread knowledge of condensation problems and of the fundamental psychrometrics and heat transfer mechanisms involved, as recently as 1989, it has been found necessary to produce a British Standard, BS 5250 (BSI, 1989) to give guidance on solving the problem. In BS 5250 graphical methods are illustrated for assessing condensation risk and advice is given on tackling condensation problems. The BS 5250 methods will not be discussed here.

Surface condensation risk

This is the most obvious sort of problem, since it can be readily observed. The calculations involved in its prediction or in designing solutions to surface condensation are relatively simple. The needs are:

1. To establish outside design conditions. For the UK, BS 5250 (BSI, 1989) suggests: average outside air temperature, T_{ao}, 5°C; average outside relative humidity, RH_o, 95%; average outside vapour pressure, p_{vo}, 0.83kPA.
2. To establish the worst inside design condition, i.e. the highest inside relative humidity, RH_i, likely to occur at the internal design dry bulb temperature/temperatures, T_{ai}, likely to be maintained.
3. To establish the dew point temperature, T_{wi}, of the inside air at temperature, T_{ai}, and relative humidity, RH_i using a psychrometric chart or tables (CIBS, 1975).
4. To establish the U values of the structural elements, in particular those that have the highest values, such as cold bridges formed by wall columns, lintels, roof beams, etc.
5. To establish the surface temperatures of building elements, T_{si}, by the method shown above;
6. To compare T_{wi} and T_{si}; and then conclude that if $T_{wi} \geqslant T_{si}$ that condensation should occur; or if $T_{wi} < T_{si}$ that condensation should not occur.

If the conclusion is that condensation should occur then improvements in the insulation (U value) or reduction in internal relative humidity must be considered.

Interstitial condensation risk

This problem is far less obvious and might not become apparent until major damage has been caused to a structure or the materials of construction. Because the assessment of risk is more complex than for surface condensation it is often neglected. The consequent problems, e.g. the occurrence of dry rot in buildings, can be very costly to remedy. The calculation procedure is as follows:

1. and **2.** As in (1) and (2) above.
3. Calculate all interface temperatures, T_1, as shown on page 206.

4. Calculate all interface vapour pressures, p_{vI}, as shown on page 207.
5. Using psychrometric tables determine the saturation vapour pressure of air at the various interface temperatures, p_{sI}.
6. Compare the values of p_{vI} and p_{sI}; and then conclude that if $p_{vI} \geqslant p_{sI}$ that condensation should occur at the interface; or if $p_{vI} < p_{sI}$ that condensation should not occur at the interface.

It should be remembered that interstitial condensation might not occur at the interface between materials, it can occur within materials. Graphical methods might prove best to analyse such situations, as described in the *CIBS Guide* (CIBS, 1986) and in BS 5502.

The amount of water that will condense on surfaces or interstitially is obviously of importance. The rate of water deposition will be related to the coincidence of the outside and inside conditions which lead to condensation and the duration of such coincident conditions. Such an appraisal can only be made if one is armed with full meteorological data. Wathes (1981) calculates that the amount of water that will be deposited due to interstitial condensation in livestock buildings is negligible.

Structures for Climate Modification

The types of structures used to modify the climate to which animals are exposed fall into three broad categories: simple shelter, climatic housing, and controlled environment housing. These categories represent very different structural forms, materials and methods of construction.

Simple shelter

This is used in applications where little more needs to be done, or can afford to be done, than to provide animals with the simplest type of protection, principally from wind and sunshine.

Windbreaks

Simple shelter from wind may be sufficient to ensure that some animals can flourish in otherwise unmodified climates. For extensive systems of grazing, or indeed for yarded animals, advantage may be taken of existing landscape features to shelter animals. An understanding of the wind flow likely to occur around natural features, e.g. hills, woods and hedges, can assist in deciding where to locate yards or corrals to take advantage of the protection such features can offer.

Alternatively, special windbreaks can be formed by deliberately planting trees and shrubs or by erecting artificial windbreaks. Caborn

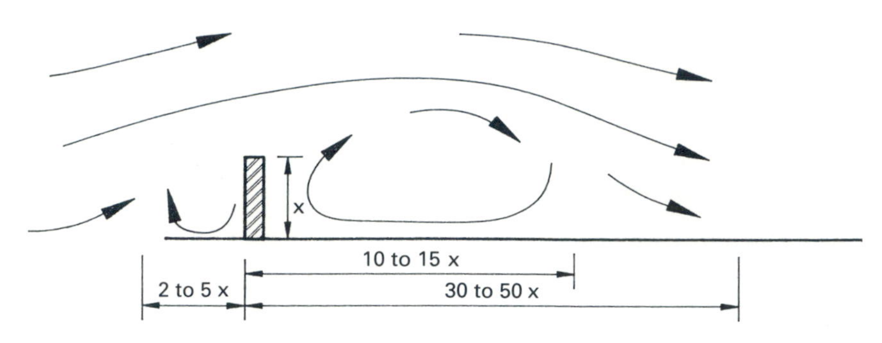

Fig. 8.4. Characteristic airflow pattern caused by a solid wind barrier (after Caborn, 1965).

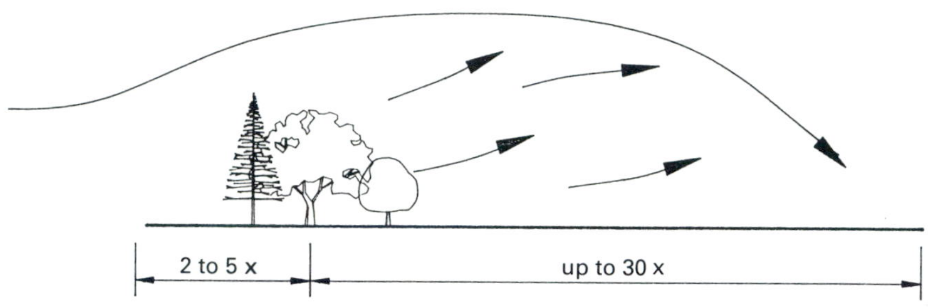

Fig. 8.5. Airflow pattern caused by a permeable wind barrier (x = height of barrier) (after Caborn, 1965).

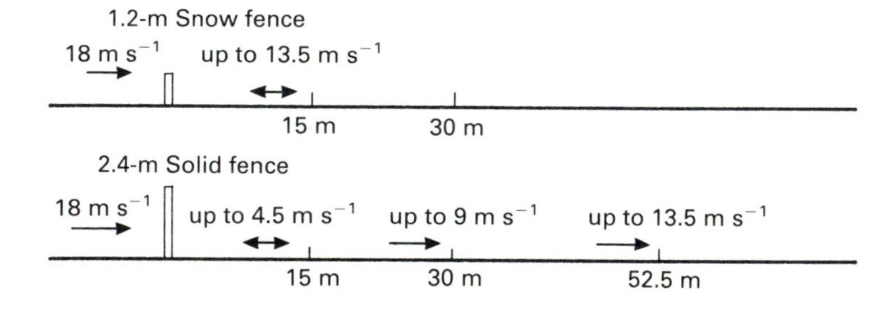

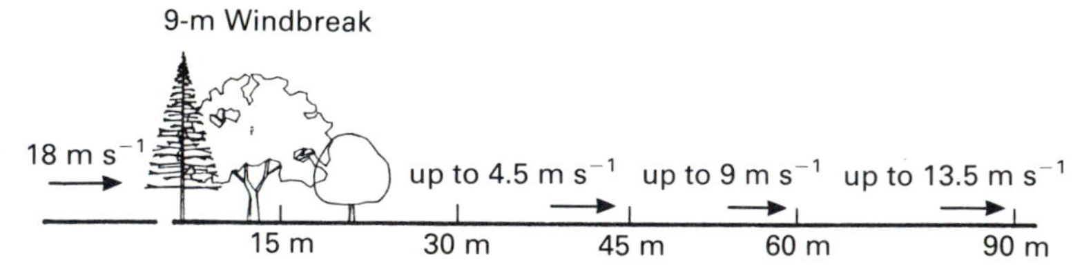

Fig. 8.6. Wind speeds that can occur in the lee of different types of wind breaks (from Boyd, 1973).

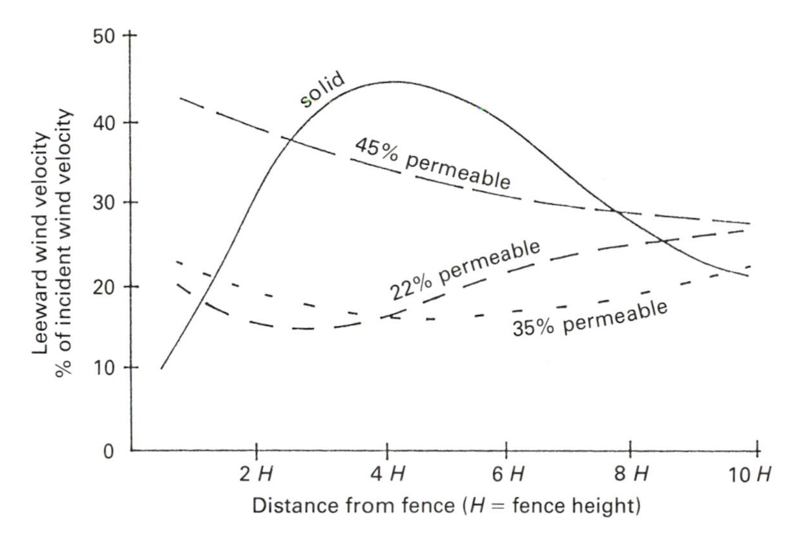

Fig. 8.7. Velocity reduction for fences of different densities (from Moysey and McPherson, 1966, in Darby, 1971).

(1965), Darby (1971), Boyd (1973) discussed the use of various forms of windbreaks, their effectiveness and airflows and speeds associated with them. Figures 8.4 and 8.5 indicate the different effects of solid and permeable wind barriers on airflow. Figures 8.6 and 8.7 indicate the speeds that might be anticipated in the lee of such windbreaks. Permeable windbreaks which allow some movement of air through the barrier, appear to be best since the high air speeds associated with solid barriers can be avoided. More recently, interest has centred on the use of windbreaks to reduce wind damage to horticultural crops and greenhouses (MAFF, 1979) and in reducing energy use in structures (Finbow, 1988; BRE, 1990). The publications cited can provide useful information which can be applied to the design of windbreaks for livestock.

Artificial windbreaks can be constructed in a variety of ways and various materials can be used to form permeable shelters. Materials can range from spaced boards to modern plastic materials in the form of nets or perforated sheets. These will be discussed later in relation to cladding of openings in climatic housing (see page 220).

Shade

In some climates, it might prove essential to protect animals from sunshine. In temperate climates, light-coloured pigs might get sunburnt outdoors. In hot climates shade might be needed by cattle to give relief from the combined effects of sunshine and high temperatures. There is little doubt

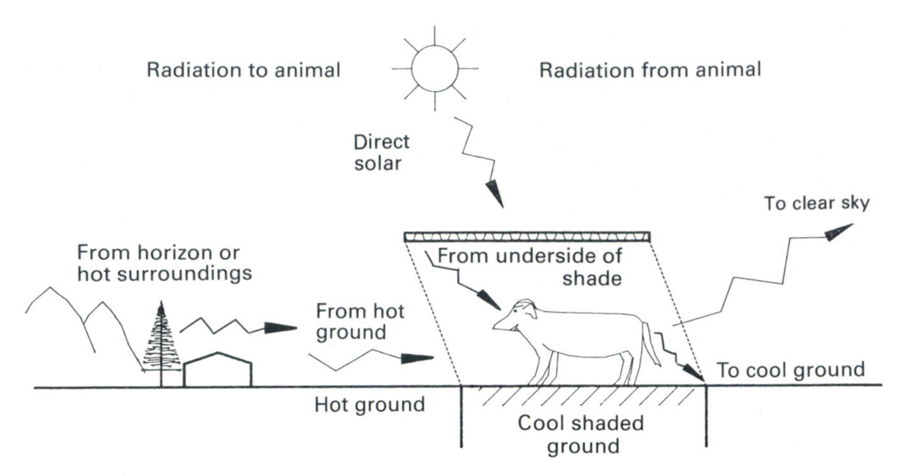

Fig. 8.8. Major paths of radiation heat exchange to be considered in the design of shades.

that shade is beneficial to all animals exposed to both high temperatures and high solar radiation. Most of the early work on shade for animals was done in California in the late 1940s and 1950s, e.g. Kelly and Ittner (1950), Kelly *et al.* (1957), Kelly and Bond (1958) and Bond *et al.* (1954, 1966). Later work has quantified effects on animal surfaces (see Chapter 5).

Figure 8.8 shows the major paths of radiation heat exchange between an animal and its surrounds when under a shade. The major consideration involved in the provision of shade are:

1. *Size of shadow.* The shadow must cover an area of ground of sufficient size to shade all the animals. Shade height will not affect the size of the shadow, but the slope of a monopitch shade might and therefore shallow slopes should be provided.
2. *Location of shade.* The shadow must cover an area of ground to which the animals have access. Animals must not be confined in such a way that they are prevented from occupying the shaded area, which will of course move during the day.
3. *Shade orientation.* The shadow beneath a shade with its long axis North–South will move over a greater area of ground than a shadow beneath a shade with its long axis East–West. The advantage of the N–S orientation is that most of the ground beneath the shade will be in sunlight for some part of the day, which will help dry up any faeces and urine. The advantage of the E–W orientation is that some of the ground beneath the shade will be permanently in the shadow and will therefore remain cooler. There are differing opinions about the best orientation, which might be dictated by the need to consider the direction of prevailing wind for cooling and ventilation purposes.

4. *Shade materials.* When a shade of any material or construction intercepts the direct solar radiation it will heat up. If the lower side of the material or construction becomes hot it will then radiate heat to the animals below. To prevent high temperatures on the underside of the shade is simply a matter of insulating the top from the bottom. It has been suggested that further advantage may be gained by making the top surface reflective (but how long it will stay so is a matter of conjecture), the bottom surface absorptive and picking materials which allow free airflow through or around them to enhance convective cooling of the shade.

The effectiveness, compared with new aluminium sheeting, of a variety of shade materials treated in different ways was measured by Kelly and Bond (1958). The results of their measurements are shown in Table 8.11. These measurements clearly demonstrate the benefits of insulation (note the figures for hay and polyethylene with an air gap), the marginal advantage that can be gained from an upper reflective surface (note the figures for white top aluminium and steel) and an absorptive lower surface (note the figures for black bottom aluminium) and the advantage of combining both (note the figures for white top, black bottom, aluminium and steel). A variety of materials and construction, from simple pole frames thatched with palm fronds to prefabricated metal frames with sheet cladding, can be used to form shades. Often the choice will be dictated by the cost and availability of materials and the other requirements of the roof, e.g. the need to be weatherproof. Natural shade provided by trees can be utilized when available. Trees can intercept a considerable amount of direct radiation, the amount varying with the amount of leaf on the tree. Deciduous trees can provide shading which varies with season. Table 8.12 indicates the order of magnitude of solar radiation passing through the canopies of some common deciduous tree species.

Climatic housing

Climatic housing is more sophisticated than simple shelter in that generally it is a properly constructed building which is weatherproof, i.e. it allows animals to be kept in dry and relatively draught-free conditions. Such buildings may or may not be insulated, will generally be naturally ventilated and do not have heating or cooling systems. No attempt is made to control inside air temperature which, while it will be modified by the structure, will follow the general pattern of outside temperature. Such housing is generally suited to ruminants, although pigs and poultry (particularly turkeys) are sometimes kept in such housing. Often the reason for housing the animals will be related to other aspects of the production system rather than a need to protect the animals from the outdoor climate. For example, in the UK, dairy cows may be winter housed to prevent poaching of grazing areas while

Table 8.11. Effectiveness of shade materials and treatments compared with new corrugated aluminium.

Material	Treatment	Effectiveness
Aluminium	Top white, bottom black	1.103
	Top natural, bottom black	1.09
	Top white, bottom natural	1.049
	Standard, untreated	1.00
	1 year old, untreated	0.994
	10 years old, untreated	0.969
Asbestos	3 mm sheet, natural	0.956
Hardboard	3 mm sheet, natural	0.942
Hay	150 mm thickness	1.203
Neoprene	Top aluminium, bottom black	1.022
	Black, thin	0.944
	Black, thick	0.933
Paper	Building, aluminium coated	0.95
Plywood	9.5 mm, top white, bottom natural	1.031
	9.5 mm, untreated	1.03
	6 mm, untreated	1.03
Polyethylene	Black film, double skinned, 50 mm air gap	1.036
	Laminated, top white, bottom black	1.028
	Black film	0.868
	Translucent film	0.774
Shade cloth	92% solid	0.926
	90% solid	0.839
Snow fence	Double layer, no openings	0.933
	Double layer, criss-crossed	0.823
	Single layer	0.589
Steel	Galvanized, top white, bottom black	1.066
	Galvanized, top white, bottom natural	1.053
	Galvanized, new, untreated	0.992
	Galvanized, 1 year old, untreated	0.985
Wood louvres	Natural	1.06
	Top natural, bottom black	1.042
	Top black, bottom black	0.97

Source: Adapted from Kelly and Bond, 1958.

Table 8.12. Solar radiation passing through the canopies of trees.

Common name	% Radiation passing	
	Full leaf	Bare branch
Elm	15	65
English oak	20	70
European ash	15	55
European beech	10	80
European birch	20	60
Horse chestnut	10	60
Lime	10	60
Silver maple	15	65
Sycamore	25	65

Source: Adapted from BRE, 1990.

ewes might be housed to enable better supervision and management of lambing. Alternatively, the building might provide better conditions than the animals require, simply because the farmer wishes to provide a better working environment for himself or his employees.

Natural ventilation

Good ventilation is of paramount importance in climatic housing, with ruminants particularly prone to respiratory ailments if good ventilation is not achieved. The basis of design of natural ventilation systems is discussed elsewhere (Chapter 7), the basic need being to provide adequately sized and located opening (inlets and outlets) in the building to allow sufficient ventilation by employing wind or thermal (stack) effects. Associated with the need to provide adequate areas of inlets and outlets is the need to prevent excessive air velocities inside the building.

The discussion here will be limited to the materials and methods that can be employed to construct inlets and outlets and to limit internal air velocities. Openings will generally need to be provided at high (outlets) and lower levels (inlets) in buildings. The size of openings required will vary considerably depending upon the species being housed, the density of stocking and the particular climatic region. The provisions that need to be made can vary from small discrete inlets and outlets to large areas of outlets at the ridge and sidewalls that can open up completely. There are numerous ways of satisfying the requirements, in fact almost every farmer will do it differently. Therefore, here are a few proven methods which can be adapted for particular circumstances.

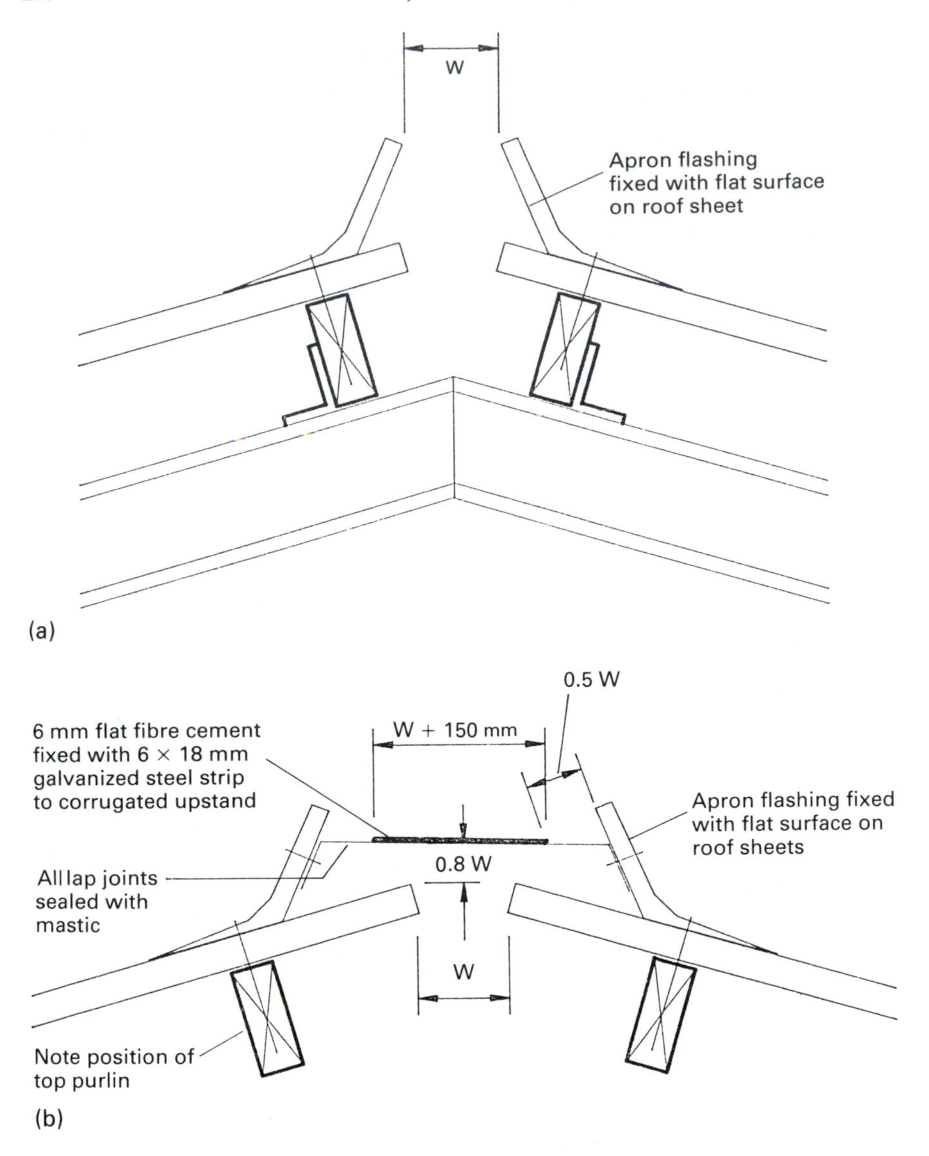

Fig. 8.9. Ridge air outlets: (a) Venturi ridge; (b) Weatherproof ridge (from Bruce, 1978). The total width, W, of the outlet is calculated from the total area of opening (see Chapter 7).

ROOF AIR OUTLETS

Ridge outlets In climates where relatively small areas of outlet will suffice, one can usually consider using horizontal openings in the roof of buildings as air outlets. It is convenient to place these in the ridge of double-pitch roofs and a variety of designs has evolved over the years. Dwybad *et al.*

(1974) and Bruce (1972, 1975) have investigated the performance of such openings. Their conclusions can be summarized as follows:

1. The simpler the design the less resistance to airflow and hence better ventilation.
2. Upstands can help prevent driven rain entry through roof openings, particularly on low pitched roofs.
3. Ridge caps increase the probability of entry of wind-driven rain and can become blocked with snow.
4. The wind pressure coefficient at the ridge is virtually unaffected by simple ridge outlet designs.

Concern about the entry of precipitation has led to many complex ridge ventilator designs, many of which simply inhibit ventilation or cause other problems. Figure 8.9(a) shows a simple design of ridge outlet and Fig. 8.9(b) an arrangement which is said to eliminate rain and snow entry.

Monitor roof outlets In hot climates large openings may be required at a high level and horizontal openings are not feasible. In such cases a monitor roof is often built to allow large vertical openings to be formed at a high level. The vertical opening can then be fitted with shutters, blinds or rotating flaps which allow the opening size to be adjusted. Figure 8.10 shows such an arrangement.

Slotted or 'breathing' roofs When refurbishing existing buildings, in wide span or multi-span installations, or when sidewall areas are limited, the use of slotted or 'Yorkshire' boarded roofs might be considered. 'Yorkshire' boarded roofs covered with profiled timber boards with gaps between them have been used for over 100 years in the UK. In the 1970s there was a revived interest in the use of such roofs, particularly since there were distinct cost benefits to be gained.

When refurbishing existing buildings, slots can be cut quite easily in existing sheet roofs. Similarly, when erecting new buildings, gaps left between adjacent sheets save on the material costs associated with 'lapping' sheets. Figure 8.11 shows examples of the methods that can be used.

When thermal effects dominate natural ventilation, the upper part of the roof acts as the air outlet while the lower part acts as air inlet. Concern about precipitation entering through slotted roofs appears to be unfounded and in-use experience has been favourable (Constrado, 1978).

Discrete roof outlets Roof outlets can of course be formed as discrete openings placed in the ridge or elsewhere in the roof of buildings. A number of commercial units, fitted with rotating flaps or louvres, are produced for other industries for smoke venting purposes. Special sheets with upstands and covers are also produced for mounting fans in roofs and these can, of

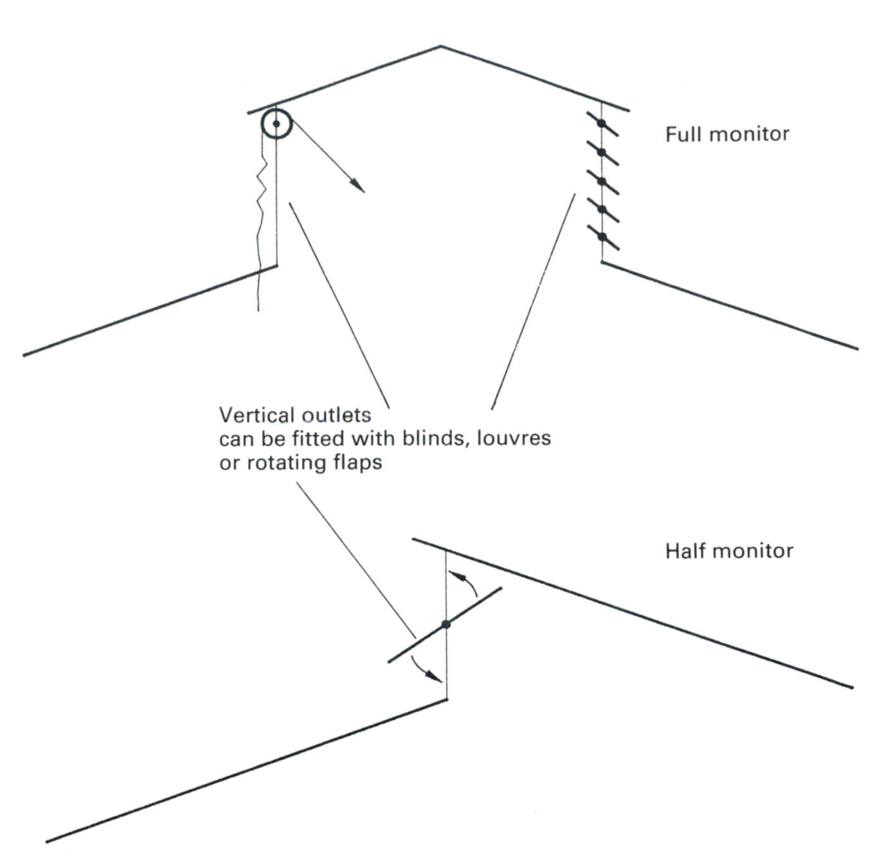

Fig. 8.10. Adjustable air outlets in monitor roofs.

course, be used without fans. Providing the correct number of adequately sized units of an appropriate design are fitted then these can obviously be used. Comparisons between open ridges and discrete chimneys suggest that there are virtually no differences in the resulting inside conditions (Choiniere *et al.*, 1988).

SIDEWALL AIR INLETS

Sidewall air inlets can be used either alone or in conjunction with roof outlets. When stack effect dominates, sidewall openings can act as both inlet and outlet, even if roof outlets are present. In such circumstances warm air flows out from the upper part of the opening and cold air flows in through the lower part. In windy conditions the windward openings will act as air inlets and the leeward openings as air outlets. Such openings may be simple unrestricted openings, variable size openings or openings covered with a perforated material of some kind. Variable openings are adjusted to vary

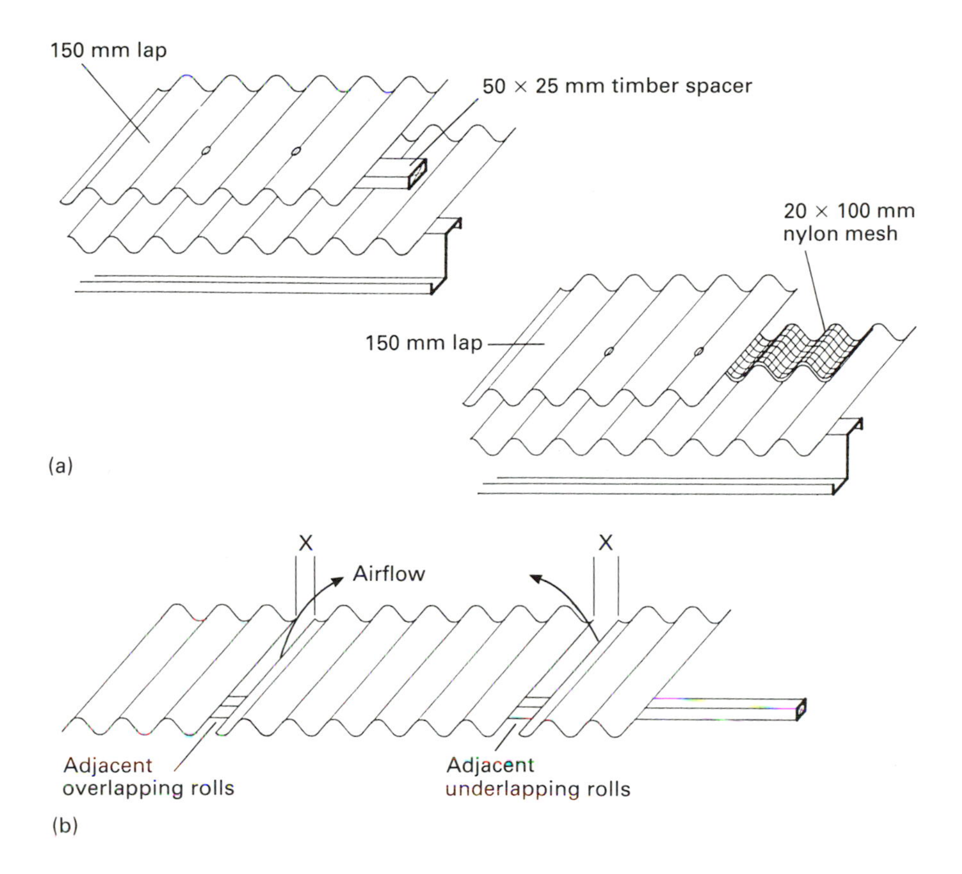

Fig. 8.11. Slotted and breathing roofs: (a) raised sheets; (b) gapped or slotted sheets.

ventilation rate with changes in outside climate while the use of perforated materials is usually intended to reduce air velocity through such openings in windy conditions, i.e. to act as windbreaks. Internal deflectors might also be used to direct and control air velocity over livestock.

Variable size openings Vertically adjustable shutters and blinds are widely used in some parts of the world to vary ventilation rate in simple structures. Theses are used to give some degree of control over temperature and may be manually or automatically controlled. Vertically adjustable shutters and blinds, particularly for deep openings, can present a very heavy load and may require a lot of power to move them. There is a variety of mechanisms that can be employed for this purpose, powered manually or motorized. Flaps pivoted at their centre of gravity considerably reduce the load to be moved, since they only need to be rotated about their pivot. Consequently much smaller motors, either connected directly to the flaps or via torque tubes, can be used.

Manually controlled systems provide only coarse control of temperature since, at best, adjustments are made only two or three times per day according to the operator's judgement of prevailing or likely weather. Automatically controlled systems which can operate continuously, usually on the basis of measured inside temperature, tend to give much better control of internal temperature.

Perforate windbreak materials A variety of materials can be used to cover sidewall openings, their efficacy in reducing inlet air velocities varying considerably with the free area (the area of voids expressed as a percentage of the total area of the material) and the physical arrangement of the voids. Carpenter *et al.* (1973) measured a range of materials used in agricultural ventilation applications to elucidate the nature of their resistance to airflow, including materials commonly used as windbreaks on air inlets in naturally ventilated buildings. The materials tested were classified as being either:

1. building components, e.g. space boarding;
2. materials with a measurable free area, e.g. perforated hardboard; or
3. materials of undefined free area, e.g. fabrics.

The airflow resistance of the materials was measured and it was concluded that the pressure drop, P, was related to the air velocity through the material by the equation

$$P = b_1 v + b_2 v^2 \tag{19}$$

where P = static pressure drop across material, mm WG (9.806 Pa); v = mean air velocity through sample, m s^{-1}. It was found that for the most resistive materials, $b_2 = 0$ and therefore the pressure drop was linear with flow. The materials for which $b_1 = 0$ were largely perforated materials and the pressure drop was proportional to the square of the flow. For other materials neither b_1 nor b_2 was zero and thus the equation is quadratic.

The term $b_2 v^2$ is a function of the kinetic energy, and it represents the destruction of kinetic energy in eddies. The contribution of this loss to the total pressure loss was seen to increase as aperture spacing increased in materials. The term $b_1 v$ arises mainly from the conversion of air from a high to a lower pressure with little energy degradation.

When selecting a material as a windbreak, it would seem to be desirable to select materials with either a value of $b_1 = 0$ or with a high b_2/b_1 ratio. The result would be a material with a low resistance to airflow at low speeds and an increasing resistance with increasing air speeds. This would seem to be a desirable characteristic in a windbreak materials. Table 8.13 lists some materials measured by Carpenter *et al.* (1973) which might be appropriate for such uses. For conventional space board (100 mm board, 12.5 mm gap)

Table 8.13. Loss factors for some windbreak materials.

Description	Free area (%)	b_2*	b_2/b_1
Expanded metal for grain	14		14.8
	15	5.1	
Extruded plastic mesh			
0.75 mm × 0.75 mm	17	0.85	
1.5 mm × 1.5 mm	35	0.29	
4.5 mm × 4.5 mm	50	0.12	
Honeycomb walling	14	1.98	
	28	0.49	
Pegboard 4.5 mm holes	3.5	43.64	
	11	7.12	
Perforated polyethylene sheet, 12.5 mm holes	1		15.5
	2	253.12	
	4	48.69	
	10	9.38	
Perforated zinc, 2.5 mm diam holes	68	0.19	
Slotted asbestos roofing	1.4	210.4	
Slotted hardboard			
25 mm × 4.5 mm slots	24	1.09	
6 mm × 4.5 mm	56		1.0
6 mm × 6 mm	70		1.0
Space boarding, 25 mm thick			
100 mm board, 6 mm gap	6	13.4	
100 mm board, 12.5 mm gap	11.1	4.84	
Wire netting	88	0.01	
Woven insect netting	57.7		0.1
	62		0.6
	64		1.0
Woven polypropylene			
551 × 551 strands m^{-1}			6.1
453 × 453 strands m^{-1}		5.2	
1575 × 472 strands m^{-1}		3.8	
1575 × 1969 strands m^{-1}			1.2

Source: Adapted from Carpenter *et al.*, 1973.

*Values of b_2 are given for materials for which $b_1 = 0$.

the air velocity inside a building with a 10 m s^{-1} wind can be calculated as follows.

$$P_v = 0.5\rho v_w{}^2, \text{ Pa}$$

where P_v = velocity pressure of wind, Pa, ρ = density of air, kg m^{-3} (1.2 approx), v_w = wind speed, m s^{-1}, then

$$P_v = 60\,\text{Pa} = 6.12\,\text{mm WG}.$$

As the wind hits the space board it will lose most of its velocity and the velocity pressure will be converted into static pressure on the space board. Assuming all the velocity pressure is converted into static pressure and that the inside static pressure is zero, then this static pressure will be the pressure across the space board. Thus from Equation (19) the mean velocity of air through the space board, U, can be found.

$$v = (P/b_2)^{0.5} = (6.12/4.84)^{0.5} = 1.12\,\text{m s}^{-1}$$

This will be the air speed in the building just inside the space board. If instead of space board, pegboard with b_2 = 48.69 were used then the resultant inside air speed would be about 0.35 m s^{-1}.

Internal deflectors Deflectors located immediately inside unrestricted openings or located elsewhere inside buildings can be used to direct airflow in the required direction. These deflectors can be used to prevent draughts on animals in cold conditions (see Fig. 8.12a) or to create, deliberately, high air speeds over animals in hot conditions (see Fig.8.12b).

Controlled environment housing

The main purpose of such housing is to control the animals' thermal environment and, in the case of poultry, the light environment. This is achieved by the use of thermally insulated structures with ventilation, heating and/or cooling systems, controlled on the basis of the monitored inside air temperature. This type of housing is used mainly for those species of animals whose production performance is most affected by climatic parameters, e.g. for pigs and poultry kept in cold and temperate climates. The capital and running costs of such housing has led to the adoption of high stocking densities in an attempt to reduce the cost per animal housed. This high stocking density makes the control of the internal environmental conditions critical if housing and welfare problems are to be avoided. When heating and/or cooling systems are required, the cost of energy is also an important consideration.

Attention must be paid to the thermal insulation of buildings to avoid excessive heat loss or gain. Insulation and vapour checks are also important in buildings where high levels of moisture production from animals can lead

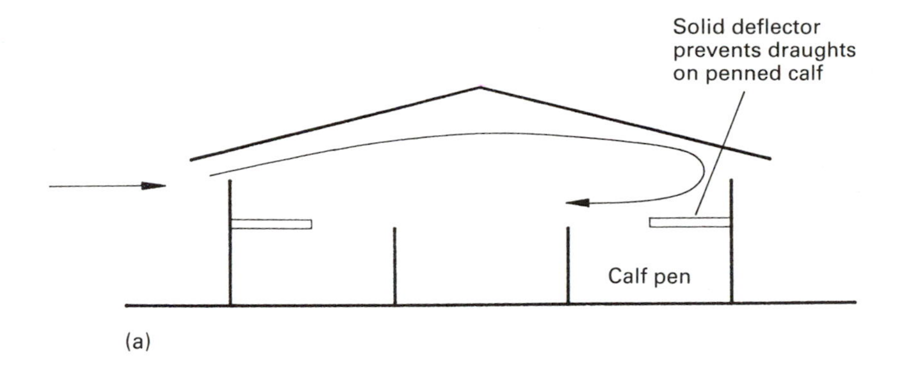

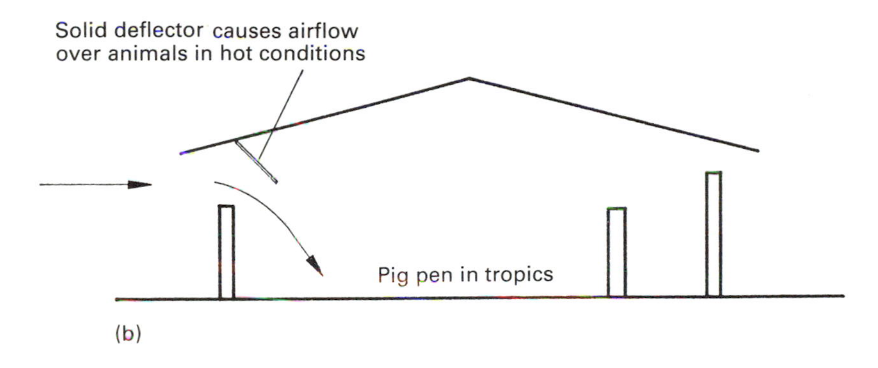

Fig. 8.12. Air deflectors to manipulate air speeds: (a) to prevent draughts; (b) to create high air speeds.

to both surface and interstitial condensation. Fan ventilation systems with a variable ventilation rate are often used as a means of controlling inside temperature. The control of ventilation in cold conditions is crucial if excessive heating costs are to be avoided. However, not only must the fan ventilation systems work properly, but excessive air infiltration (due to outside wind and temperature effects) must also be prevented. This requires attention to weather tightness of the structure and draught stripping of doors and windows. These features, however, make provision for, and warning of, failure even more critical.

Thermal insulation

Fabric heat losses and solar heat gain have been discussed previously (page 190) as has the problem of condensation (page 207). That the thermal

Table 8.14. Insulation materials for building structures.

Material	Typical conductivity ($W m^{-1} K^{-1}$)	Comments
Blocks and screeds – lightweight, load-bearing		
Aerated and foamed concrete	0.10–0.50	Few fire
Aerated pulverized fly ash	0.18–0.29	or vermin
Expanded clay aggregate	0.11–0.21	problems
Sintered clay aggregate	0.34	
Foamed blast furnace slag	0.21	Permeability
Pumice aggregate	0.25	can lead to
Vermiculite aggregate	0.14	some problems
Boards – rigid, extruded, expanded or foamed		
Ceramic fibre	0.030–0.037	Performance in
Glass fibre	0.033–0.049	fire can be a
Isocyanurate	0.022–0.023	problem
Mineral wool	0.034–0.040	
Polyurethane	0.022–0.039	Vermin can
Polystyrene	0.028–0.039	cause severe
Polyvinyl chloride	0.027	damage to some
Wood fibre	0.040–0.060	of these
Foams – foam in situ *and spray*		
Ceramic fibre	0.041–0.28	As for boards
Isocyanurate	0.023	
Mineral fibre/wool	0.038–0.097	
Polyurethane	0.023	
Urea formaldehyde	0.032	
Vermiculite	0.094–0.209	
Granular fills – loose and blown in situ		
Cellulose	0.032	As for boards
Cork	0.036–0.040	
Mineral wool	0.036–0.048	
Polyurethane	0.032	
Polystyrene	0.032–0.043	
Vermiculite	0.065–0.072	
Mats and quilts		
Ceramic fibre	0.030–0.037	Vermin can
Glass fibre	0.038–0.049	cause severe
Mineral wool	0.034–0.037	damage

insulation of structures is most important in respect of controlling these, will be obvious. It will also have become apparent that good insulating materials will be characterized by their low 'k' value and well-insulated building components by their low 'U' value. There are many types of insulation material available, the vast majority of them being manufactured materials. Some derive their thermal characteristics from the properties of the basic material from which they are made, others from air or other gases which are trapped within the structure of the material. The form of the materials can vary considerably. Table 8.14 summarizes the types of insulating materials generally used in buildings.

Many of these insulation materials can be made up into composites, i.e. they can be bonded to other materials at the manufacturing stage to make boards or cladding sheets. By combining materials, composite materials can be manufactured which have all the properties required, e.g. thermal insulation, structural strength, fire resistance and low surface spread of flame, low vapour permeability, weather resistance, durability and so on. Insulation materials can also be incorporated into building units such as hollow concrete blocks, e.g. filling the voids with a foam insulation. While industry has made available a whole new range of modern manufactured insulation materials, there are problems associated with these.

Modern 'plastic foam' insulation materials can give rise to major fire hazards: some burn rapidly, others melt and some produce toxic and voluminous quantities of smoke. The surface spread of flame, combustibility and smoke production of a material should be carefully considered. British standard, BS 5502 (BSI, 1990a), sets out requirements for the fire performance of livestock buildings, the requirements varying with the ease of rescuing animals in the event of fire and the amount of bedding likely to be in use. The designation of the roof covering required and the surface spread of flame rating for the walls and ceiling in accord with BS 476 (BSI 1958, 1971) is set out.

Insulation materials are particularly prone to damage from vermin, rodents, birds and insects. Severe damage can be done to such materials by birds and rodents that use the materials for nesting and chew, scratch, tear, burrow into and move such materials. Mat and quilt insulation may be bundled up against the purlins in buildings, leaving large areas of the roof uninsulated. Board materials can be riddled with tunnels. The problem is severe and the best solution appears to be an effective pest eradication scheme.

More recently concern about ozone depletion and global warming has raised the issue of the use of chlorofluorocarbons (CFCs) in the manufacture of some 'foam plastics'. CFCs are used as blowing agents in the production of polyurethane and isocyanurate foams, extruded and expanded polystyrene and phenolic foams. CFCs are a major contributor to the low thermal conductivities of the final product. The Montreal Protocol called for a 100% phasing out of CFCs by the year 2000, while the European Community has brought forward its CFC ban to 1 July 1997. Manufacturers are currently developing CFC-free alternatives. These might have some disadvantages, not least the lack of a period of comprehensive testing before use.

Floor insulation

Insulation of floors in livestock buildings is important for two different reasons:

1. To limit the fabric heat loss from the building via the floor.
2. To limit the heat loss from animals to the floor.

Insulation to reduce fabric heat loss via floors The loss of heat through the floor of buildings has been discussed previously. In most buildings, even those occupied by people, ground floors are not insulated. This is because the U value of an uninsulated floor is generally much lower than the U value of an uninsulated wall or roof or even double glazed windows. To provide floor insulation has not appeared to be cost effective when compared with roof or wall insulation.

The need for and methods of providing insulation in ground floors has largely arisen in countries with cold climates, where the freezing of the ground down to 1 metre or more can cause problems. In more recent years, in an attempt to reduce energy usage other countries have started to consider ground floor insulation, e.g. in the UK, the 1990 revised Building Regulations require ground floors to have a maximum U value of $0.45\,W\,m^{-2}K^{-1}$. However, because of the size of floor slabs in most livestock buildings, this value can usually be achieved without any insulation.

Where ground floor insulation is deemed necessary for livestock buildings, the first thing that should be considered is the use of edge insulation to achieve the desired U value. Figure 8.13 shows a number of ways in which such edge insulation can be easily and economically installed. It should be noted that when insulation is used below ground it should have the following characteristics: very low water absorption, high resistance to ground contaminants, high compressive strength. Extruded polystyrene is the most commonly used material for this job.

Insulation to reduce animal heat loss to floors Bruce (1977) discussed the conductive heat loss from animals lying on floors and developed a model for heat loss from an animal to the floor. He cited the earlier work of Mount (1967) in justifying his model. Bruce postulated that the major heat transfer path was from the animal to the floor, then laterally through the floor material to the air surrounding the animal. The thermal resistance of the floor, R_f, is a significant factor in such heat loss. Floors can be considered to

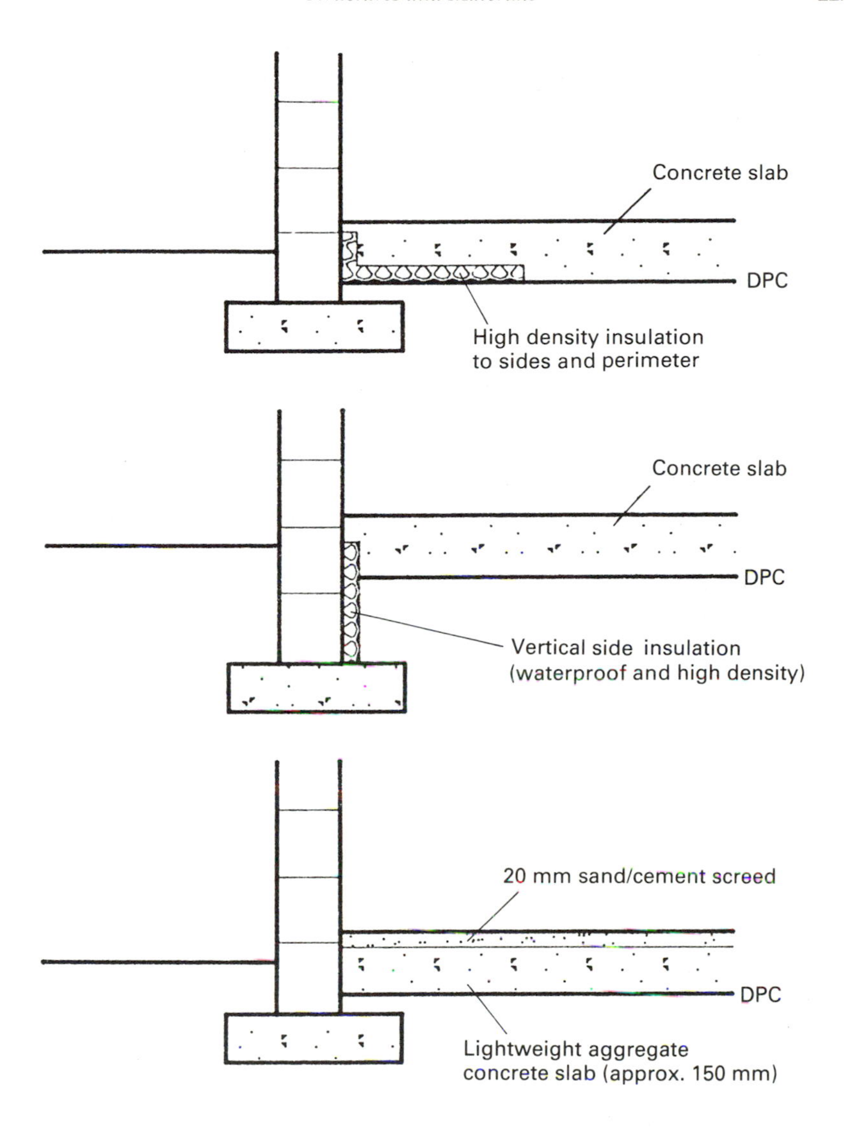

Fig. 8.13. Insulation of ground floors.

be thermoneutral if R_f is equal to the thermal resistance of the air boundary layer surrounding the animal, R_a. Animals lying on thermoneutral floors will lose the same amount of heat as during standing. Floors on which animals lose less heat than when standing, i.e. $R_f > R_a$ can be considered as thermo-positive and floors on which animals lose more heat than when standing, i.e. $R_f < R_a$ can be considered thermo-negative.

Using a physical model to simulate a 45 kg pig, Bruce measured the heat loss from the model on various types of floors and calculated the floor

Table 8.15. Thermal resistances* of various floors.

Type of floor	Thermal resistance R_{f45} ($K m^2 W^{-1}$)
Thermoneutral floor	
45 kg pig standing ($R_{f45} = R_a$)	0.12
Bedding materials on concrete	
38 mm dry redwood chips on concrete	0.71
60 mm dry straw	0.66
17 mm dry straw	0.46
17 mm wet straw	0.23
12 mm dry straw	0.17
Various concrete floor constructions	
3 mm topping on 50 mm expanded polystyrene	0.73
6 mm topping on 50 mm expanded polystyrene	0.46
20 mm cement/sand topping on no-fines aggregate	0.17
16 mm rubber cow mat on concrete	0.11
50 mm cement/sand topping on 50 mm expanded polystyrene	0.10
12 mm K board on concrete	0.078
Concrete slats 100 mm wide, 19 mm gap, 17 mm deep	0.052
Dense concrete floor	0.04
Slurry covered concrete floor	0.031
Non-concrete floors	
Wooden slats 58 mm wide, 10 mm gaps, 70 mm deep	0.23
Expanded metal	0.12
T bar metal slats 24 mm wide, 12 mm gap	0.067
Ground conditions	
250 mm growing grass after rain	0.13
Muddy ground	0.044

Sources: Bruce, 1977; Barnes, 1984.

*Based on measurement with model of 45 kg pig with 20% of body in contact with floor.

thermal resistances, R_{f45}, as measured by the model. Table 8.15 shows the thermal resistances of floors as cited by Bruce and others (Barnes, 1984). It can be clearly seen from the table that the best way to reduce the thermal conductivity of a floor is to insulate it as near the top as possible, i.e. use some form of bedding on the floor, or use insulation with a minimal thickness of topping over. Of course the use of bedding might not be possible, because of cost or some other constraint. When toppings as thin as 3–6 mm are to be used, then these cannot be of cement/sand screeds because of their lack of structural strength. Special reinforced toppings will need to be used.

It must be remembered that the heat loss from animals to floors can be compensated for by reducing heat loss elsewhere, i.e. by increasing the air temperature and saving on heat loss by convection. Furthermore, the need to reduce floor heat loss will be most important in young newborn animals.

Roof and wall insulation

There is very little difference between insulating the walls and roofs of buildings since the same insulating materials and forms are used for both. It is important to ensure that the continuity of insulation is maintained to avoid cold bridging. Wetting of insulation must be prevented and moisture transfer through the materials needs to be minimized if interstitial condensation is to be avoided. There are numerous publications available, from manufacturers and others, which give guidance on installing thermal insulation. BRE (1989) has published a most useful report which discusses the risks involved and how they can be avoided at the installation stage.

Weatherproofing and vapour checks

Rain

The techniques for weatherproofing livestock buildings are no different from those used for other structures. Traditional and newer methods of construction and the skills of building workers are based to a great extent on the proven methods of construction which provide adequate weatherproofing. The techniques for preventing water ingress, i.e. the prevention of rain ingress (normal or driven), the prevention of moisture transmission (damp) through building elements and the provision of adequate drainage are extensively covered in many other publications.

Air infiltration

The other aspect of weatherproofing which is important is the control of air infiltration due to temperature and wind effects. Such air infiltration can have significant effects on the ability to control temperature in livestock buildings and on the cost of heating and cooling. In recent years interest in the problems of air infiltration has increased enormously because of its importance in the energy use of buildings.

Most work on air infiltration has been related to industrial, commercial and domestic buildings: however, much of this is applicable to livestock buildings. Ferguson (1982) reported on work on air infiltration in warehousing and light industrial buildings. He identified the major sources of air leakage in buildings as being:

1. Wall and roof cracks, particularly at the intersection of walls, floors and roofs. He cited Shaw (1980) who had identified floor/wall joints, windows and window sills as the major leakage sources in outside walls.

2. Windows, where leakage occurs around the sash of operable windows and around the frame.
3. HVAC systems, where leakage can occur around louvres and poorly fitting dampers, and via chimneys and supply ducts.
4. Exterior doors, where leakage is a function of the fit and the frequency of use.

Having established that airflow through cracks was the dominant source of air leakage, Ferguson suggested that the following measures might be considered:

1. Windows and doors should be fitted tightly and all joints should be caulked or weather stripped.
2. Where possible, fit a continuous vapour barrier on the warm side of thermal insulation. This is a very effective means of reducing air leakage for walls and around windows and frames.
3. For masonry walls, the use of foamed-*in-situ,* low vapour permeability insulation is effective in sealing most cracks.
4. Potential leakage openings at wall/roof intersections should be given careful attention when detailing their construction, for example the use of butyl rubber gaskets could be considered.
5. To reduce air infiltration through exterior doors a variety of techniques might be adopted. For extensively used entrances these might include the use of air curtains, plastic strip door curtains, slight pressurization of the entrance or automatic door closers.

WATER VAPOUR AND VAPOUR CHECKS

In buildings a variety of proven techniques is adopted to prevent water vapour movement from regions of high to low vapour pressure, the most simple of which is a well-jointed polyethylene membrane placed as close to the 'warm, humid' interior as possible.

The problems caused by moisture and their remedies are exactly the same in animal housing as in human habitations. Problems can arise because of lack of care by building workers, relaxations of standards for agricultural buildings and the more severe working environment, in agriculture, for materials. These circumstances require that greater not less attention be paid to the installation of vapour checks.

Degradation of Materials in Livestock Housing

It would take considerably more space than is available here to discuss fully the selection and properties of materials, the problems of corrosion and rotting in buildings and the methods of protection that can be used. Here, only those problems that occur because of the particular conditions that arise in livestock houses, can be discussed.

Factors contributing to degradation of materials

In relation to the structure and materials used in livestock buildings a number of problems can arise which are caused by the nature of the housing used:

1. *Condensation.* Surface and interstitial condensation and wetting of materials can occur. Moisture ingress into equipment, particularly electronic controls can cause failure and malfunction.
2. *Contaminants.* The practice of storing faeces and urine in tanks and pits can give rise to gaseous contaminants such as hydrogen sulfide and ammonia; dust from animals, feed, bedding and other sources can reach high aerial concentrations; biological organisms such as bacteria, viruses, mites and spores can reach high aerial concentrations and may pollute building surfaces; faeces and urine can build up on and around surfaces and structural components. Such contaminants can cause corrosion and decay problems and may lead to malfunction of equipment. (See Chapter 6)
3. *Vermin.* The shelter afforded by livestock buildings, together with a readily available supply of food makes such buildings particularly attractive to vermin, e.g. mice, rats and birds. These vermin can cause severe damage to the building materials and structure as well as transporting disease.
4. *Animal damage.* Housed animals can cause damage to the building. This may be due to the force they can exert by pushing, leaning or standing on building elements; they can cause impact forces due to kicking, stamping or butting; they can also cause damage by gnawing, chewing, pecking or rubbing.

The design of the structure and the selection of materials used will need to be carefully considered in the light of the above problems in addition to the normal design parameters such as structural strength, stability, weatherproofing, etc.

Corrosion and decay

A number of factors can contribute to the failure of materials. Those related to the environmental conditions within livestock buildings largely affect either corrosion or rotting.

Corrosion of metals

This is a rather loose term used to describe the deterioration of metals under adverse environmental conditions, which usually occurs at the boundary between a metal and its environment. The corrosion product can delay further corrosion, by forming an impervious barrier to the environment, e.g. the oxide coating on aluminium. Alternatively the corrosion process can continue until failure occurs.

Most corrosion involves an electrochemical reaction in the form of a corrosion cell, i.e. an anode, a cathode and an electrolyte. Under suitable conditions materials will dissociate into their ionic state and ions will pass from the anode to the cathode, where they will be deposited. The electrical potential to cause a corrosion cell may be created by local differences in composition of metals, by two different metals in contact with an electrolyte, or local differences in the electrolyte.

Such corrosion reactions require an electrolyte, invariably a liquid, and require free supply of oxygen to the electrolyte. The electrolyte is normally water, but may vary depending on what is dissolved in the water. Materials like urine, faeces and stored slurries will obviously vary considerably from normal water. Condensation in conjunction with soluble gases, e.g. ammonia and hydrogen sulfide, or in conjunction with dust which might contain aggressive salts, e.g. chlorides or sulphates, may form electrolytes which can cause corrosion of normally impervious materials such as aluminium.

Decay in timber

Rotting is caused by the action of biological organisms on materials. Living organisms such as fungi and moulds found growing on wood use it as a source of nutrients and break down its structure. Most fungi and moulds require relatively high moisture contents (> 20%) in the material on which they live, such conditions only occur when buildings are damp or wet. Moulds in particular are associated with surface condensation.

Selection of materials

Most livestock buildings are framed structures, composed of a main structural frame of steel, timber or concrete, sidewalling of masonry or sheet or board cladding and a roofing of sheet cladding or tiles. Insulation is either in the form of rigid boards or quilts attached inside the exterior cladding. Internal lining may be the insulation board or some other sheet material.

Main frame

Technically there is little difference between the major materials used; capital cost more often than not is the deciding factor. When large clear spans are required, steel tends to be the most economic material to use. In small buildings timber and steel are of similar cost. Concrete frames can be competitive, but rarely in wider span buildings.

Thermally, timber has some advantages due to its lower thermal conductivity which can help reduce condensation problems caused by thermal bridging. Concrete buildings tend to have a greater thermal mass and can modulate the amplitude of temperature variations.

Claddings

The choice of cladding materials includes timber in board form, metals, plastics, fibre-cement, in sheet form and other materials such as clay, stone, slate and wood in tile form. Of these, timber is the only material used which can contribute significantly to a building's thermal insulation.

A considerable amount of condensation can form on sheet materials, particularly thin metal and plastics sheets. The problem is largely found in uninsulated buildings, where it is associated with inadequate ventilation and warm moist air, e.g. steam from mixing of warm liquid feeds coming into contact with a cold cladding. Where roof sheets contact purlins, side and end laps on sheets and joints at flashings are considered to be high risk areas for corrosion. Newer, deep profile sheets have led to thinner materials without loss of strength. Consequently, when corrosion occurs penetration is more rapid.

There appears to be much less of a problem with fibre-cement sheets which are thicker, absorb some of the condensate and do not corrode. Few condensation problems are found with tile roofing probably because with all its joints there is plenty of ventilation to remove moisture.

Failure and life of materials

There is little information on the comparative life of materials used in livestock buildings as opposed to their use in other situations. However Martin *et al.* (1985) reported the results of a postal survey carried out on piggeries in Australia. The survey questioned farmers about the replacement, the actual life and the expected life of materials in use. The conclusions from the survey are set out below for the materials used in the construction of roofs and walls. Materials for floors, fixtures and equipment, which were also included, are not discussed here.

1. *Roofing materials*

(a) *Roof framing* – timber, painted steel and galvanized steel were all in extensive use. Timber appeared to be a better material than steel, being less frequently reported as a short life material. Generally there were few problems with any roof framing.

(b) *Roof purlins* – these were predominantly of timber which gave no problems. Painted and galvanized steel were significantly worse with more problems reported.

(c) *Roof claddings* – these were predominantly galvanized steel, which had a poor performance (19.5% short life and 10.6% replacement). Both asbestos cement and aluminium cladding were significantly better. Painted steel appeared to have an even shorter life than galvanized steel.

(d) *Roof insulation* – polyurethane foam was the most commonly used insulation followed by aluminium foil, fibreglass and expanded polystyrene. Many roofs were not insulated at all in more temperate states. Polyurethane foam was the best performer having significantly fewer reports of short life than fibreglass, expanded polystyrene and aluminium foil. Polystyrene foam needed replacing most often.

2. *External walling materials*

(a) *External walls* – these were mainly of concrete, in precast panel, block or cast *in situ* form, and galvanized steel, a few were of brickwork. The incidence of short life was significantly greater in galvanized steel than the other materials except for precast panels. Many walls were a mixture of materials with concrete at animal level and galvanized steel cladding above.

(b) *Wall opening coverings* – these were of three main types, i.e. meshes to keep out flies and birds, awnings to provide shade and blinds, louvres or shutters to control ventilation. While information was limited, the indications were that canvas was a better material than polypropylene for blinds and aluminium was a better material for awnings than galvanized steel. Galvanized steel was the most common louvre material and had performed satisfactorily, as had aluminium shutters. Painted steel and plastic-on-steel shutters did not appear to be promising.

Mills (1984) also reported on an investigation of roofing materials in cubicle houses for cattle. The work involved investigations on 36 farms with a cubicle building, roofed with a variety of metal roofing products, i.e. aluminium, aluminized steel, galvanized steel, externally painted steel and plastic coated steel. The buildings had been in use for between 2 and 13 years. The investigation revealed that 19 of the roofs were corroded, the degree of corrosion varying from staining to severe rusting. A high tensile galvanized steel roof in one building had been replaced after only 8 years. The following factors were identified as contributing to the high rate of corrosion:

1. *Poor ventilation.* Only one of the buildings investigated appeared to have adequate ventilation. Based on ventilation calculations current at that time, one building had 90%, seven buildings 40–65% and the rest 10% or less of the recommended minimum ventilation requirements. This would obviously add considerably to the condensation and corrosion risk.

2. *Corrosion barriers.* None of the buildings had corrosion barriers between the roof sheets and the purlins, even where timber purlins had been treated with copper chrome arsenic preservative, for which corrosion barriers are recommended.

3. *Collection of condensate.* Condensate collects at purlins, sheet side and end laps due to natural drainage and capillary action and moisture can remain trapped for a long time. Corrosion was identified in these areas.

4. *Siting.* There appeared to be a striking similarity between the incidence of corrosion and the 'Atmospheric Corrosion of Zinc' map for the UK.

These findings tend to illustrate the need for attention to overall design, e.g. proper provisions for ventilation and selection of sheet materials appropriate to the site, and detailed design, e.g. the use of sealants on sheet laps and corrosion barriers on purlins. Too often livestock farmers' thinking is dominated by capital cost with little or no consideration of subsequent maintenance and replacement costs.

Selection, protection and use of materials

Standards and guidance

Clear guidance to the selection, performance and use of materials in agricultural buildings is given in BS 5502 (BSI, 1990b). This standard highlights the hazard and factors affecting the durability of materials, the measures that should be taken to protect materials and the factors affecting the use of them. It cites many other standards which pertain to either specific materials, protection or preservation treatments and installation techniques.

The characteristics of materials used in building services, the environments to which they might be exposed, the types of corrosion that can occur, precautions to be taken when using materials and the protection of materials, are discussed in a BSRIA handbook (BSRIA, 1987). This publication also has a comprehensive bibliography of related publications. For those with an interest in the use of materials this will prove a useful starting point.

Vermin proofing

Keeping birds, insects, mice, rats and other pests out of livestock buildings is a virtually impossible task. However, a number of precautions can be taken to proof new and existing buildings, the objective being to keep buildings as free from pests as possible. These precautions are largely concerned with aspects of detailed design and as such require to be discussed at length and in detail. Such a discussion is not possible here, therefore the following texts are cited for those wishing to pursue this topic: Jenson (1979), BRE (1980), Canada Plan Service (1985), Hall and Grigg (1990).

Costs and Benefits of Materials and Structures

Costs of materials and structures

These are various cost guides available which give the basic costs of materials, complete structures and rates for various types of work in the buildings industry. In the UK, E & F.N. Spon Ltd are well known for their publications in this field. For agriculture buildings the *Farm Building Cost Guide* (MacCormak, 1991) is the best known, readily available UK publication. While government departments (Ministry of Agriculture, Fisheries and Food) have cost information on a computerized database, they no longer publish the information for use by others. Information can, however, be bought through their consultancy services.

Information from any cost guide is always likely to be inaccurate. By the time cost information is collected and published, the costs of materials, labour, etc., are very likely to have changed. The effects of location, quantity discounts, transportation costs and other such variables will also significantly affect the final price.

Cost–benefit appraisals

Rarely do livestock farmers carry out anything other than a cursory appraisal of buildings or of investments made in the upgrading of buildings. However, this is not surprising since a full appraisal will require skills and knowledge beyond the scope of most farmers and there is very little published information to guide farmers. A rational appraisal will need to address the following points:

1. *The response of the animals* to those parameters that housing can influence, i.e. largely the thermal environment to which the animals are exposed. Such responses will need to be described in a quantifiable way in terms of production parameters, e.g. growth rate, mortality, feed conversion efficiency, if any economic evaluation is to be made.

Other aspects of the husbandry or housing system might also need to be considered, e.g. the risk of disease as it might be influenced by air quality or the waste disposal system, or the welfare of the animals as it might be influenced by group size or stocking density. These aspects might prove to be more important than thermal performance.

2. *The performance of the building* in respect of the thermal parameters or energy inputs to be controlled must be evaluated. While the thermal performance and energy consumption of existing buildings can be measured and the results can highlight problems, the performance of new or improved buildings will need to be predicted.

3. *The climate to which a building is exposed* will influence its performance.

Any prediction of a building thermal performance or energy use will require some description of the climate. Either data for a typical climatic year or some appropriate derived index are needed.
4. *The costs of deficiencies in the thermal performance* of buildings can be valued in terms of extra production costs (e.g. heating, cooling, feed use or reduced output). The capital cost of measures taken to prevent or correct such deficiencies will then need to be judged against the subsequent saving in production costs.

Various measures will give different levels of improvement and different levels of cost effectiveness. Therefore, guidance is required to aid strategy decisions. Such decisions can be about the efficacy of various measures taken at the design stage prior to constructing buildings or both the efficacy and sequencing of improvements to existing buildings.
5. *Some method of financial appraisal* will be required to compare the costs and benefits involved. One or more of a variety of well-established techniques can be used, depending on a producer's preference or particular circumstances.

Any method of appraisal needs to allow the rapid evaluation of a variety of measures that might be taken. Therefore computer 'spreadsheet' programs, which are simple to use and can run through a variety of options very quickly, are most useful.

Optimum economic level of insulation

Various authors have discussed the optimum economic thickness of insulation for livestock buildings and have discussed methods that might be used. Wathes (1981) discussed these methods and, concentrating on the method developed by Carpenter and Randall (1975), arrived at some general conclusions about the optimum thickness of insulation for pig and poultry housing. Any conclusions drawn in such papers about the optimum economic thickness of insulation inevitably reflect the monetary prices prevalent at the time of writing.

Example cost–benefit appraisal

To illustrate a method of cost–benefit appraisal an example is show below. It illustrates how all the five points outlined above are covered. Notes are added at various stages to explain the procedure.

Example Building
The building concerned is a dry sow house for 200 sows, the sows are individually housed, in gated stalls with concrete floors, and are fed 1.5 kg day^{-1} of food of 12.0 MJ kg^{-1} energy density. The building is continuously stocked with pigs of an

average weight of 175 kg. Air speed over the pigs should not exceed 0.3 m s^{-1} in cold conditions.

The building is old, it is poorly insulated with an overall U value of 2.0 W m^{-2}°C^{-1} and has a heat loss factor, h_f (see page 196), of 2920 W °C^{-1}. With a building volume of 1445 m^3, the minimum ventilation rate that can be achieved is 3 air changes per hour and the building is draughty with an average air speed of 1 m s^{-1} at pig level. The building can be heated using a gas-fired warm air system with an efficiency of 65%. The building is obviously too cold for the pigs.

The building is located on a farm in southern England

Questions

The farmer wishes to know:

1. Is it cheaper to heat the building or give the pigs extra feed in cold weather?
2. What benefit is to be gained by insulating the building to reduce the heat loss factor?
3. What benefit will there be in renewing the ventilation system to achieve the correct minimum ventilation rate and to stop draughts?
4. What is the most cost-effective way to improve the building?

Appraisal method

1. Animal response

For the housing and feeding conditions described the pigs have the following temperature requirements

Lower critical temperature (LCT) of sows = 23.2°C
Upper critical temperature (UCT) of sows = 34.7°C

and they will require an extra 0.11 g feed °C^{-1}.day^{-1} to compensate for temperatures below the LCT.

If the draught over the pigs is reduced the LCT and UCT will become 21.1 and 33.4°C respectively and the extra feed required will be 0.11 g feed °C^{-1}.day^{-1}

The pigs will produce 43.5 kW of heat

2. Building performance

The thermal performance of the building is most readily predicted in terms of *temperature lift*, T_l, i.e. the amount the inside temperature is raised above outside temperature by heat gains to the building, excluding heating. Such heat can be produced by animals, lighting, motors, etc., internally and by solar gain to the structure.

In this example the only internal gain considered is pig heat and it is reckoned only 80% (Bruce, 1981) of this will be available as sensible heat to warm up the air in the building. Solar gain is negligible in winter.

Temperature lift can be evaluated from a consideration of the heat gains and fabric and ventilation heat loss factors for the building. Thus for this building, as it exists, with ventilation at its minimum rate in cold conditions then:

Pig heat available to warm air in building = 43,500 × 0.8 W
Fabric heat loss factor h_f = 2920 W °C^{-1}
Ventilation heat loss factor h_v = (3 × 1445)/3 = 1445 W °C^{-1}
T_l = 8°C (approx.)

As improvements are made to the insulation and ventilation, the values of h_f and h_v will change and different values of T_l will result.

3. Climate to which building is exposed

There will be some outside temperature below which the building will require heating if the temperature inside is to be maintained at the LCT. Alternatively, the temperature inside will drop and the sows will need extra feed. This outside temperature can be considered to be the *outside base temperature,* T_b, and can be found by subtracting T_l from the LCT of the pigs. Thus if $T_l = 8°C$ and LCT = 23°C (approx.) then $T_b = 15°C$.

From climatic data one can find out by how much and for how long temperatures are below this base temperature in a typical year. In the UK such information is widely published for 17 areas as *degree-days* (Energy Efficiency Office, 1987), to a base temperature of 15.5°C, in trade magazines and elsewhere (CIBS, 1982). The values published are on a monthly basis derived from

$$\text{Monthly degree days} = \Sigma\ \text{month}\ [T_b - 0.5(T_{max} - T_{min})]$$

where $T_b = 15.5°C$, T_{max} = daily maximum temperature, °C, T_{min} = daily minimum temperature, °C, and on an annual or heating season basis which is derived by adding together the appropriate monthly totals.

To obtain figures to bases other than 15.5°C, one must work from raw meteorological data or use some conversion method (CIBS, 1988; Schoenau and Kehrig, 1990) to obtain the values from the published data.

The degree-days for this example to the differing bases that will occur depending on the insulation and ventilation of the building are shown in Table 8.16.

4. The cost of deficiencies in thermal performance

(a) Feed

The amount of extra feed each sow requires, Feed_i, to compensate for cold conditions in the building is $0.11\,\text{g}\,°\text{C}^{-1}.\text{day}^{-1}$. This will need to be multiplied up by the number of sows, *N*. Whenever the outside temperature drops below T_b then it will be matched by a corresponding drop inside the building. Therefore, the inside will effectively have the same number of degree-days below the LCT as the outside temperature has below T_b. Thus

$$\text{Annual extra feed use} = \text{Feed}_i \times N \times \text{degree-days below } T_b$$

The extra amounts of feed required for the building with various insulation and ventilation options is shown in Table 8.16.

(b) Heating

To maintain the sows' LCT, heating will be required in the building any time the outside temperature drops below T_b. The rate of heating required will be directly related to the temperature difference between the inside temperature required (sows' LCT) and the outside temperature. The heating energy use will be related to both the rate of heating, the duration for which it is required and the efficiency, η, of the heating system (including its controls). Thus

$$\text{Annual heating energy use} = (h_f + h_v) \times \text{degree-days below } T_b \times \eta$$

The annual energy use required for the building with various insulation and ventilation options is shown in Table 8.16.

Table 8.16. Evaluation of energy and feed use in sow house with various improvements.

Improvement option	LCT of sows (°C)	Temp. lift (°C)	Base temp. (°C)	Degree days	Heating energy use (kWh)	Extra feed use (tonnes)
1. *Do nothing*	23	8	15	2,000	322,338	44
2. *Insulate* to achieve overall *U* value ($W m^{-2} °C^{-1}$) of						
(a) 1.0	23	12	11	1,050	169,228	23
(b) 0.5	23	16	7	440	70,914	10
3. *Improve ventilation* to achieve correct minimum air change rate and air speed over pigs	21*	9	12	1,370	220,802	30
4. *Combination of 2 and 3*						
2(a) & 3	21	14	7	500	80,585	11
2(b) & 3	21	19	2	55	8,864	1

*Ventilation improvement by reducing draughts over the sows results in a lower LCT.

Table 8.17. Financial appraisal of building improvement options.

Option	Capital cost (£)	Cost of heat (£)	Cost of feed (£)	Saving on heat (£)	Saving on feed (£)	Payback on heat (years)	Payback on feed (years)
1. *Do nothing*	0	17,357	6,600	0	0	0	0
2. *Insulate*							
(a) 1 $W m^{-2} °C^{-1}$	7,525	9,112	3,450	8,245	3,150	0.91	2.39
(b) 0.5 $W m^{-2} °C^{-1}$	10,845	3,818	1,500	13,539	5,100	0.80	2.12
3. *Improve ventilation*	1,500	11,889	4,500	5,468	2,100	0.27	0.71
4. *Combination of 2 and 3*							
2(a) & 3	9,025	4,339	1,650	13,199	4,950	0.68	1.82
2(b) & 3	12,345	477	150	16,880	6,450	0.73	1.91

5. Financial appraisal

Such an appraisal will require that monetary costs associated with improvements to the building and with heating and the provision of extra feed be established for the period under consideration. A variety of financial appraisal methods can be used, which might require guesses and forecasts of future price trends and other economic factors. For this example, a simple method, i.e. Payback is used. The method simply divides the value of the annual benefits into the capital cost of the proposed improvement, the result is a figure in years which indicates how long it will take to recover the initial investment. Based on the temperature lift and degree-days, the amounts of feed and energy used with the various building insulation and ventilation options have been evaluated, the results are shown in Table 8.16. Based on an energy cost of 3.5p per kWh for propane and a feed cost of £150 per tonne, Table 8.17 summarizes the monetary costs and savings and the payback associated with the various options.

6. Answers to farmer's questions

Table 8.17 provides the answers to the original questions posed. Dealing with the questions in sequence:

– *Is it cheaper to heat the building or give the pigs extra feed in cold weather?* It is obvious that giving the pigs extra feed is far cheaper than heating the building in all the circumstances described.

– *What benefit is to be gained by insulating the building to reduce the heat loss factor?* Insulating the building will reduce heating or extra feed costs; however, the best payback is when the building is improved to an overall *U* value of $0.5 \mathrm{W\,m^{-2}{}^{\circ}C^{-1}}$. There will still be a need to provide heat or extra feed in cold weather.

– *What benefit will there be in renewing the ventilation system to achieve the correct minimum ventilation and to stop draughts?* Improving the ventilation system will reduce heating or extra feed costs and will give a much better payback than improving the insulation. There will still be a need to provide heat or extra feed in cold weather.

– *What is the most cost-effective way to improve the building?* In monetary terms the first thing to do is to give the sows extra feed and avoid the use of heating in cold weather. Secondly, if improvements are to be made, tackle the ventilation system first since this will give a very quick return in cost savings. The insulation level should then be improved to achieve an overall *U* value of $0.5 \mathrm{W\,m^{-2}{}^{\circ}C^{-1}}$. These improvements should pay for themselves in terms of cost savings in about two years. If both the ventilation and insulation are improved as suggested above then there will be very little requirement for extra feed or heat.

Conclusions

This chapter has shown that there is a wealth of information on the design, materials and construction of livestock buildings. Despite this, farmers are continually beset with environmental problems in buildings. Many of these are due to ignorance, on the part of farmers, building manufacturers and suppliers, of the requirements of livestock, the performance characteristics of materials, construction standards and housing recommendations.

Most producers do no more than compare the capital cost of materials, buildings and associated equipment when erecting or refurbishing livestock buildings. This concern about minimizing capital costs leads to buildings which do not perform adequately. Very rarely is a proper environmental design or a cost–benefit appraisal undertaken and when it is the approach and data used are often suspect.

Many of the new developments in materials and construction technology are aimed at reducing construction costs for buildings for humans. These are often seized on by the suppliers of farm buildings, who see an opportunity to maintain or increase market share by reducing the cost of their product. Unfortunately, such developments have rarely been subjected to testing in a rigorous farm situation and suppliers often have little experience of the materials and construction methods. Consequently, durability and design life may well prove to be considerably shorter on-farm than was anticipated and materials and structures fail.

Undoubtedly lack of attention to such matters has contributed to animals being housed in conditions which are abhorrent to some laypeople. This has resulted in regulations intended to safeguard animal welfare. Currently new 'improved' livestock building design, in developed countries, is being driven mainly by animal welfare considerations. Too often such considerations override other considerations to the detriment of the farming operation. Additionally, building technology which is appropriate in developed countries might be misplaced in developing countries or in different climates.

Little improvement will be made in livestock buildings until farmers, building manufacturers and suppliers, livestock specialists, welfarists and others recognize the need to adopt a rational, integrated approach to their design. This integrated approach must encompass animal health and welfare, management and husbandry, materials and construction technology, energy and pollution, and economic considerations.

References

Anderson, B.R. (1990) The U value of ground floors: application to building regulations. BRE Information Paper IP 3/90. Building Research Establishment, Garston, Watford, England.

ASHRAE (1967) *Handbook of Fundamentals*. American Society of Heating, Refrigeration and Air-conditioning Engineers, New York.

Barnes, M.M. (1984) Insulated floors for piggeries. Cement and Concrete Association, Farm Note 3, Wexham Park, Slough, England.

Bond, T.E., Kelly, C.F. and Ittner, N.R. (1954) Radiation studies of painted shade materials. *Journal of Agricultural Engineering* 35, 389–392.

Bond, T.E., Kelly, C.F., Morrison, S.R. and Perrira, N. (1966) Solar, atmospheric and terrestrial radiation received by shaded and unshaded animals. *Transactions of the American Society of Agricultural Engineers.* Paper No. 66, p. 47.

Boyd, J.S. (1973) *Practical Farm Buildings.* The Interstate Printers and Publishers Ltd, Danville, Illinois.

Bruce, J.M. (1972) Open ridges for natural ventilation – a review. *Farm Building Progress* 32, 11–14.

Bruce, J.M. (1975) The open ridge as a ventilator in livestock buildings. Scottish Farm Buildings Investigation Unit, R & D Studies No. 6, Aberdeen.

Bruce, J.M. (1977) Conductive heat loss from the recumbent animal. Scottish Farm Buildings Investigation Unit, R & D Studies No. 8, Aberdeen.

Bruce, J.M. (1981) Ventilation and temperature control criteria for pigs. In: J.A. Clark (ed), *Environmental Aspects of Housing for Animal Production.* Butterworths, London, pp. 197–216.

BRE (1980) Reducing the risk of pest infestation: design recommendations and literature review. *BRE Digest* 238. Building Research Establishment, Garston, Watford, England.

BRE (1989) Thermal insulation: avoiding risks. BRE Report. Building Research Establishment, Garston, Watford, England.

BRE (1990) Climate and site development Part 3: Improving micro climate through design *BRE Digest* 350, Part 3. Building Research Establishment, Garston, Watford, England.

BSI (1958) BS 476: Part 3: External fire exposure roof test. British Standards Institution, London.

BSI (1971) BS 476: Part 7: Methods for classification of the surface spread of flame of products. British Standards Institution, London.

BSI (1989) BS 5250: Control of condensation in buildings. British Standards Institution, London.

BSI (1990a) BS 5502: Part 23: Code of practice for fire precautions. British Standards Institution, London.

BSI (1990b) BS 5250: Part 21: Code of practice for selection and use of construction materials. British Standards Institution, London.

BSRIA (1987) *Building Services Materials Handbook.* Building Services Research and Information Association, E. & F.N. Spon, London.

Caborn, J.M. (1965) *Shelter Belts and Windbreaks.* Faber and Faber, London.

Canada Plan Service (1985) Rodent and bird control in farm buildings. Plan M-9451, Canada Plan Service, Ottawa.

Carpenter, G.A., Moulsley, L.J. and Boothroyd, D.N. (1973) The resistance to airflow of some materials used for ventilation in agriculture. NIAE Dept. Note DN/FB/235/3020, National Institute of Agricultural Engineering, Silsoe, Beds., England.

Carpenter, G.A. and Randall, J.M. (1975) The interpretation of daily temperature records to optimise the insulation of intensive livestock buildings. *Agricultural Meterology* 15, 245–255.

Choiniere, Y., Munroe, J.A., Desmarais, G., Renson, Y. and Menard, O. (1988) Minimum ridge opening widths of an automatically controlled naturally ventilated swine barn for a moderate to cold climate. Canadian Society of Agricultural Engineers. Agricultural Institute Annual Conference, Calgery, Alberta.

CIBS (1975) *CIBS Guide C1 & 2: Properties of Humid Air, Water and Steam.* Chartered Institution of Building Services, London.

CIBS (1978) *CIBS Guide A1: Environmental Criteria for Design.* Chartered Institution of Building Services, London.

CIBS (1979a) *CIBS Guide A5: Thermal Response of Buildings.* Chartered Institution of Building Services, London.

CIBS (1979b) *CIBS Guide A9: Estimation of Plant Capacity.* Chartered Institution of Building Services, London.

CIBS (1980) *CIBS Guide A3: Thermal Properties of Building Structures.* Chartered Institution of Building Services, London.

CIBS (1982) *CIBS Guide* A2: *Weather and Sola Data.* Chartered Institution of Building Services, London.

CIBS (1986) *CIBS Guide A10: Moisture Transfer and Condensation.* Chartered Institution of Building Services, London.

CIBS (1988) *CIBS Guide B18: Owning and Operating Costs.* Chartered Institution of Building Services, London.

Constrado (1978) *Spaced Steel Roofing for Farm Buildings.* Construction Steel Research and Development Association, Croydon, Surrey, England.

Darby, D.E. (1971) Snow and wind control for farmstead and feedlot. Canadian Department of Agriculture, Ottawa, Ontario.

Davies, M.G. (1986) A critique of the environmental temperature model. *Building and Environment* 21, 155–170.

Davies, M.G. (1988a) Heat loss from rooms: Comparison of determination methods. *Building Services Engineering Research and Technology* 9(2), 69–78.

Davies, M.G. (1988b) Environmental temperature: Validity as a room index temperature model. *Building Services Engineering Research and Technology* 9(2), 79–82.

Dwybad, I.R., Mylo, A.H., Johnson, C.E. and Mol, D.L. (1974) Ridge ventilation effects on model building ventilation characteristics. *Transactions of the American Society of Agricultural Engineering* 17, 366–370.

Energy Efficiency Office (1987) *Degree Days.* Fuel efficiency booklet, Department of Energy, London.

Fanger, P.O. (1972) *Thermal Comfort. Analysis and Applications in Environmental Engineering.* McGraw-Hill Book Co., New York.

Ferguson, J.E. (1982) Air infiltration in warehousing and light industrial buildings. Buildings Energy Technology Transfer Publication No. 82.06, Canadian Department of Energy, Mines and Resources.

Finbow, M. (1988) In: Dodd, J.S. (ed.), *Energy Saving Through Landscape Planning: Vol. 3. The Contribution of Shelter Planning,* HMSO, UK.

Hall, J. and Grigg, J. (1990) Rats in drains. Building Research Establishment Information Paper, IP 6/90, Garston, Watford, UK.

Holmes, M.J. (1988) Heat loss from rooms: Comparison of determination methods. *Building Services Engineering Research and Technology* 9(2), 69–78.

Jenson, A.G. (1979) *Proofing of Buildings Against Rats, Mice and Other Pests.* Ministry of Agriculture Fisheries and Food, HMSO, London.

Kelly, C.F. and Bond, T.E. (1958) Effectiveness of artificial shade materials. *Journal of Agricultural Engineering* 39, 758–759.

Kelly, C.F. and Ittner, N.R. (1950) Thermal design of livestock shades. *Journal of Agricultural Engineering* 601–606.

Kelly, C.F., Bond, T.E. and Ittner, N.R. (1957) Cold spots in the sky may help cool livestock. *Journal of Agricultural Engineering* 38, 726–729.

Lacy, R.E. (1971) An index of exposure to driven rain. *BRE Digest* 127. Building Research Station, Garston, Watford, England.

McArthur, A.J. (1990) Thermal interactions between animal and micro climate: Specification of a 'standard environmental temperature' for animals outdoors. *Journal of Theoretical Biology* 148, 331–343.

MacCormak, J.A.D. (1991) *Farm Buildings Cost Guide 1991.* Centre for Rural Building, Aberdeen.

MAFF, (1979) *Windbreaks.* Ministry of Agriculture, Fisheries and Food Publications, Pinner, Middlesex, UK.

Martin, K.G., Wrathall, L.S. and Spencer, J.W. (1985) *A Postal Survey of Intensive Pig Accommodation in Australia. Part 2: Performance of Materials* CSIRO, Division of Building Research, Highett, Victoria, Australia.

Milbank, N.O. and Harrington-Lynn, J. (1974) Thermal response and admittance procedure. *BSE* 42, 38–51.

Mills, B.C. (1984) Investigation of corrosion to metal roof sheets on low cubicle buildings MAFF Note: RD/FBS/22. Ministry of Agriculture, Fisheries and Food Publications, Pinner, Middlesex, UK.

Monteith, J.L. and Unsworth, M.H. (1990) *Principles of Environmental Physics,* 2nd edn. Edward Arnold, London, pp. 214–215.

Mount, L.E. (1967) The heat loss from new-born pigs to the floor. *Research in Veterinary Science* 8, 175–186.

Moysey, E.B. and McPherson, F.B. (1966) Effect of porosity on performance of windbreaks. *Transactions of the American Society of Agricultural Engineers* 9, 74–76.

Prior, M.J. (1985) Directional driving rain indices – computation & mapping. BRE Report 59. Building Research Station, Garston, Watford, England.

Schoenau, G.J. and Kehrig, R.A. (1990) A method of calculating degree-days to any base temperature. *Energy and Buildings* 14, 299–302.

Shaw, C.Y. (1980) Methods of conducting small scale pressurisation tests and air leakage data of multi-storey apartment buildings. *American Society of Heating, Refrigeration and Air-conditioning Engineers Transactions* 86, 1.

Wathes, C.M. (1981) Insulation of animal houses. In: Clark, J.A. (ed.), *Environmental Aspects of Housing for Animal Production.* Butterworths, London, pp. 379–412.

Housing Systems

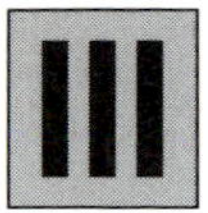

9 Poultry Housing

D.R. Charles, H.A. Elson and M.P.S. Haywood
ADAS Nottingham, UK

Historical Background

Poultry are very sensitive to temperature, light and air change rate, and the biological and cost consequences of suboptimal environments are severe, as described in Chapter 1. This is one important reason why there have been more elaborate controlled environment housing and ventilation systems developed for poultry than for any other class of farm stock.

In temperate countries, particularly Europe and the US, high capital, low labour, controlled environment intensive production units became the dominant style of production during the great expansion period of the poultry industry during the 1950s to 1970s. A glance at some of the tables of requirements and responses in Chapter 1 will reveal that this emphasis was fully economically justified. Furthermore, the precise control of temperature developed during that period was probably beneficial to animal welfare since the comfort temperature is likely to be within the thermoneutral zone, which is somewhere between 24 and 27°C for a well-feathered adult hen. However, by the late 1980s and early 1990s a market-led swing, at least in Northern Europe, had begun towards simpler less intensive systems for reasons of consumer preference and perception of bird welfare. The history of the swings in popularity of egg production systems in the UK illustrates these changes, and is given in Table 9.1. It may be assumed, when reading this table, that virtually all layers in cages will have been in what was referred to as controlled environment. Broilers, turkeys and most breeding stock have, however, almost all been kept on litter throughout this period, mainly in controlled environment houses.

The need for precise control of temperature, lighting and ventilation was far from the only reason for the dominance of controlled environment.

Table 9.1. Systems of egg production in the UK, percentage of national flock in four different systems.

Year	Battery cages	Litter or barn	Free range
1951	8	12	80
1963	27	56	17
1965	53	37	10
1966	67	25	8
1980	95	4	1
1990*	85	3	12

Source: Adapted from data in the Museum of the British Poultry Industry.

*Estimate only.

There were also some powerful practical operational reasons. Large numbers of birds began to be concentrated into small areas for reasons of land, labour and capital economy before controlled environment was developed. Indoor systems became possible once vitamins, particularly vitamin D, were understood.

Battery cages came into serious use about 1933, and were then usually one tier high and constructed of timber and wire netting (though poultry cages of sorts go back to Roman times), mainly with a view to getting the birds out of contact with their own droppings though also for the purposes of recording individual performance. In the UK the end of poultry feed rationing in 1953 boosted the development of larger units of tiered cages.

Problems soon became apparent and the technology of environmental control began to be applied to their solution. The concentration of birds at higher stocking density meant that their ventilation had to be consciously calculated and designed. The moisture respired by the birds began to be associated with condensation and wet litter, and eventually insulation was added to the specification. It was found that this led to better ventilation and air quality. It was not long before natural convectional ventilation gave way to the more reliable controllable systems based on electric fans (though interestingly 30 years later there are now very controllable versions of natural ventilation).

Supplementary lighting for egg production was understood in the 1930s, but by 1958 it was sufficiently refined to have stimulated the elimination of windows and total reliance on electric lighting. This in turn led to tighter limits to the design of air inlets and outlets, which made possible the full exploitation of the high temperatures found to be ideal by the early 1970s.

This evolution did not always happen smoothly. Lighting patterns had been in widespread use for a long time before it was discovered that they had been failing due to inadequate light proofing, and it was as late as the 1980s before it was demonstrated that temperature control required rather more attention to detail than that which it had been afforded. These developments were reviewed by Charles (1988) and Appleby *et al.* (1992).

Structural Constraints

The need to provide precise temperature control at a fairly high temperature while yet providing enough air to maintain air quality dictates that for intensive houses in cold and temperate climates insulation is needed. The amount depends on the climate, the stocking rate and the local economics: in Europe and the US a thermal conductance of $U = 0.4\,W\,m^{-2}\,°C^{-1}$ or better is usually necessary. Chapter 8 gives the thermal properties of materials. In hot climates, and even in hot clear weather in temperate climates, such standards are also necessary, both for welfare and for performance, in order to minimize solar heat gain. Wilson (1988) found that at $U = 1$ solar gain was up to $30\,W\,m^{-2}$ in old buildings. At $U = 0.4\,W\,m^{-2}\,°C^{-1}$ the corresponding value may be as low as $5\,W\,m^{-2}$.

In cool climates the air in a poultry house is usually at a high enough humidity to form condensation within unprotected insulants, therefore a vapour check is necessary, either as a protective layer or inherent in the insulant. This has been a standard recommendation for 30 years but is not always applied (see also Chapter 8).

Building dimensions and configurations are constrained not just by the number of birds to be housed but also by several operational details. The height of the building may be affected by the need to incorporate a manure pit, by the need for a minimal height to eaves for working convenience, by the height of battery cages and associated equipment, or by the height of other fittings, systems or equipment.

Broiler and turkey houses may require a clear span design in order to facilitate cleaning and catching.

Internal surfaces usually need to be smooth for cleaning (see also Chapter 6). External surfaces, colour, appearance and design are increasingly important in the interests of good relations with neighbours. Feed bins should be inconspicuous as well as functional. The site may require screening for reasons of shelter and the improvement of ventilation controllability and also for aesthetic reasons.

The choice of structural strengths and the design of structural members is dictated by the weights of birds, food, water and equipment to be carried. However, there are now so many competitive companies fully experienced in the design and erection of poultry houses, usually prefabricated, that the farmer is scarcely ever likely to need to undertake the detailed calculation of these structural matters, though a design specification in terms of the environment to be achieved should be stated when seeking bids. The site will usually require preparations including levelling, the provision of roads, water, electricity and drainage, and these days landscaping.

Having specified the above constraints, the choice of building materials depends on price and local tradition. Prefabrication in materials such as glass fibre is rare, but laminated structures in which the insulant is part of the cladding are increasingly popular.

Housing and Production Systems

Housing systems used in the poultry industries (Figs 9.1–9.4) of developed countries are mainly of the high capital, low labour type, and the designs used are superficially very numerous. However, in principle there are only a few generic types of housing and systems. They have been developed to meet certain constraints and specifications. Table 9.2 provides a classification, based on the structures of the systems, Table 9.3 gives a summary of design criteria and Table 9.4 summarizes ventilation rate requirements.

Battery cage design

Since there is a highly competitive worldwide market in proprietary laying cages (see Fig. 9.1) it is not necessary for users to design their own cages in detail. However, it is usual to tender against a specification, which, apart from the constraints outlined in Table 9.2, should include the following points:

1. Structural strength adequate to support the weight of birds, feed, eggs, water and droppings over the useful life of the cages without failing or sagging.
2. Absence of gaps, snags, sharp edges and corners, and traps where birds can be caught.
3. At least 10 cm per bird linear allowance of waste-free feeder, with dispensing equipment distributing the feed uniformly to all cages (in temperate climates at a low level in the trough).
4. In temperate climates one nipple drinker per five birds, with access to at least two from each cage, but for hot climates a more generous allowance.
5. The cage floor to be free of snags or sagging, slopes to be as suggested in Table 9.2. Eggs should roll freely to the collection point, but their rolling should be arrested gently. Collection of eggs may be manual or mechanized.

Ventilation system detail

Chapter 7 contains more detail, and Figs 9.5 and 9.6 show examples of two important components of a ventilation system satisfactory for many

Table 9.2. Systems and design constraints.

Stock	Production system	Principal design constraints: Reason	Principal design constraints: Numerical value	Manure handling	Ventilation (see Chapter 7)
Laying hens	Battery cages (Fig. 9.1)	Welfare codes EC Directive Performance	Numbers per cage usually 3–5 allowing at least 450 cm^2/bird 10 cm/bird feeder	Belt or scraper	Various, particularly HSJ, ACNV
			At least 40 cm high over 65% of the area and 35 cm high at any point. Maximum floor slope 8° or 12° depending on mesh shape	Deep pit (high rise) or stilt (Figs 9.2 and 9.3)	Various, particularly HSJ perforated ceiling
	Non-cage intensive				
	1. Deep litter (rare)	Welfare codes	Max 7 birds m^{-2} 17 kg m^{-2}, 1 nest/5 birds	Tractor and fore loader or specialist vehicle	
	2. Aviary	Welfare codes Performance Marketing Regulations (EC only)	Max 25 birds m^{-2} 17–20 recommended 1 nest/5 birds	Belt or deep pit	Various

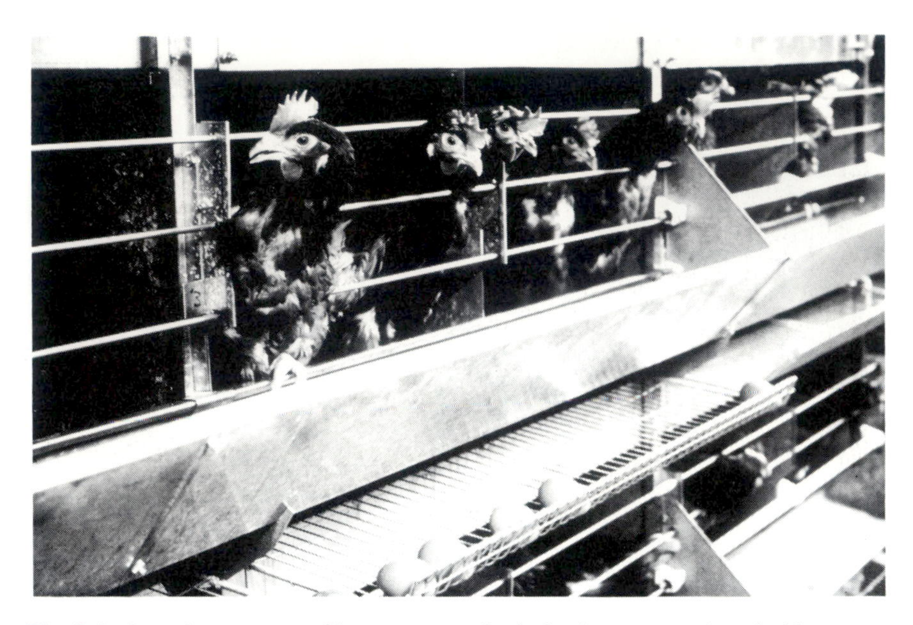

Fig. 9.1. A modern system of battery cages for laying hens, reproduced with permission of Holt Studio Ltd.

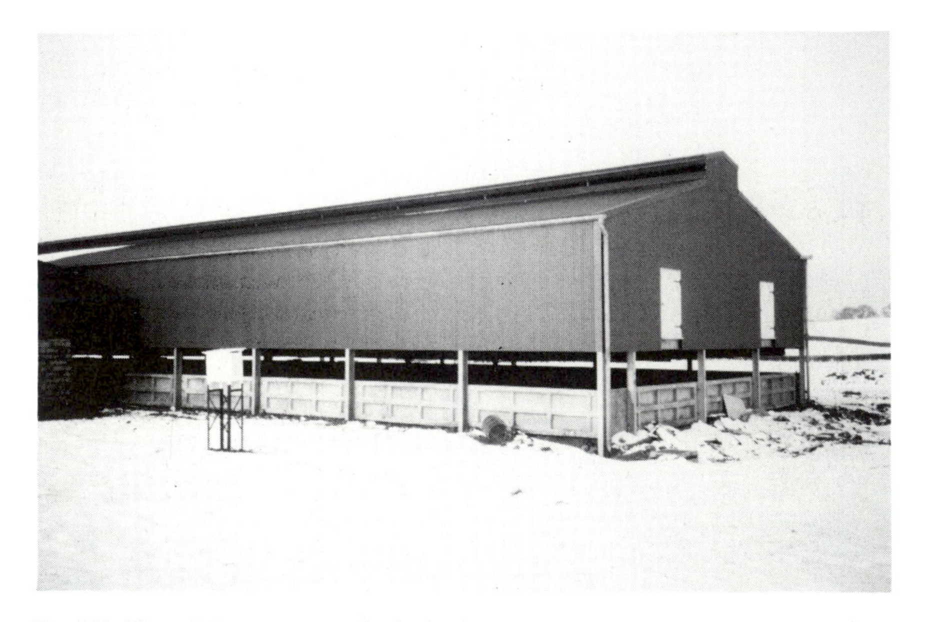

Fig. 9.2. The stilt house system for laying hens.

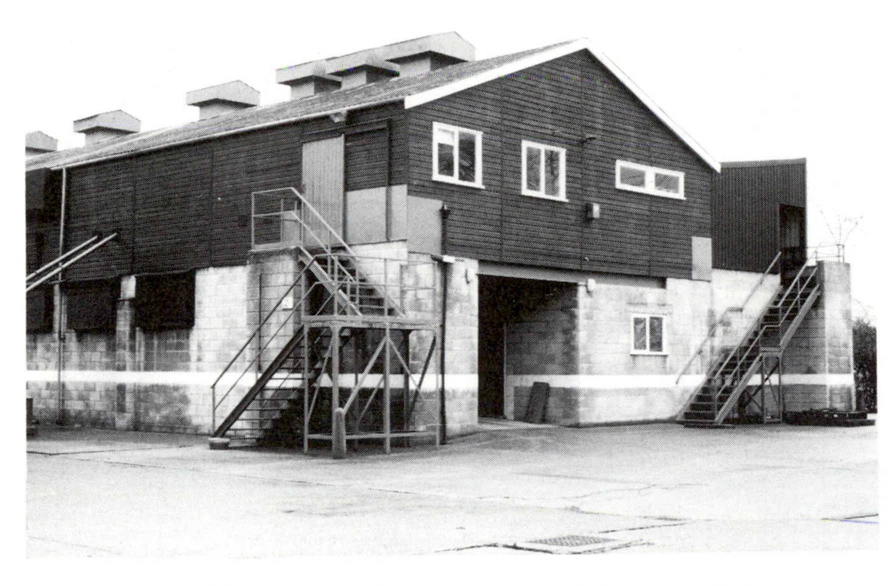

Fig. 9.3. A deep pit laying house with manure storage below, also called a high-rise in some countries.

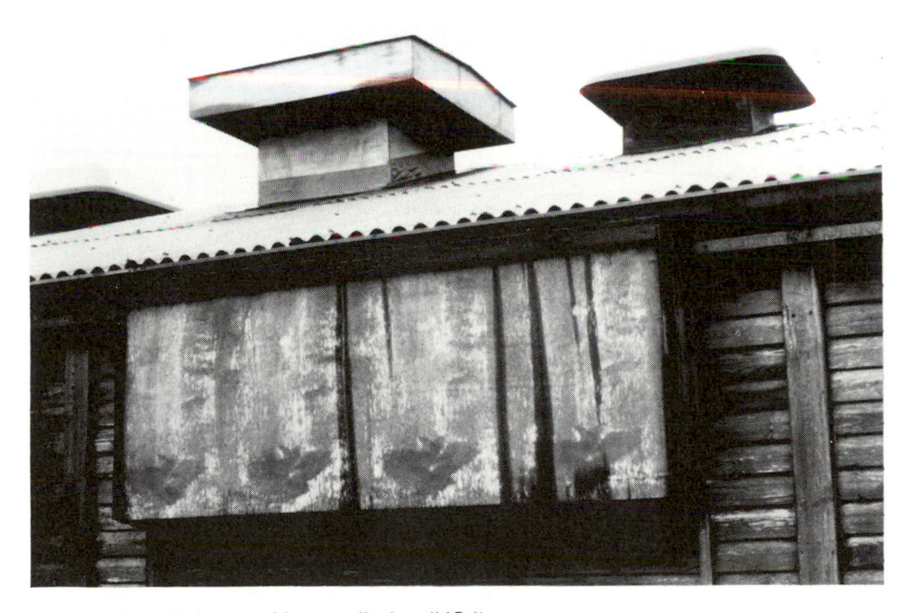

Fig. 9.4. The high speed jet ventilation (HSJ) system.

Table 9.2. continued

Stock	Production system	Principal design constraints		Manure handling	Ventilation (see Chapter 7)
		Reason	Numerical value		
	3. Perchery (barn)	Ditto	Ditto At least 15 cm perch per bird	Belt or deep pit (Fig. 9.3)	Various, particularly HSJ, ACNV
	4. Deep litter with perforated platforms or perforated floors (wire or plastic mesh or slats)	Ditto	Maximum 11.7 birds m^{-2}	Ditto	Ditto
	Free range (housing may be any of above except cages)	Ditto	Ditto but continuous daytime access to pasture at a maximum of 1000 birds per ha	Ditto	Ditto
Replacement pullets	Cages	Welfare codes Production requirements	250 $cm^2 kg^{-1}$ liveweight	Usually belt or scraper	As above, but also polythene duct systems
	Litter	Ditto	17 $kg m^{-2}$	Litter disposal. Sometimes 1/3 floor area as droppings pit	Various, particularly HSJ, ACNV

	Perchery, aviary (barn)	Ditto	$17\,kg\,m^{-2}$	Belt, scraper and litter removal	Various, but often ACNV or similar
Broilers	Litter	Welfare codes Production requirements Specific quality assurance schemes	$34\,kg\,m^{-2}$ Feeders and drinkers well distributed. Drinkers cup or nipple and drip cup or multidirectional nipple, bell shaped. Brooding equipment at up to 5 W/bird (see Chapter 8)	Tractor and fore-loader or special vehicle	Various, particularly HSJ (Fig. 9.4)
Broiler and layer parent stock	Cages	Only for AI (except grandparents)			Various
	Litter	Welfare codes	$17\,kg\,m^{-2}$	Often 1/3 floor area as droppings pit	Various
Turkeys (breeders)	Cages	Only for AI			
	Litter	Welfare codes	$515\,cm^2\,kg^{-1}$	Tractor and fore-loader or special vehicle	Various, but usually simple natural
Growing turkeys	Pole shed	Welfare codes Simple accommodation often adequate	$410\,cm^2\,kg^{-1}$	Litter disposal	Simple open sided often adequate

Table 9.2. continued

Stock	Production system	Principal design constraints		Manure handling	Ventilation (see Chapter 7)
		Reason	Numerical value		
	Controlled environment	Welfare codes Suitable for birds destined for lower value trade	$260\,cm^2\,kg^{-1}$	Litter disposal (see Chapter 1)	Various, particularly HSJ

Notes

1. Chapter 7 gives detailed recommendations for ventilation systems. The systems in the table mainly refer to those for cool and temperate climates. See below and also Chapter 1 for further information on housing for hot climates.

Abbreviations: HSJ = high speed jet. Figure 9.6 shows some design criteria.
ACNV = automatically controlled natural ventilation.

2. Welfare codes are for UK only. Codes of Recommendations for the Welfare of Livestock, revised 1990.

3. For EC countries the Council Directive Laying Down Minimum Standards for the Protection of Laying Hens Kept in Cages, sets constraints on design.

4. Performance constraints refers to requirements as reviewed in several other chapters.

5. For EC countries space allowance is $450\,cm^2$ per bird (Directive 88/166/EEC).
For UK only the Welfare of Battery Hens Regulations (1987) requires the following:
$1000\,cm^2$ per bird for 1 bird per cage
$750\,cm^2$ per bird for 2 birds per cage
$550\,cm^2$ per bird for 3 birds per cage
$450\,cm^2$ per bird for 4 birds or more per cage.

6. For EC countries the Egg Marketing Regulations impose design constraints on non-cage systems.

N.B. Regulations are constantly changing and R and D progress is rapid. Readers should seek professional advice on current requirements.

Table 9.3. Some design criteria for poultry housing, environment and systems.

Feature	Current recommendations	Reasons	Sources of further information
Ventilation rate	Maximum for warm weather $1.5 \times 10^{-3} m^3 s^{-1} kg^{-0.75}$	Remove metabolic heat in warm weather	Chapter 1 Table 9.4
	Minimum for cold weather $1.6 \times 10^{-4} m^3 s^{-1} kg^{-0.75}$	Maintain air quality	Chapter 1 Table 9.4
Ventilation systems	Systems must be engineered to achieve the requirements of the birds as described in Chapter 1. Where precise control is appropriate, e.g. layers and broilers in temperate and cold climates, and where the gross margin analysis justifies the capital (see Chapter 1) then wind and light proofing are required	To achieve the requirements independently of weather if appropriate	Chapter 1 Chapters 7 and 8
Inlet and outlet equipment	Wind and light proof if precise control is appropriate. Very simple equipment is adequate where biological and economic requirements do not justify precise control		Figs 9.5 and 9.6 Chapter 7
Ventilation control	Generally thermostatic devices where precision is needed		Chapter 7
Temperature	Layers As optimized by models, but often 21–22°C		Chapter 1
	Brooding – pullets 32–35°C at day old reduced 2°C per week. Use chick behaviour as the guide	Meet changing thermal competence of chicks	

Table 9.3. continued

Feature	Current recommendations	Reasons	Sources of further information
	Brooding – broilers 31°C at day old, reduced to 21°C at 17–21 days. Cooler for radiant systems. Use chick behaviour as the guide		Chapter 1
	Broiler finishing 18–24°C as optimized by models	Optimize margin over feed, provide comfort	Chapter 1
	Broiler breeders 18–20°C		
	Turkeys 12–20°C depending on market	Optimize margin, provide comfort	Chapter 1
Photoperiod	Layers – light proofed houses – 8 h to 18 weeks, then increased to 17 h, usually by weekly steps of 15–20 min; or 4 × 1 h steps from 18 weeks followed by weekly 15 min steps to 17 h, or to 18 h in hot climates	Stimulate ovulation	Chapter 1
	Windowed open houses, or poorly light proofed houses 23 h at day old reduced to natural light at 18 weeks, then step up		
	Broilers – often long days of up to 23½ h, but intermittent now debated		Table 9.5 Chapter 1
Light intensity	Layers – 10 to 20 lux for all birds		This chapter
	Rearing – unimportant provided not bright rearing followed by dim laying		

	Broilers – bright at first, then declining		See Table 9.5
Insulation	*U* Value 0.4 W m^{-2} °C^{-1} or less. Vapour check on the inside essential		Chapter 8
Broiler feeders	Versions of chains or pans	Supply feed to appetite but with minimal waste	
Broiler drinkers	Nipples and drip cups – several versions available	Supply water *ad libitum*, but with minimum waste, thereby keeping litter drier (cold climates)	
	For hot climates (particularly hot and dry) large drip cups needed	Encourage water intake and head wetting (hot climates)	
Nesting systems	Litter, plastic, plastic turf and various mechanized systems are available		
Laying cage design			
Cage floors	Flexible floors of moderate slope better than rigid steep slope floors. If welded wire steep slopes are used, they should have a horizontal collecting cradle	To minimize shell damage	
Anti-egg eating baffle plates	Should be designed so that birds can grip them, e.g. rods or slats – or shallow sloping plate	To avoid egg eating	
Feeding systems	Use a deep trough with waste prevention lips and keep the level of feed in the trough low	To minimize waste (particularly in cold climates)	

Table 9.3. continued

Feature	Current recommendations	Reasons	Sources of further information
	Some alternatives are hopper/trough, spiral, sleeve, grid, disc, and chain feeders. Check metal troughs regularly for rusting and repair if necessary to avoid feed wastage		
Drinking systems	Nipple or cup drinkers at 1 per 10 birds. It is necessary to allow access to 2 such drinkers from each cage	To achieve good performance while minimizing water wastage	
	In hot climates cups or troughs are preferable to encourage water intake		
Cage fronts and sides	These should be as smooth and as open as possible to minimize abrasion and feather wear		
Laying cage shape	Shallow or reverse cages increase capital cost per bird without consistently improving bird performance		
Effect on house stocking rate	For high stocking rates use vertical or semi-stepped cages several tiers high. These may necessitate mechanical manure handling and provision for inspection. Medium stocking rates are achieved with fully stepped cages and low stocking rates with flat deck (single tier) cages. In both of these, frequent manure handling can be avoided		

Manure handling and storage	Vertically tiered cages require mechanical manure handling – most other systems allow or assist manure to fall by gravity onto a conveyor or into a pit In the latter case the drier the manure the better, because there is less weight to move and odour problems are reduced. In-house manure drying systems help by allowing warm exhaust ventilation air to pass over the manure, which builds up in all columns with a high surface area
Broiler litters materials for raised floors and perches	Various alternative litters to wood-shavings have been tested. Most, including chopped straw, chopped newspaper, sand and mixtures of these with shavings have proved acceptable. Metal or wooden slats covered with a foam cushion and encased in tough PVC or welded wire with plastic cushioned overlay can be used as raised floors – and avoid the need to use litter
Feeding systems for turkeys	Pan tube and bulk hoppers are often mechanized. Chain feeders are not popular because of the carcass damage they cause
Alarms and back-up ventilation	Alarms are essential to both welfare and financial risk, and mandatory in EC. Back-up ventilation can be combination of generators and failsafe

Fig. 9.5

N.B. Regulations are constantly changing and R and D progress is rapid. Readers should seek professional advice on current requirements.

Table 9.4. Poultry ventilation rates.

			Requirements			
			Maximum		Minimum	
Stock	Age (days)	Weight (kg)	m^3s^{-1} per 1000 birds	Fans per 1000 birds	m^3s^{-1} per 1000 birds	Fans per 1000 birds
Pullets and layers, including breeders	–	1.8	2.3	0.9	0.25	0.10
	–	2.0	2.5	1.0	0.27	0.11
	–	2.2	2.7	1.1	0.29	0.12
	–	2.5	3.0	1.2	0.32	0.13
	–	3.0	3.4	1.4	0.36	0.15
	–	3.5	3.8	1.5	0.41	0.16
Broilers	7	0.17			0.04	0.02
	14	0.43			0.08	0.03
	21	0.80			0.14	0.05
	28	1.25			0.19	0.08
	35	1.74			0.24	0.10
	42	2.23			0.29	0.12
	49	2.68	3.1	1.3	0.33	0.13
Turkeys	–	0.5	0.9	0.4	0.10	0.04
	–	2	2.5	1.0	0.27	0.11
	–	5	5.0	2.0	0.53	0.21
	–	10	8.4	3.4	0.90	0.36

Source: Recalculated and updated from values given by Charles (1981).
≈ 610 mm fans per 1000 birds at 70 Pa working resistance in a modern ventilation system.

purposes. There is a highly competitive market in both complete turnkey package houses and in the key components, so that detailed design by the user is not normally necessary, though as for cages a specification is useful. This should list the tolerances to be accepted in temperature control, light control, ventilation capacity and control, *U* value and brooder capacity where relevant. Values for all of these can be found in other chapters, e.g. ventilation rate recommendations are given in Chapter 1. However, a brief summary may be useful at this juncture.

Air change rate

A suitable maximum ventilation rate is $1.5 \times 10^{-3} m^3 s^{-1} kg^{-0.75}$. This is roughly 1 × 610–630 mm fan per 1000 layers or broilers. The minimum is a little over one-tenth of the maximum. Chapters 1 and 7 explain the

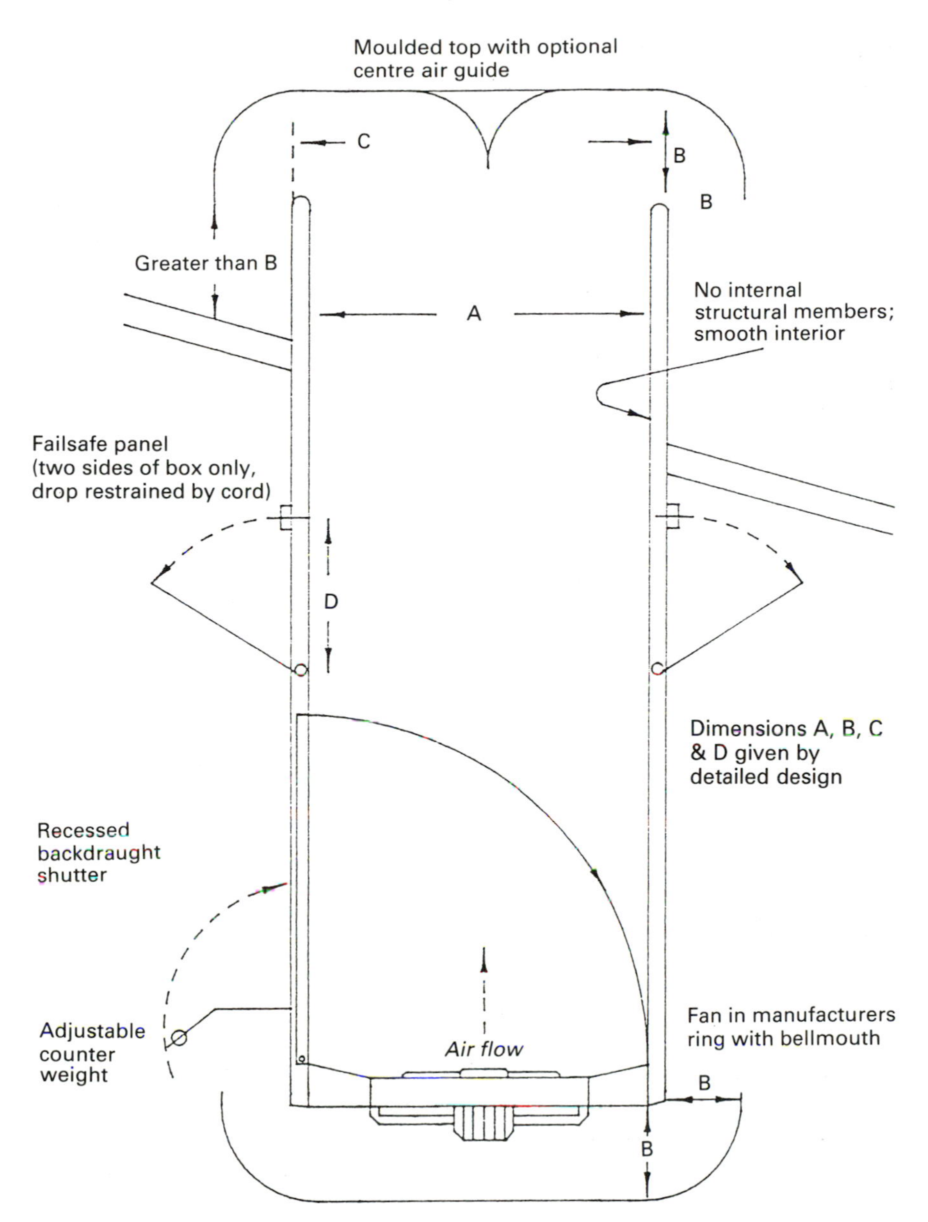

Fig. 9.5. Fan box with failsafe.

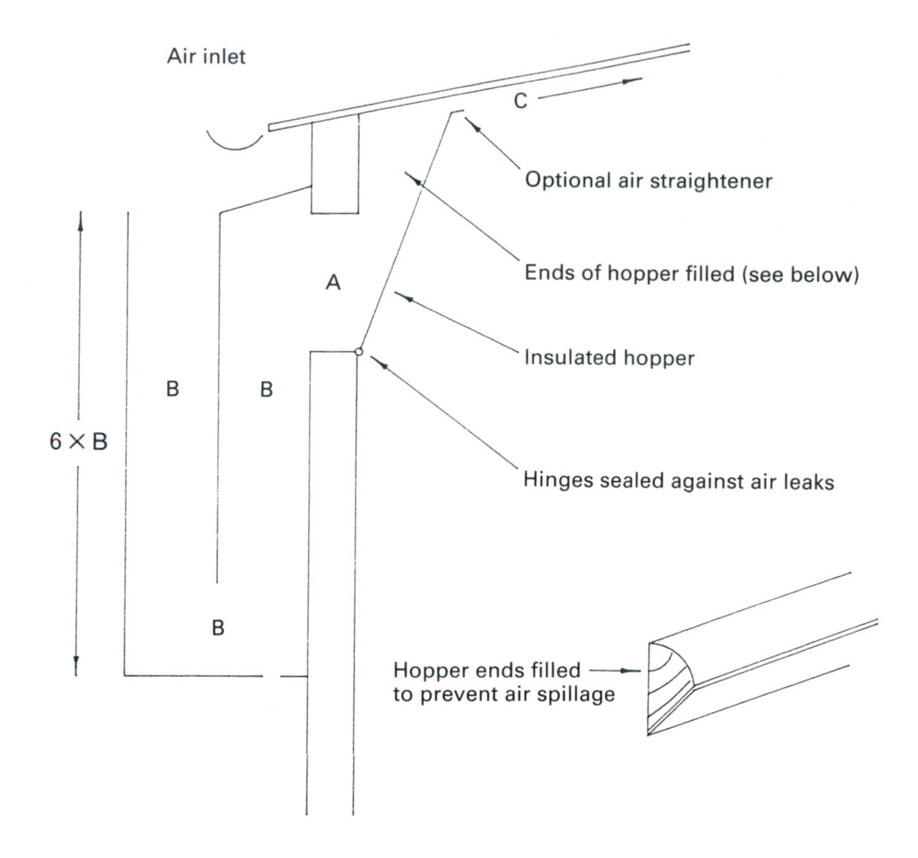

Fig. 9.6. A typical light and wind baffled air inlet. Dimensions A, B and C require detailed calculation, but typically result in airspeeds of 3.7, 4 and 5 $m s^{-1}$ respectively.

principles behind these values, which should not be used without further reference to these chapters. For growing broilers and turkeys it is necessary to recalculate the minimum ventilation rate requirement daily in order to set the system controls. Precision is worth while, because excessive air will be associated with high heating costs and inadequate air with poor air quality and all its consequences, some of which are very serious both to welfare and to commercial operations.

Equipment

This includes feeders, feed bins and distribution equipment, drinkers, and nests where appropriate. As for the items above they are all readily available at competitive prices, though usually the house supplier is treated as the main contractor in new installations.

Types of feeder

1. Manually filled open troughs are suitable for low capital high labour installations, which means small units in some countries.
2. Systems for cages employing an open trough but equipped with a travelling hopper or conveyor of some kind are desirable. It has been found necessary to limit the feed depth and to protect the feed against flicking in order to reduce waste. This is important since in most countries feed is a high proportion of the total cost of production.
3. There are distribution systems based on various conveyors for battery cages, and for floor systems there are two main systems – chain feeders running in continuous troughs or pans supplied by overhead or adjacent conveyors in pipes.

Types of drinker

For battery cages nipple drinkers are the most popular but for floor systems there are cups, valves, nipples and nipples with drip cups (whose size depends on class of stock), bell-shaped drinkers and troughs, each of which occurs in several versions.

Electrical equipment and lighting

Engineering detail is beyond the scope of this chapter, but a few specific points, relevant to poultry, may be helpful in addition.

Power supply and capacity

Supply to the house must be adequate for lighting, electric motors associated with feed distribution, egg collection equipment, ventilation fans and equipment. None of these are large loads, and power consumption is not a large proportion of production costs, so while electrical efficiency is important it is not as important as adequate specification for the job. Typically, fan motors are about 0.5 kW per 1000 birds, lights about 2–5 $W m^{-2}$, and feeder and equipment motors about 0.5–1 kW each, serving up to perhaps 10,000 birds per motor. Total supply capacity should exceed the sum of these because starting loads of motors are about 20% higher than running loads.

Voltage drop over the length of the wiring installation should not exceed that decreed by local regulations, e.g. in the UK no more than 2.5%. Of course all these values should be checked with the supplies of the equipment and all installations should be carried out by a qualified electrician. Supplies to the site must be satisfactory to the electricity supply company.

Lighting

LAYING HENS

At least 10 lux of white light is generally agreed to be necessary, but recent evidence on the subject is confusing. In order to achieve this for all birds, typical installations include 25–40 W tungsten filament lamps at 3 m centres, suitably shaded to prevent excessive intensity at the top tier of battery cages. Alternatively, 20 W 0.6 m fluorescent tubes at 5 m centres can be used, though great care should be taken to prevent very high intensities shining on the nearest birds. Shading can be designed to achieve this, but when commissioning a new house it is wise to check for reasonable uniformity using a light meter, and adjusting the angle and fit of the lamp shades. There is not perfect agreement about the suitability of fluorescent light for layers, and according to the most complete experiment on the subject the electrical savings are about equal to the cash value of a small increase in feed intake.

BREEDERS

The design constraints are similar to those for layers, except that it seems to be particularly important to avoid bright patches of intensely illuminated litter.

Table 9.5. A typical lighting scheme for broilers.

Age (days)	Maximum intensity (lux)
0	40
1	40
2	30
3	20
4	20
5	20
6	10
7	10
8	3.5
9	3.5
10 to end	2.5

BROILERS
At day-old, 15–40 lux is usually provided, often reducing to much lower intensities later, at least in countries adopting light tight housing.

Considerable care with the orientation and position of the fittings is needed in order to achieve these intensities, and from day 8 the light sources need to be lifted up and are hung on chains.

Alarms, failsafes and generators

The need for these items of equipment is partly dictated by technical and commercial requirements, and partly by animal welfare requirements. In addition, in the UK there are British Standards applying. Table 9.2 alludes briefly to some of these things, but much more detail is available in Chapter 15. There are, however, some simple technical constraints, which have had some influence on the statutory guidelines and which are important enough to merit brief mention in this chapter.

Alarms should generally respond to off-limits temperature, rather than, for example, to power failure, since temperature is the most reliable single indicator of failure of the ventilation equipment, even though that failure may be for any one of several possible causes. When the ventilation fails there is a build-up of temperature, ammonia, carbon dioxide, humidity, and many lesser pollutants, but high temperature is reliably related to all the others and is detectable by simple reliable equipment.

Back-up ventilation systems, including failsafe systems (Fig. 9.7) and stand-by generators, are usually designed to an air change capacity capable of preventing metabolic heat causing house temperature to exceed 5°C above outside temperature. This has been shown to be associated with acceptable control over air composition, at least for the purposes of an emergency, and in temperate climates to be associated with a very low meteorological probability of disaster due to the coincidence of hot still humid weather and maximum bird air requirement.

Brooders and heaters

There are two different principles of brooding young chicks and poults. As explained in Chapter 1 quite high temperatures are required for the first few days, but they may be arrived at by various combinations of convected and radiant heat. Charles (1986) reviewed the earlier literature, since when Alsam and Wathes (1991a,b) have provided more information.

Systems employing a high radiant component may be used to provide a focus of heat under the heater while running the room dry bulb air temperature at 21–25°C in the interests of fuel economy. Convectional systems, miscellaneously called blown air or whole house systems, heat the whole space to the brooding temperature as required on that day (see

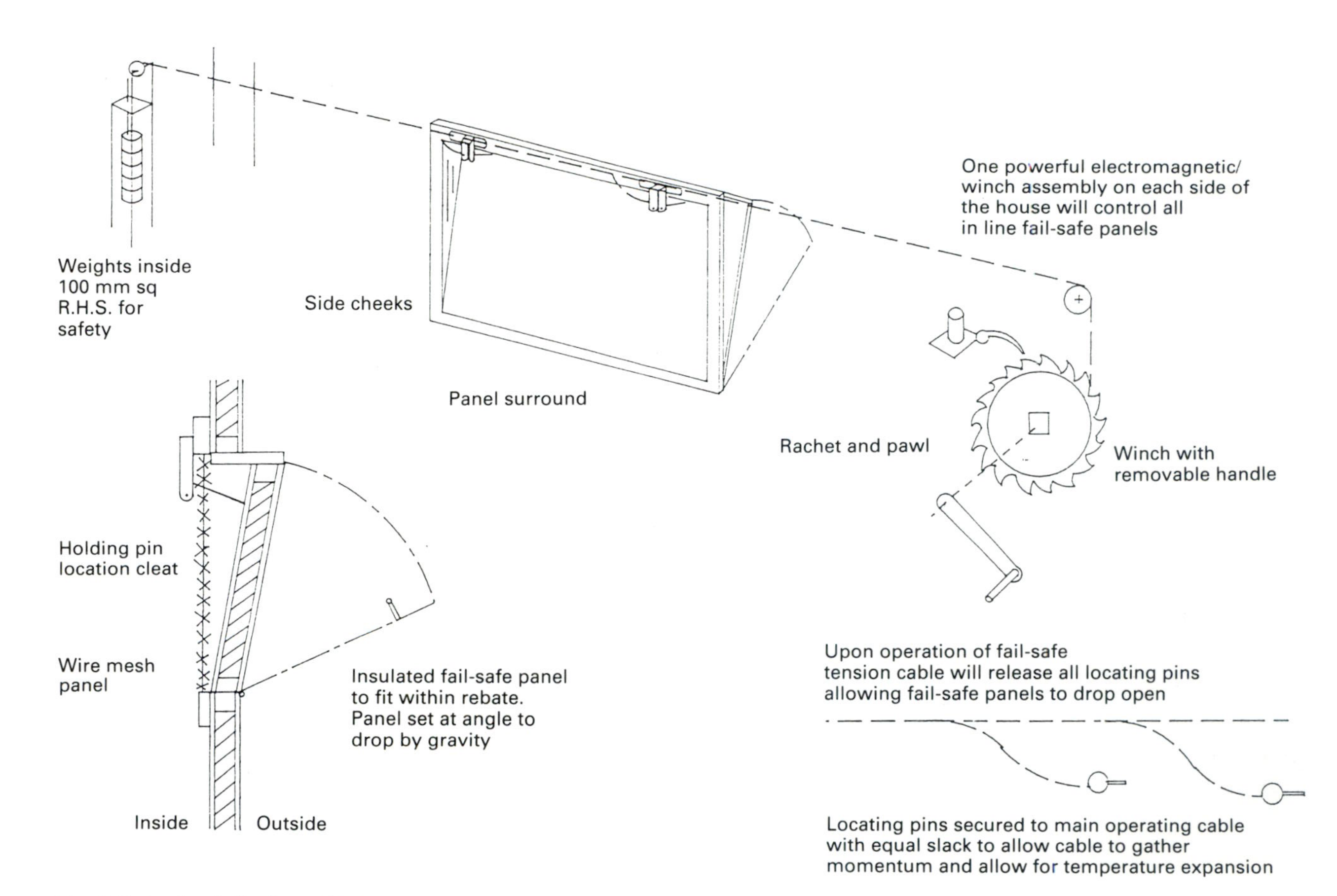

Fig. 9.7. In-line failsafe system.

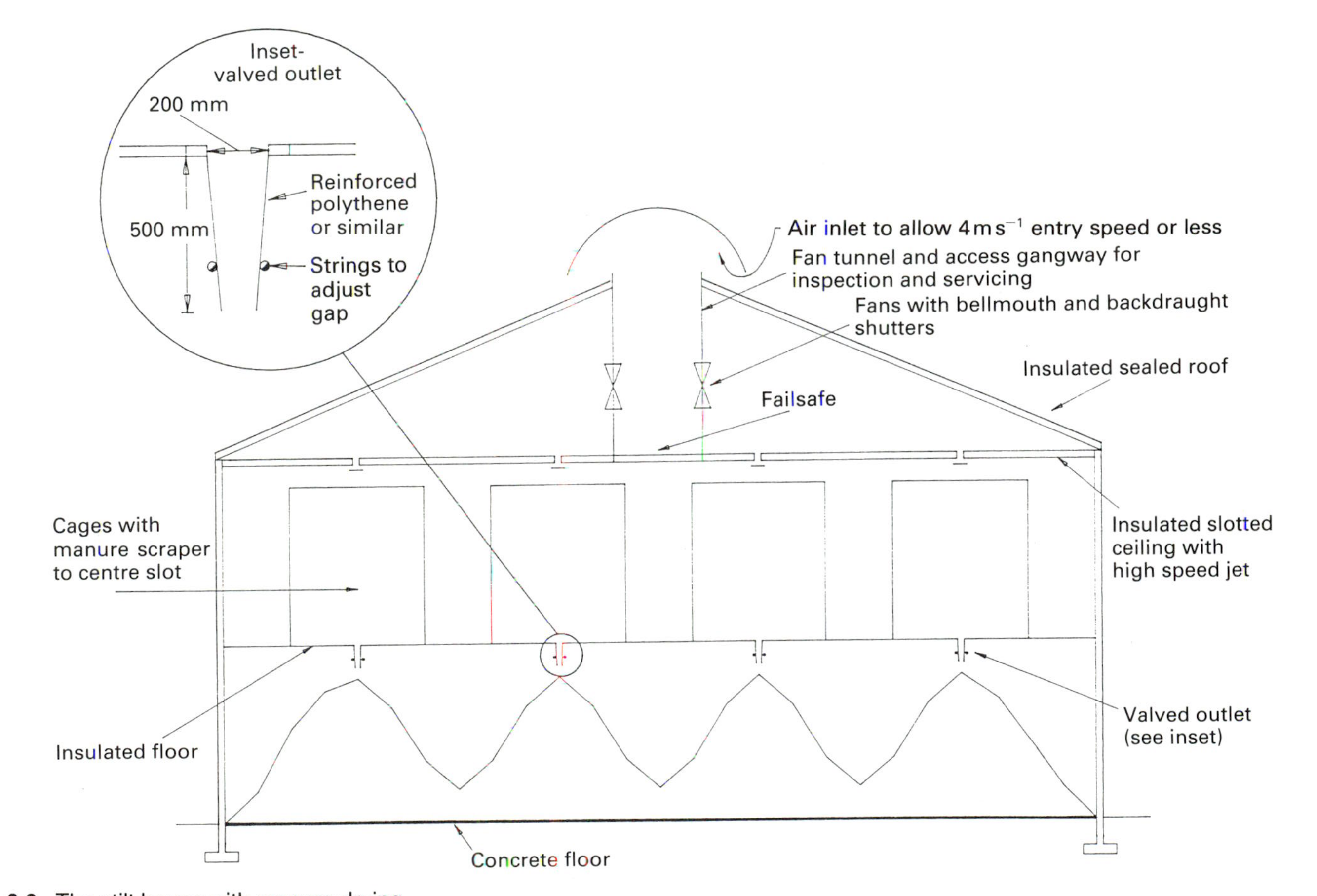

Fig. 9.8. The stilt house with manure drying.

Chapter 1). Both systems, or combinations of the two, have been shown to be biologically acceptable and to sustain chick growth.

Radiant systems are potentially cheaper to run, and give the birds an element of choice of temperature, but they involve large numbers of relatively small modules in large houses. Some may consider this less convenient to operate. The percentage of the heat which is radiant is very variable between designs. Whole room heaters inevitably consume a little more fuel since the whole house is warmed, but they permit the use of low numbers of heaters even in very large houses. The capacity of heater required depends on circumstances and professional advice should be sought for the calculations, but as a rule of thumb an allowance of about 4–10 W per chick will often suffice.

Manure drying

In many countries one of the problems facing poultry producers is disposal of manure, since there is growing concern abut the pollution of water by leachates. The housing and ventilation system shown in Figs 9.2 and 9.8 has recently been developed to provide drying of manure, by virtue of reuse of the metabolic heat. At the time of writing there were about 350,000 layers housed in the system, with a biological performance ranking among the best in the world. Readers should seek professional advice before installing, since attention to detail is important.

References

Alsam, H. and Wathes, C.M. (1991a) Thermal preference of chicks brooded at different air temperatures. *British Poultry Science* 32, 31–46.

Alsam, H. and Wathes, C.M. (1991b) Conjoint preferences of chicks for heat and light intensity. *British Poultry Science* 32, 899–916.

Appleby, M.C., Hughes, B.O. and Elson, H.A. (1992) *Poultry Production Systems: Behaviour, Management and Welfare.* CAB International, Wallingford, UK.

Charles, D.R. (1981) Practical ventilation and temperature control for poultry. In: Clark, J.A. (ed.), *Environmental Aspects of Housing for Animal Production.* Butterworths, London.

Charles. D.R. (1986) Temperature for broilers. *World's Poultry Science Association Journal* 42, 249–258.

Charles, D.R. (1988) Defining the environment. In: *Progress in Poultry Production.* Royal Agricultural Society of England, pp. 7–14.

Wilson, E.A. (1988) Surface energy exchange in poultry houses. Unpublished thesis. University of Nottingham.

10
Pig Housing

A.T. SMITH
ADAS Wolverhampton, UK

Historical Background

Pig production in many countries gradually developed from a cottage industry with a large number of small herds to a highly specialized industry with a smaller number of comparatively large herds. The changing structure of the industry in England and Wales is illustrated in Table 10.1. Prior to the 1960s simple housing was common with little modification in type between production stages. Indeed the clear stratification between production stages only developed during the 1960s as large enterprises and specialist producers became more common.

Increasing specialization brought improved skills with a desire to utilize them to maximum effect. Housing designs became tailored to the specific needs of production stages to optimize labour use and eliminate the laborious tasks which were associated with general-purpose accommodation. The combination of specialized producers, economically dependent on a sole commodity, and the ever-fluctuating economic returns forced the pursuit of ever higher productivity.

Sow stalls grew in popularity as they were perceived as a convenient method of caring for large numbers of animals while attending their individual needs. Feed levels could be accurately controlled and health problems detected early. Tether stalls had particular application in the conversion of existing buildings in the late 1960s and early 1970s, as they could be accommodated where structural dimensions did not facilitate the use of full stalls.

Farrowing facilities also became increasingly specialized during this time, as long-term trials demonstrated lower mortality levels in crates compared to traditional free farrowing pens which provided very limited

Table 10.1. The changing pattern of sow herd structure in England and Wales.

	Percentage of total sows and gilts		
Size of herd (sows and gilts)	1962	1972	1987
1–9	32.4	10.0	2.4
10–19	22.9	11.1	2.6
20–29	12.2	9.0	2.5
30–49	13.4	14.6	5.5
50–99	11.6	24.0	14.3
100 and over	7.5	(31.3)	(72.6)
100–199	–	18.4	25.3
200 and over	–	12.9	47.4
No. of sows and gilts ('000)	678.2	778.9	710.3
No. of herds	82,789	37,995	11,877
Av. no. of sows and gilts per herd	8.2	20.5	59.8

Source: MAFF, annual data.

control (Robertson *et al.*, 1966). Crates also require less space than traditional pens and the resulting increase in stocking density, together with insulation of the structure and ventilation control, creates a warmer environment for the newly born piglets. An additional benefit of the fixed crate system is the reduction in labour involved in cleaning. Crates in fixed positions ensure that effluent is concentrated in one place in each pen and hence easily removed, particularly when perforated floors are also incorporated. Thus the single pen farrowing system was replaced with rooms of crates, reducing labour and increasing piglet survival rates simultaneously.

Intensive pig production may be classified by the types of construction of particular housing systems. These can be considered in terms of fully insulated, 'controlled environment' buildings in which the pig has limited scope to select its environment, and those buildings incorporating kennels, in which the thermal environment is subject to control in the lying area only. The design of the latter is largely governed by a combination of structural requirements and pig behaviour. The proportion of herds adopting a whole house 'controlled environment' approach varies with production stage while 'kennel housing' remains an important form of pig housing in the UK (Table 10.2; Smith, 1987). Kennel housing persists to a greater extent in the UK than in other countries because of the temperate climate and the availability of straw. Other factors include cyclical profitability of pig production and a predilection for home-based construction of buildings.

Table 10.2. Proportion of kennel housing.

Stage of production	Whole house (% herds)	Kennel type (% herds)
Dry sows	52	48
Farrowing and lactation	93	7
Post-weaning	44	56
Follow-on	17	83
Finisher	41	59

Factors Influencing Housing Design

Climate

Pigs are sensitive to temperature and their responses can be detected in both performance and behaviour. However, their ability to modify heat loss through behavioural changes makes them extremely adaptable, and they can thrive in a wide range of circumstances. Their performance response to changing temperatures depends on all the components of the environment. Pigs kept individually on unbedded floors and a controlled level of feeding have little opportunity to use their behavioural repertoire to cope with changing climatic environments. By contrast, group housed pigs fed *ad libitum* with a generous space allowance and free access to a sheltered, insulated lying area have great scope to manipulate their behaviour in response to temperature changes. Consequently, the former require a closely controlled thermal environment unlike the latter in a temperate climate such as that in the UK. This explains, in part, why optimum pig performance is obtainable in a wide range of housing types.

The clear implication is that many interdependent components are important in the provision of a satisfactory environment for pigs. Air temperature, although of prime importance, needs to be considered in the context of all the thermal components (see this volume, Chapter 5).

Current production systems involve early weaning which has the potential to raise sow output by shortening the breeding cycle. Unfortunately, early weaning leads to a temporary decline in energy intake in piglets thereby creating a severe drop in metabolic heat output (MAFF, 1982). Counteracting this deficit requires high air temperatures (Fig. 10.1) which are most reliably achieved in fully insulated, controlled environment buildings incorporating supplementary heating. Early weaned pigs are also susceptible to enteric diseases and therefore benefit from accommodation with a high standard of hygiene. This requirement is met by the use of fully

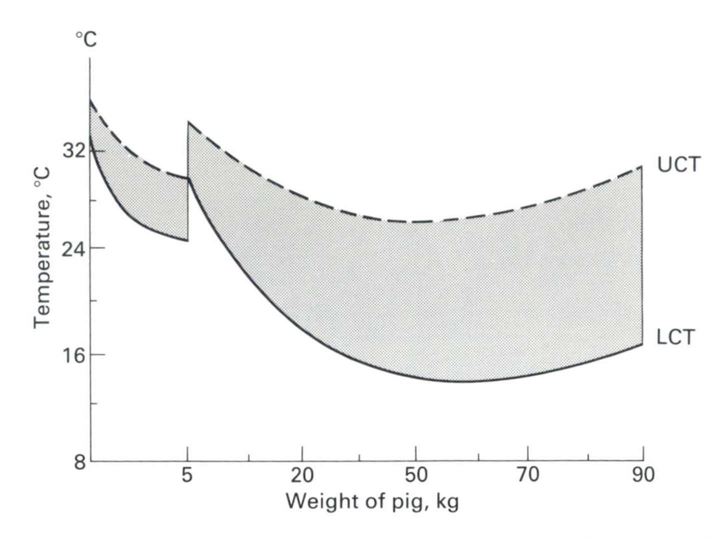

Fig. 10.1. The effect of early weaning on critical temperature: UCT, upper critical temperature; LCT, lower critical temperature.

perforated floors and an all in, all out, system of management, as found in flat deck housing.

Lighting

The level of lighting needs to be considered in terms of the law, the welfare codes (Chapter 15), the pigs' requirements and those of the stock keeper.

The legal requirements are aimed at stock inspection and are satisfied quite easily. With regard to the pig, Baldwin and Start (1985) have shown that pigs prefer light rather than dark, and dim rather than bright light. Very high levels of light intensity are associated with increased levels of activity. Light intensities between 1 and 50 lux apparently satisfy the pig.

Breeding

The effect of animal breeding on housing did not begin to have a major impact until the 1980s, after a successful national breeding programme aimed at improved carcass quality and economy of production. The success of the programme in the UK can be judged by the changes in average backfat thickness of the slaughter generation over a 17-year period (Fig. 10.2). Pigs produced under the programme could now be fed *ad libitum* without accumulating an excessive thickness of backfat. In effect, their appetite no longer exceeded their capacity to convert feed into acceptable proportions of lean and fat.

Furthermore, the use of entire males for meat production, which now

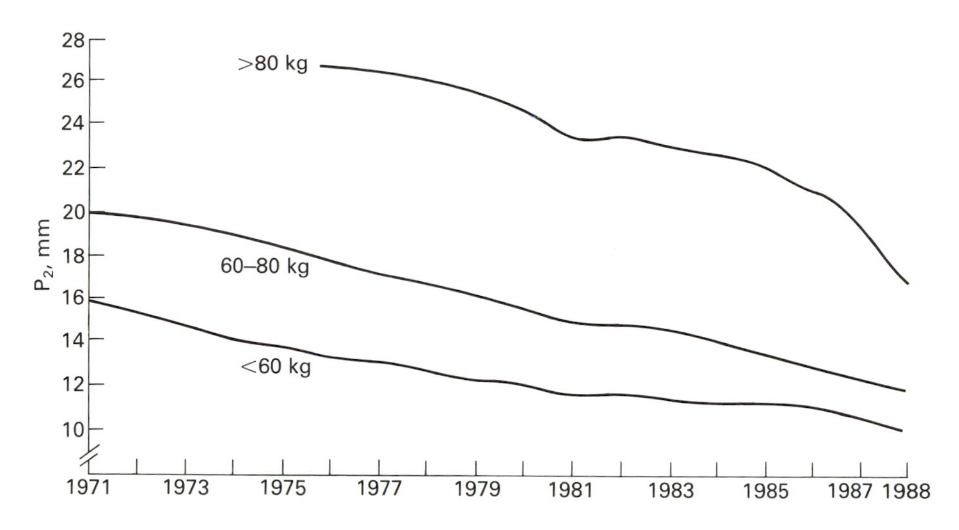

Fig. 10.2. The changing level of backfat in British pigs (1971–1988).

accounts for 85% of males slaughtered, has also reduced backfat and limited appetite. The incidence of boar taint has been kept to a very low level by the comparatively low slaughter weights prevalent in the UK.

Ad libitum feeding removes the necessity for all pigs to be fed simultaneously, and hence trough space requirement is greatly reduced. This simplification eliminates a major constraint on pen shape, which is otherwise dominated by the need to provide sufficient trough space for all pigs to be fed together. Floor feeding can be used to avoid this constraint, but at the cost of reduced feed conversion efficiency. All pigs cannot be fed *ad libitum* because of genetic variation, differing carcass specifications and market weights. Housing design must be sufficiently flexible to cope with changing requirements.

Local resources

Local resources also play a part in housing design. In some cereal growing areas in the UK systems involving the use of generous straw bedding persist, despite the trend to slatted floors and slurry elsewhere. Similarly, systems have been developed in dairying areas to utilize milk by-products. Good drainage is particularly important in these designs because urine output is inevitably high. Shortage of skilled labour has often meant the introduction of fully slatted systems to minimize laborious tasks.

Public opinion

There has been a steady growth in public opinion against pig production systems which are perceived to be highly restrictive, harmful to the environment, or which constitute a health hazard. Concerns over animal welfare were aroused in the late 1960s and led to the publication of the Codes of Recommendations for the Welfare of Pigs (MAFF, 1983; see also this volume, Chapter 15).

Growing concern over environmental issues also affects pig production via greater control over activities which could give rise to either air or water pollution. The siting of enterprises and management of effluent is now subject to greater constraints.

The implications for the pig industry are far reaching. Not only is there a requirement to minimize odour because of its offensiveness, but also to reduce emissions of specific pollutants such as ammonia. Ground and water pollution may also arise from poor manure management during storage, handling and land application. The challenge to the industry is to manage its affairs in such a way as to minimize harmful effects on the environment, e.g. by devising diets of optimum protein content which minimize urea excretion.

The implications for pig housing of anxiety over food safety, are far reaching. Concern about the misuse or abuse of drugs increases the emphasis on the need for maintenance of health through good management, husbandry and housing practices. In essence this requires that the overall strategy should be aimed at minimizing stress, which lowers resistance to disease, and minimizing the risk of pathogen challenge.

The above concerns have led to consumer demand for products that are perceived to be healthy and produced under good welfare and environmentally friendly conditions. The major retail organizations have responded to this demand by marketing 'branded pig meat products'. A guarantee is given of the product's source and the production methods employed, in particular the type of housing. These developments usually increase the production costs, which must be related to the likely returns. An essential element of this development is that it should safeguard the real welfare of the pig. The long-term success will be influenced by the realism of the production constraints imposed.

Legislation

Of particular concern in relation to pig housing design are the Welfare of Livestock Regulations 1990, (MAFF, 1990) the Welfare of Pigs Regulations 1991 and the Welfare of Livestock (Intensive Units) Regulations 1978 (amended with effect from 1/1/92), which specify particular requirements in housing (see also Chapter 15). Specified requirements include alarm systems to warn of failure of mechanically controlled ventilation systems with alternative means of ventilation; accommodation for sick animals; adequate lighting for stock inspection; well-drained lying areas, and secure and safe structures and fittings.

The Welfare of Pigs Regulations 1991 prohibit tethering or the very close confinement of pigs. Existing systems can continue in use until 1999 but the erection of new stall or tether systems is banned.

Structural constraints

There are two fundamentally different approaches to pig housing in the UK and many variations on those two general concepts.

Controlled environment systems

These are insulated structures which contain the whole pen and have a measure of ventilation control. A wide range of materials is in general use, from insulated concrete blocks to multi-component prefabricated panels. The target insulation value is $0.5\,W\,m^{-2}°C^{-1}$ or less (Chapter 8).

Controlled environment buildings frequently fail to meet specifications in practice for a range of reasons:

1. The characteristics of the ventilation system are not in accord with pen layout.
2. The ventilation system is inadequately designed, installed, maintained or managed.
3. Inadequacies in metabolic heat output are not compensated for by supplementary heat.
4. The overall design or management fails to take full account of pig behaviour.

Kennel systems

The alternative to controlled environment housing is the kennel, sited in the open or within uninsulated structures. Kennel systems provide pigs with: (i) a warm lying area; (ii) a second area in which they can feed, dung and exercise but without control over air temperature. Long-term comparisons of the performance of weaners in flat decks and kennels show no significant differences (Table 10.3, NAC 1979–1984).

Sows kept in kennels under range conditions have a higher feed maintenance requirement, despite access to a warm lying area. This is to be expected since pigs outdoors can cover substantial distances, often under muddy and windy conditions. The energy required for both thermoregulation and physical activity will often be substantially higher than in intensive or semi-intensive systems.

Kennel systems evolved in the absence of lightweight insulants. They decrease structural heat losses by reducing surface area. Roofs are lower and only cover the lying zone of the pen. Kennels are only fully effective when

Table 10.3. Weaner performance in two types of housing.

	Flat decks	Kennels
Number of pigs	14,238	6,047
Average weight in (kg)	6.15	6.03
Average weight out (kg)	16.9	16.45
Average daily gain (g)	319.6	320.1
Average feed : gain	1.40	1.39
Average mortality (%)	1.2	0.93

Source: NAC 1979–84.

ventilation rate is controlled by good structural design, manipulation of the ventilation openings, and correct stocking density. Kennel systems are low cost since they can be erected outdoors, or fitted within uninsulated general-purpose type structures. The latter may add value to a farm unlike specialized pig buildings.

Housing variations

NURTINGER SYSTEM

Probably the ultimate in the kennel concept is the Nurtinger system (Schwarting, 1989), which relies on well-insulated kennels (beds) of an appropriate size and shape such that the occupants breathe cool fresh air while keeping their bodies warm. All the pigs are able to lie side by side in a long narrow box with their snouts protruding through the flexible material in the side (Fig. 10.3).

OPEN-FRONTED MONOPITCH

This variant utilizes good structural design to obtain some of the advantages of kennels and of an insulated structure with controlled ventilation. Each pen is open only to the exterior. This is the simplest form of pig housing, is low cost and, given good management, allows excellent pig performance.

STRAW YARDS

These follow neither principle but rely on an abundance of straw and pig behaviour to achieve thermal comfort in the lying area (minimum 1.5 m^2 total per finishing pig). They are invariably erected in uninsulated buildings. Although growing in popularity, performance is unlikely to be optimum in the absence of kennelled lying areas.

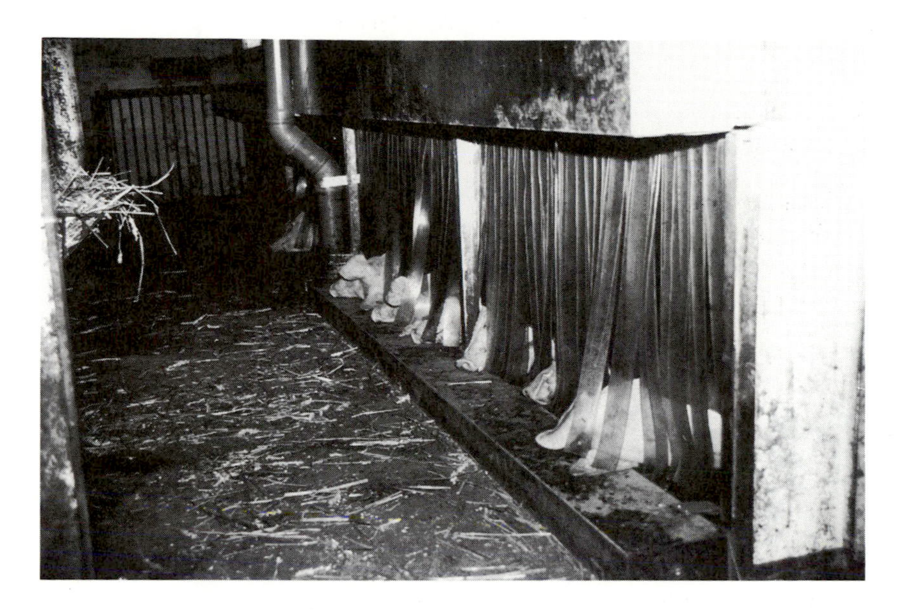

Fig. 10.3. Nurtinger beds for weaners.

Choice of ventilation system

The principles of ventilation design and the characteristics of the major ventilation systems are discussed in detail in Chapter 7.

Successful pig housing is heavily dependent on selection of a ventilation system which matches the specific requirements of the pigs at a given stage of production. A number of alternative systems are available.

Failure to understand the key role of ventilation may create many problems in practice, in relation to control of the thermal environment. If pigs are closely confined, e.g. sows in farrowing crates, and their physical environment inhibits the expression of their full behavioural repertoire, then the emphasis must be on accurate and stable temperature control to prevent stress and deficiencies in performance. If pigs have freedom of movement and a rich physical environment, then their need for thermal comfort will dominate their behaviour patterns (Fraser, 1985). The emphasis in these circumstances is to design a thermal environment which favours the desired behaviour. In practice the thermal needs of closely confined pigs are usually recognized but certainly not always met. The needs of less intensively housed pigs are much less often perceived and probably much less often fulfilled.

Table 10.4 lists the major features of ventilation systems required in various housing types. When the objectives of the housing system are

Table 10.4. Selection of ventilation design.

	Flat decks	Tier and cages	Weaner kennels	Farrowing crates	Free farrowing	Sow stalls	Sow yards	Part slatted growers	Fully slatted growers	Straw yards
Uniform temperatures	Yes	Yes	No	Yes	No	Yes	No	No	Yes	No
Temperature gradients	No	No	Yes	No	Yes	No	Yes	Yes	No	Yes
Low air speeds throughout	Yes	Yes	No	Yes	No	Yes	No	No	Yes	No
Differential air speeds	No	No	Yes	No	Yes	No	Yes	Yes	No	Yes
Independent air speed control	No	No	No	No	No	No	No	Yes	Yes	No

Table 10.5. Implications of waste management systems.

Floor type	Relative space required	Temperature gradient	Pen shape constraints	Air quality*	Pen hygiene*
Fully slatted	100	No	No	Poor	Good
Part slatted	104	Yes	Yes	Moderate	Moderate
Part scraped	104–120	Yes	Yes	Moderate	Moderate
Deep bedded	245	Yes	No	Good	Moderate
Sloping	100–110	Yes	Yes	Good	Moderate
In situ composting	160	No	No	Good	Moderate

* Variations in day-to-day management within individual systems have a major influence.

matched to the characteristics of the ventilation system the choice usually becomes quite limited; making the choice is then greatly simplified.

Alarms and alternative ventilation

All ventilation systems which rely on automatic equipment require alarms to warn of system failure. In addition, the buildings must be equipped with alternative means of ventilation to ensure that any system failures do not result in unnecessary distress.

Waste management systems

The choice of manure management system has a direct influence on space requirements, air quality, pen hygiene and overall building design. It also has implications for the choice of ventilation system. Separate lying and dunging areas necessitate warm and cold zones and hence temperature gradients, whereas fully slatted systems can function satisfactorily with uniform temperature distribution.

The major implications of waste management systems are summarized in Table 10.5.

Feeding system

Feeding regime

In sequential feeding, pigs are fed either *ad libitum* from self-help hoppers or restricted quantities via a computer-controlled feeder. There is no requirement for a particular pen shape. There is some scope for variation in siting the feeding point, but the primary consideration should be to create an undisturbed lying area and ample space for manoeuvring near the feeder. Pigs will normally choose to rest for 75–80% of time, but feeding activity in the pen may take up to 50% or more of time depending on the ratio of pigs to feeding places.

If pigs are fed a restricted quantity then trough spaces should match the number of pigs. This regime has important implications for pen shape and total space. Space requirements are minimized where feeding occurs in the lying area. Straight troughs result in long narrow pens, while round troughs require square pens. Floor feeding removes pen shape constraints but invariably increases feed wastage.

Feed type

The use of concentrates allows maximum flexibility in pen design. The use of bulky feeds has been limited during the period of increasing intensivism.

The likelihood is that the use of such feeds will increase in future. The major implications for pen design are that large dispensers are required and the feeding period will be prolonged. It is desirable to avoid provision of bulky feeds in the lying area

Feeds which contain a high water content raise urine output, and should not be fed in solid-floored lying areas because of spillage. Where this cannot be avoided, floor slopes should be pronounced and be designed to minimize the spread of spillages.

Water delivery systems

The provision of an adequate water supply is crucial to the well-being of the pig. Water requirements of pigs vary considerably depending on air temperature, humidity and feed ingredients but are normally around 2.5 times the weight of dry food consumed. The manner in which water is provided can influence both accessibility and waste. The former has important implications for welfare and performance, and the latter for effluent management.

Drinkers should always be sited well away from lying areas, and in a manner which eases access and limits unnecessary waste. Drinkers should be set at an angle of 15 to 20° to the horizontal, slanted upwards at a height which creates an appropriate upward drinking angle (Gill and Barber, 1990). Side barriers ensure that pigs stand straight on to the drinker which helps to reduce water wastage. Low flow rates reduce performance and increase competition, while high rates increase waste (Barber *et al.*, 1988). The ratio of drinkers to pigs is subject to Welfare Code guidelines of one drinker to ten pigs. More may be needed for simultaneous feeding, which creates higher peak demands for water than *ad libitum* feeding (Hepherd *et al.*, 1983). Water troughs are more flexible, but require sound design and a high standard of management to maintain hygiene.

Implications of the use of straw

The Codes of Recommendations for the Welfare of Pigs (MAFF, 1983) strongly recommend systems in which straw or similar material is provided in the lying area. Bedding, especially straw, is advised because 'it contributes towards the needs of the pig for thermal and physical comfort, and satisfies some of its behavioural requirements'.

The implications for waste management draw attention to the increasing space requirements normally associated with straw-based systems. Other implications of straw use include running costs, labour requirements, and perhaps animal and human health.

Thermal comfort

The influence of including bedding straw, as one means of reducing heat loss to the floor, is well established (Bruce and Clarke, 1979). Straw also allows pigs to create 'nests' as protection against draughts. However, alternative bedding materials and floor designs are available with insulation values similar to those of straw.

Physical comfort

Physical comfort might be construed to be important to an animal that spends 75–80% of its time lying down. The extent to which straw contributes to this potential need depends on temperature (Fraser, 1985; Mertz, 1988), as confirmed by practical experience. If cold, pigs choose a straw bed, and if hot, they reject it. This suggests that thermal comfort is a more compelling motivator than physical comfort. Pigs can differentiate between floor types, and newly weaned pigs prefer plastic coated mesh, perforated metal, glass fibre slats, or plastic panels to wire mesh when given a choice of perforated floors (Farmer and Christison, 1982; Marx and Schuster, 1982). In a review of work on flooring for pigs, it was concluded that pigs' floor preference is determined by void: solid ratio, surface temperature, traction and friction (Kornegay and Lindemann, 1984).

Behaviour requirements

Pigs have a strong tendency to root and chew, and straw serves as a focus for this activity. Given the opportunity, pigs will spend much time on these activities. Newly weaned pigs kept in flat decks showed a markedly greater tendency towards massaging, sucking and nibbling other pigs than those on straw (Van Putten, 1981). Provision of straw to confined pigs generally reduces tail biting and other anomalous behaviours (Fraser, 1985). There seems little doubt that environmental enrichment by provision of straw enables pigs to express 'natural' behaviour patterns (see Chapter 4). However, alternative environmental enrichment solutions are possible where the use of straw is impractical.

Running costs

The use of straw inevitably increases costs: however, it also has a value as manure. Traditional straw-bedded systems use about 650 g of straw per kg liveweight gain (Smith, 1981) compared to 60–125 $g\,kg^{-1}$ liveweight gain in the 'straw flow' system (Bruce, 1990). There is a strong incentive for building designers to give careful consideration to the type of straw-based system. Costs of handling straw within buildings are unknown. Modern equipment and well-designed layouts can do much to limit the labour required. Time spent littering down with straw in a traditional open-fronted piggery is about 30 min per 100 pigs per week (Meneer, 1977, personal communication).

Health and safety

Studies carried out in a number of countries have revealed that pig stock keepers have a high incidence of respiratory disease (Donham *et al.*, 1984; Watson and Friend, 1987), which is probably related to the level of airborne contaminants, including dust. Straw clearly provides a further source of pollutants, which may impose additional burdens on the stock keepers (and pigs). However, critical levels have yet to be established (see Chapter 6).

Space requirements

Trough space

Traditionally, trough space has been allocated on the basis of shoulder width for restricted fed stock while normally one feeder place is provided for each four or five pigs on *ad libitum* feeding. Shoulder barriers are more effective than increased trough space in reducing aggressive encounters (Baxter, 1986). The commercial introduction of the single space feeder in place of multi-space feeders calls into question the space allocation required for *ad libitum* feeding. A number of trials have shown that pig performance has not been diminished but often enhanced by such feeders (Walker and Overton, 1988). The ratio of pigs to feeder spaces can be as high as 20 to 1 without affecting performance (Morrow and Walker, 1991). These feeders have fairly well protected sides which resemble shoulder barriers. The question of the real influence of such feeders on pig behaviour has not been fully resolved although very high pig to feeder ratios change feeding patterns and increase aggressive interactions. One feeder place shared by 10–12 pigs appears to provide both acceptable behaviour and performance.

Feeding space for dry sows varies from one place per sow for simultaneous feeding up to one place for every 45 sows or more on sequential feeding. Higher ratios are possible with multi-pen systems.

Total space

The total space required in any system of housing depends on which criteria are used. The UK Codes of Recommendations for the Welfare of Pigs (MAFF, 1983) proposed space allowances – based on liveweight – for lying areas which were close to the then current commercial practice. The Codes also state that space is required for exercise and dunging. Lying space

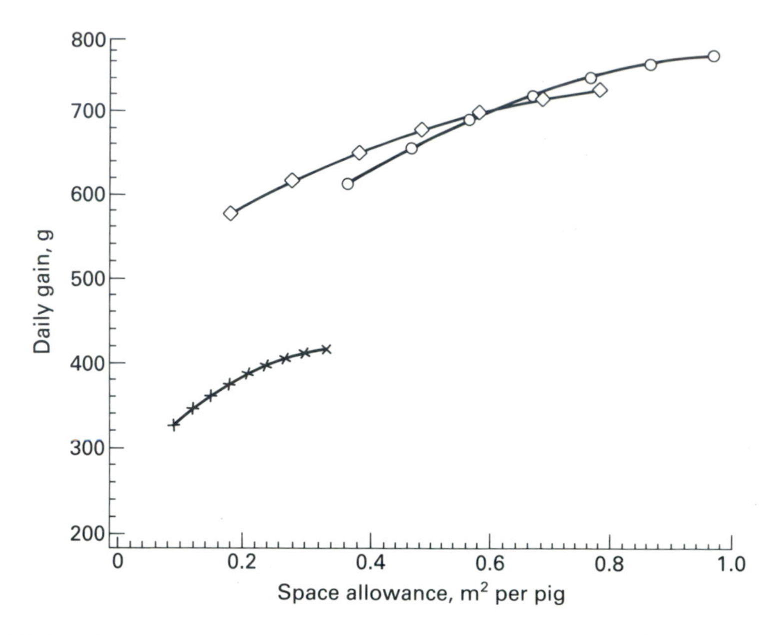

Fig. 10.4. Relationship between space allowance and growth rate (from Kornegay and Notter, 1984).

requirements were given an improved scientific foundation by the use of allometry (Petherick, 1983). Other space requirements include the needs for specific activities such as mating, farrowing, thermoregulation and feeding behaviours as well as those associated with establishing dominance.

Many trials have been undertaken to determine effects on performance of space restriction and have usually, but not invariably, shown a deterioration in performance as space allowances have been reduced (NRC, 1984, 1989; Kornegay and Notter, 1984 (see Fig. 10.4); Hunt, 1987).

Stocking density trials have often produced results confounded by group size and/or trough space. A trial to eliminate those variables and establish a response curve for growth rates of finishing pigs at different space allowances on fully slatted floors was undertaken at ADAS Terrington Experimental Husbandry Farm (Edwards *et al.*, 1988). Growth rate increased with space allowance (A, m^2) with the minimum value required represented by $A = KW^{2/3}$ (where $K = 0.027$ and W = liveweight, kg). In commercial practice the slightly higher value of $K = 0.030$ should be adopted as a minimum.

Space allowances must also take account of possible adverse effects on behaviour. It has been established that reducing space allowance can increase agonistic activity (Ewebank and Bryant, 1972). It is clear that total space allowance must not be divorced from environmental quality, which may be enriched by the provision of bedding, rooting material or even

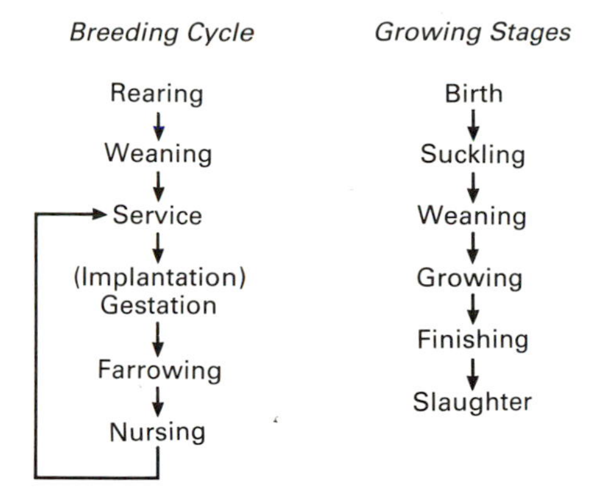

Fig. 10.5. Stages of pig production.

'toys'. The Edinburgh family pens are an example of enrichment (Stolba, 1981), but even relatively minor modifications, such as hides, have been shown to have important effects on behaviour (McGlone and Curtis, 1985).

Production Stages

Modern pig production systems, including housing, have evolved through the commercial objectives of maximum output at least cost. The production stages are shown in Fig. 10.5. The breeding cycle involves the distinctly separate stages of service, pregnancy, farrowing and lactation, while the growing stage is normally subdivided into weaners, growers and finishers. A single but complex pen can be used from birth to the slaughter, as in the Edinburgh family pen, but it is not yet commercially viable (Stolba, 1981). In its original form it apparently satisfied behavioural needs but was demanding on management and labour use as well as leaving scope for improvement in pig performance. Nevertheless, it demonstrated the difference between systems born of commercial pressure and those aimed at the pig's requirements.

The design of pig buildings is constantly evolving and there is no doubt that some of the principles demonstrated in the family pen project will find their way into commercial production.

General principles

The following general principles need to be addressed for all stages of production:

1. *Space.* Sufficient space to allow normal behavioural activity is a basic welfare requirement. Performance declines as space is reduced (Kornegay and Notter, 1984).

2. *Thermal comfort.* This includes air temperature, air speed, floor surfaces and all the other components of heat exchange. Thermal balance influences resting behaviour and hence greatly affects overall activity and pen use (Geers *et al.*, 1986; Marx *et al.*, 1989).

3. *Feed and water.* Nutrition must be adequate to sustain health and well-being. Fresh water should be freely available.

4. *Stimuli.* Appropriate stimuli should be provided to allow the expression of the normal behavioural repertoire (van Putten, 1981; Simonsen, 1990).

5. *Light.* Intensity and duration should be appropriate to establish indigenously induced biphasic rhythms of activity (Schrenk, 1981).

These criteria are focused on the pigs. In order to function in the commercial world consideration must also be given to:

- The economic viability of the enterprise.
- The health, safety and job satisfaction of the workers.
- The impact on the external environment.

In all commercial enterprises the following should have a high priority at all production stages:

- Capital and running costs within the economic constraints of the business.
- Manure management designed to avoid water pollution and curtail odour nuisance.
- Safeguards for workers health.

The fundamental requirement in all pig enterprises is good husbandry. This is well understood by good stock people but has also been quantified (Hemsworth *et al.*, 1981).

In addition, each production stage has specific requirements as shown below.

Service stage

1. Provide optimum stimulation for gilts and sows to promote early and pronounced oestrus (Tilbrook and Hemsworth, 1990).

2. Provide appropriate space to allow normal mating behaviour to take place (Petchey and Hunt, 1990).

3. Minimize the likelihood of physical or thermal stress following service and throughout the implantation period.

4. Focus the attention of the stockkeeper on this key production area.

Gestation stage

Separate housing may be provided from immediately post-service or from up to one month after service (implantation stage) or the service section may be contained within the gestation building. The essential requirements remain similar.

1. Allocate accurately the nutrients to maintain reproductive efficiency without waste.
2. Provide means of combating the hunger normally created by pronounced reduction in feed level (Lawrence *et al.*, 1988).
3. Minimize aggression by due regard to group dynamics.

Farrowing and lactation

1. Minimize piglet mortality by providing an appropriate thermal and physical environment.
2. Maximize sow comfort by providing appropriate space and thermal environment.
3. Ensure sufficient flexibility to cater for the rapidly changing needs of the growing piglets.

Combining farrowing and lactation facilities into one pen is common practice. It is, however, a practical compromise which is not necessarily optimum for either stage.

Post-weaning stage

The needs of weaners are dictated by the age of weaning. In natural weaning the process is completed at between 7 and 14 weeks of age. In those circumstances piglets have gradually acquired the habit of eating dry food and suffer no sudden energy deficit at weaning.

In artificial weaning systems the sudden removal of the dam's milk creates an energy deficit while the digestive system adjusts to the solid feed.

1. Provide elevated thermal environment to balance reduced metabolic heat production after weaning.
2. Provide a high standard of pen hygiene to reduce pathogen challenge while the immune system is vulnerable.
3. Minimize physical, social and climatic stressors.

Growing and finishing stage

The precise requirements depend on the genetic make-up of the pig, the type of feed provided and market demand.

1. Provide a feed delivery regime that optimizes performance while producing a carcass quality that meets market requirements.
2. Provide facilities to separate the sexes where appropriate.

Current Housing Options

Pre-pubertal gilts

SPECIAL REQUIREMENTS

- Sexual stimulation (1 m separation from mature boar).
- Controlled feeding.

DESIRABLE PROVISIONS

- Temperature gradient.
- Access to hard (concrete) exercise area.
- Group size < 12.
- Space: lying $> 0.66\,m^2$ per sow; feeding $0.37\,m \times 1.3\,m$.

Note: Many different layouts are satisfactory.

In-pig gilts

SPECIAL REQUIREMENTS

- None.

DESIRABLE PROVISIONS

- Temperature gradient.
- Access to hard (concrete) exercise area.
- Group size < 12.
- Space: lying area $> 0.75\,m^2$ per sow; feeding $> 0.39\,m \times 1.38\,m$.

Dry sows

Individual confinement layouts are already well documented and basically consist of rows of sows secured by tether or stall each with an area of $2.1\,m \times 0.6\,m$. In temperate climates the stalls are invariably contained within controlled environment buildings.

Group housing is the focus of attention in the UK since the banning of new installations featuring close confinement.

In seeking to establish new systems it is important to focus on the needs of the sow at every stage from weaning to farrowing. A specific housing

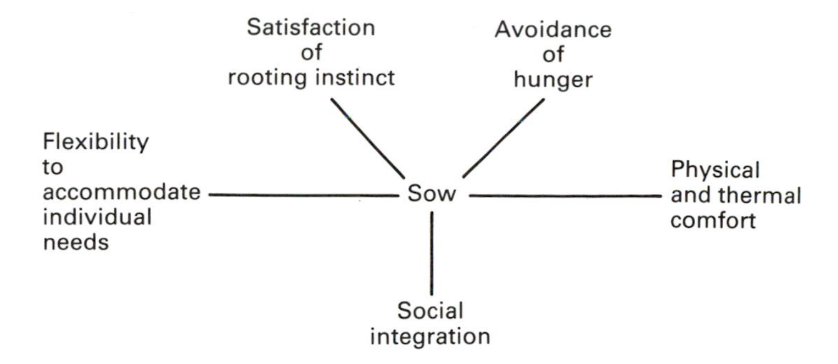

Fig. 10.6. Key considerations in selecting a group housing system for dry sows.

system may meet those needs at specific stages but not at others. Accurate feed allocation is less important during the service period and in mid-pregnancy than it is in early and late pregnancy. Aggressive interactions are more likely to have serious consequences during implantation and in late pregnancy. Appropriate space to allow the establishment of hierarchy dominance is most important when new introductions take place.

Taking all those factors into account it is clear that a good housing system may feature different components at the different stages between weaning and farrowing.

SPECIAL REQUIREMENTS

- Minimize aggression – particularly during implantation and late pregnancy.
- Combat hunger (low feed level).
- Provide thermal and physical comfort.
- Satisfy rooting instinct.

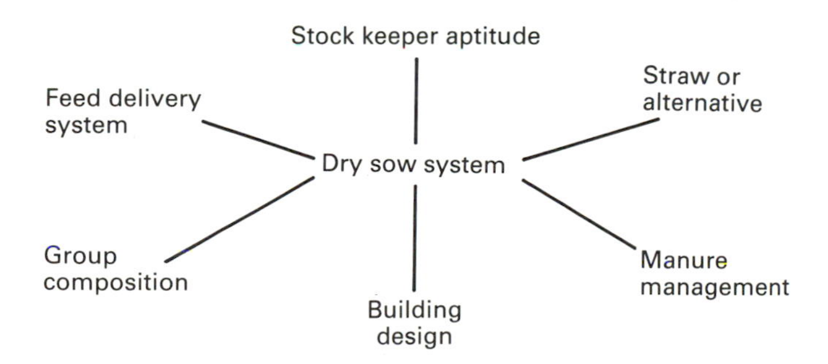

Fig. 10.7. Key components in selecting a group housing system for dry sows.

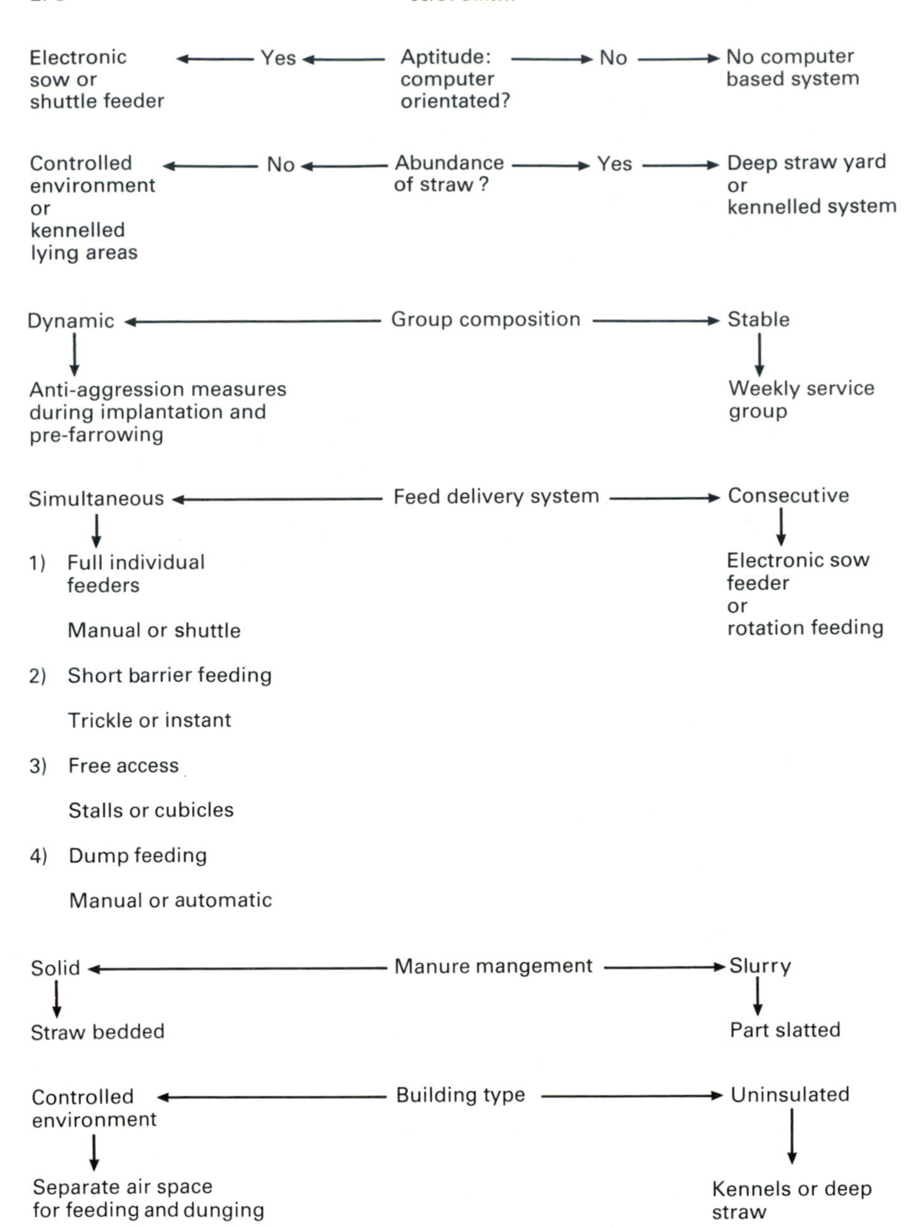

Fig. 10.8. Options for selecting a group housing system for sows.

DESIRABLE PROVISIONS

- Accurate feed allocation.
- Facility to cater for sows which require a different feed level or protection from other sows.
- Create quiet lying areas by arranging feeding, drinking, and dunging activities well away from lying areas.
- Flexible layout to allow group size adjustment.

The key considerations to be taken into account to satisfy the sow's needs are shown in Fig. 10.6.

The key components involved when selecting a new group housing system are shown in Fig. 10.7. The main options which will influence selection within the components are considered in Fig. 10.8.

Many permutations are possible. Examples of possible layouts for sequential feeding with electronic sow feeders (Fig. 10.9) or for simultaneous feeding with short feed barriers (Fig. 10.10) are illustrated. The combination of short barrier feeders (Fig. 10.11) and Nurtinger beds for sows could well form the basis of another alternative dry sow system.

Farrowing sows

SPECIAL REQUIREMENTS

- Physical protection for piglets.
- Thermal comfort for piglets.
- Protection from high temperatures for the sow.
- Access to separate thermal environments for the sow and piglets.

DESIRABLE PROVISIONS

- Freedom for the sow to nest build.

The farrowing crate is in almost universal use throughout intensive pig production. Appropriate layouts consist of crates contained within pens measuring approximately 2.4 × 1.6 m. In modern layouts the number of crates per room relates to the weekly farrowing numbers so that all-in and all-out systems of occupation can be implemented. Currently, considerable R & D effort is being devoted to farrowing systems in which the sow is not restrained. The essential features are a system of rails to prevent overlying; freedom for the sow to leave the 'nest' for dunging, feeding and drinking and a secure and comfortable refuge for the piglets (Fig. 10.12).

A successful system should achieve piglet survival rates similar to crates, be safe for the stock keeper and avoid the laborious tasks associated with traditional free farrowing systems.

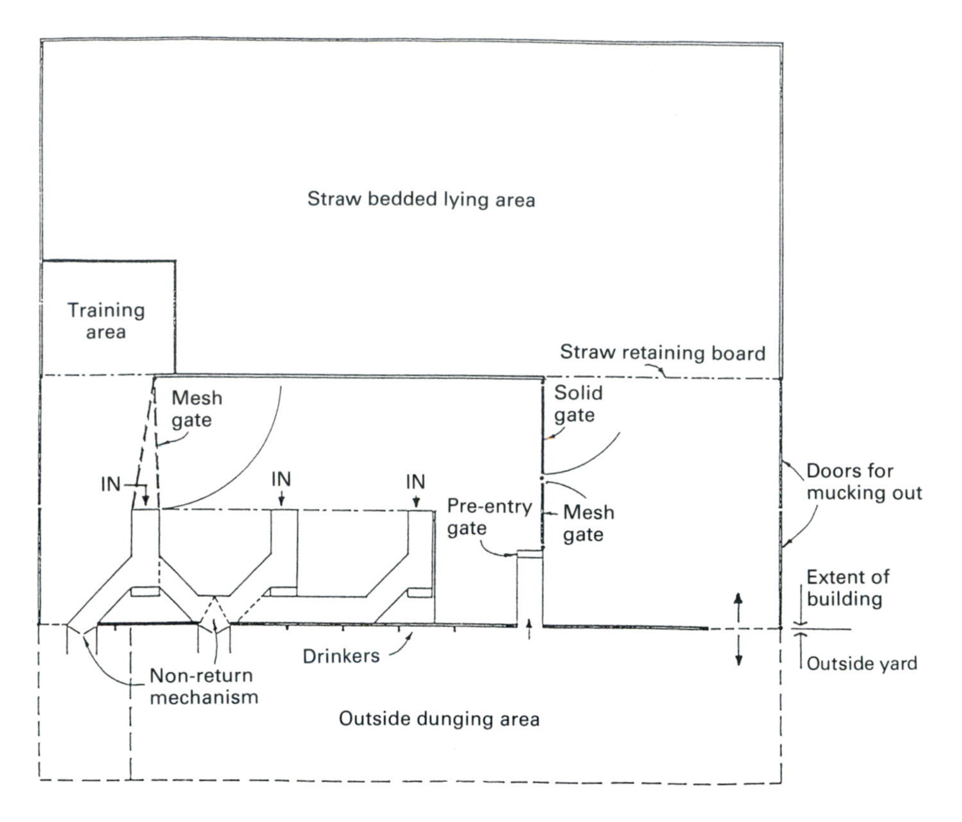

Fig. 10.9. Dry sow housing system incorporating electronic sow feeders.

Lactating sows

SPECIAL REQUIREMENTS

- Similar to those for farrowing but much less demanding.

DESIRABLE PROVISIONS

- Facilities to allow natural mixing of contemporary litters.

Current practice is to utilize farrowing facilities for the full lactation period. This is a high cost approach when farrowing crates are used and therefore tends to create pressure towards earlier weaning.

Three developments in lactation practice appear probable:

1. Free farrowing systems will be used throughout the lactating period.
2. Free farrowing systems will be modified after 7 to 10 days to create a community lactation facility as currently used at the Dutch Welfare Farm at Hengelo in The Netherlands (Fig. 10.13).

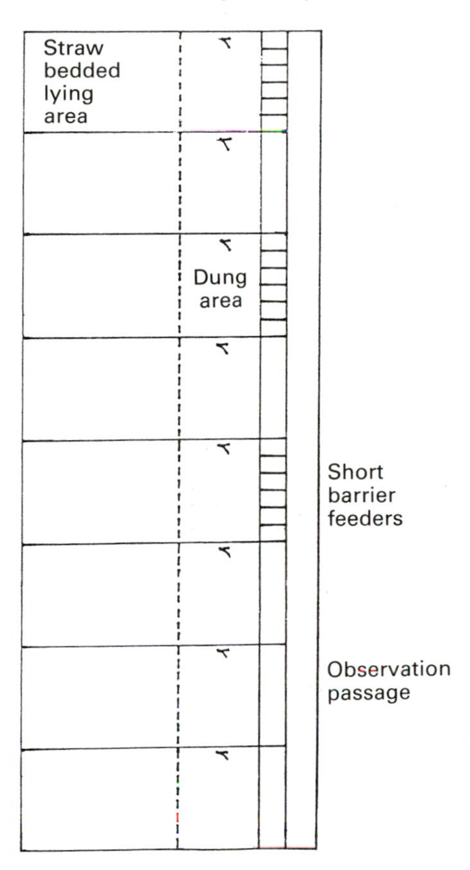

Fig. 10.10. Dry sow housing system featuring small yards and short barrier feeders.

3. Farrowing crates will be used for farrowing but sows and litters will be moved to a community lactation facility after 7 to 10 days.

Weaners

SPECIAL REQUIREMENTS

- High and stable temperatures if early weaned. High standard of air and surface hygiene if early weaned.

DESIRABLE PROVISIONS

- Use of bedding or access to substrate.
- Utilization of thermal gradients to influence lying and dunging behaviour.
- Weaning delayed until at least 3½ weeks.

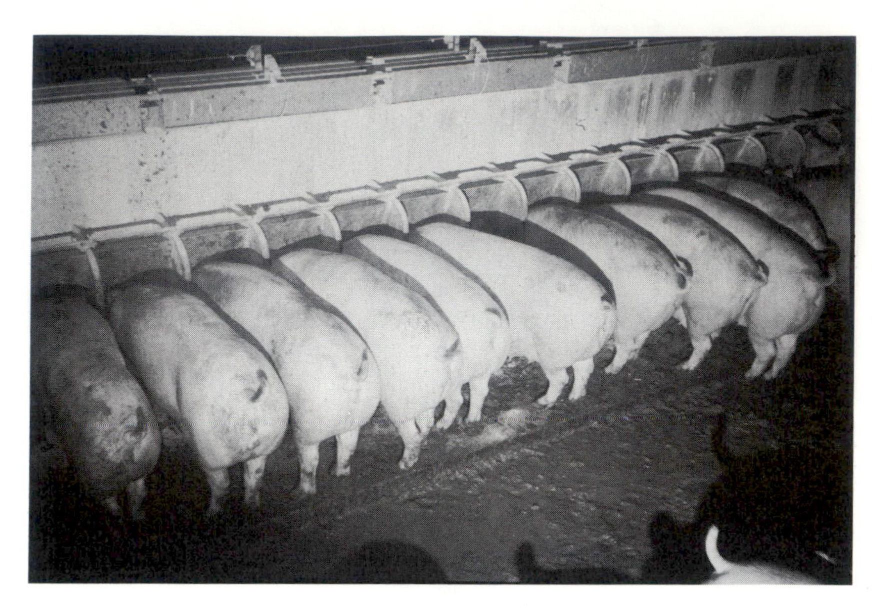

Fig. 10.11. Short barrier feeders for dry sows.

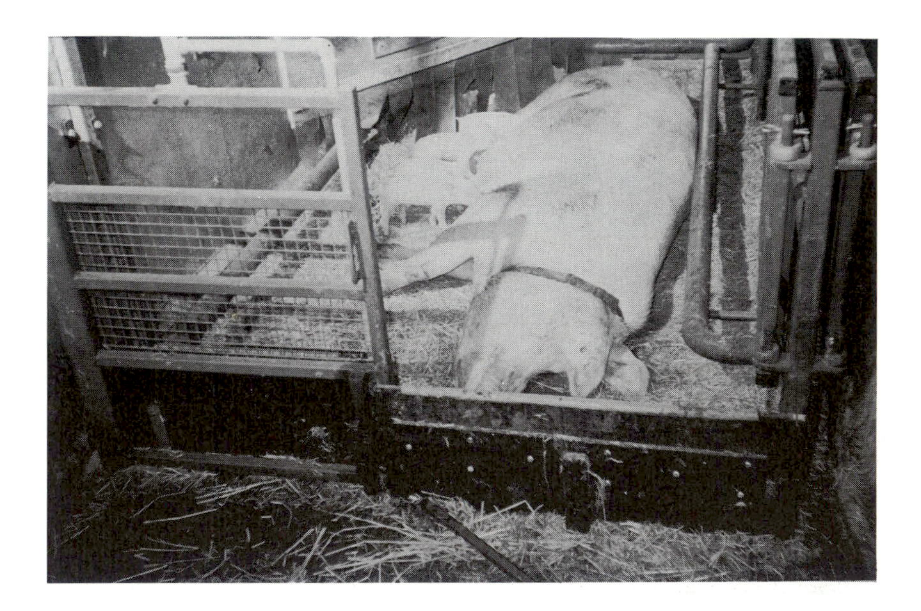

Fig. 10.12. Farrowing facilities without restraint.

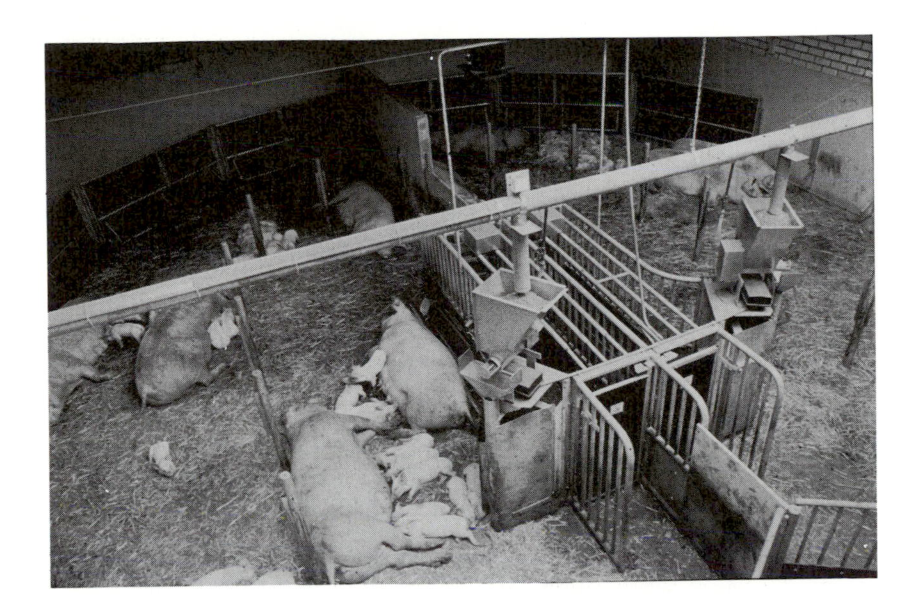

Fig. 10.13. Community lactation facility at the Dutch Welfare Farm, Hengelo.

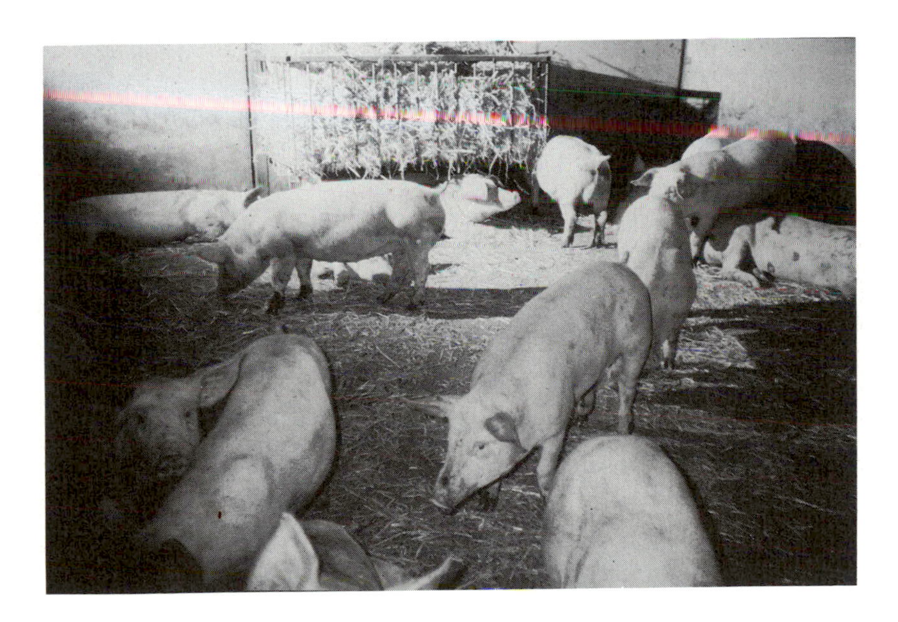

Fig. 10.14. Straw flow system for growing pigs.

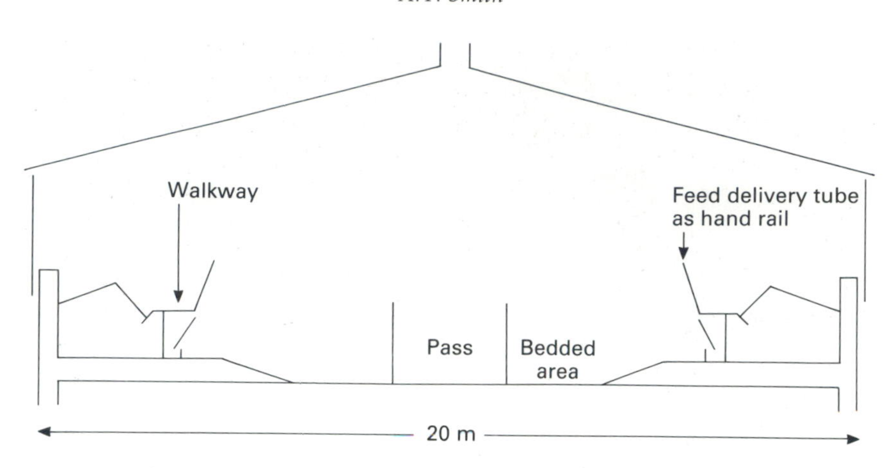

Fig. 10.15. Kennelled accommodation in conjunction with deep straw yards.

Late weaning eases the accommodation specifications required for the newly weaned pig. Much later weaning lowers output by reducing the frequency of farrowing unless sows are successfully served while lactating. This is certainly possible as was demonstrated in the family pen system, although it has yet to be shown that it can be done sufficiently reliably in commercial practice. Currently popular systems of housing, such as flat decks, will undoubtedly continue in use for some time.

The main alternatives which vary in their appeal according to geographical location and circumstances include:

1. Kennelled accommodation in conjunction with slatted dunging areas.
2. Insulated monopitch incorporating part-perforated floors and automatic natural ventilation control.
3. Kennelled accommodation in conjunction with sloping floors and straw flow (Fig. 10.14).
4. Kennelled accommodation in conjunction with a deep straw yard (Fig. 10.15).
5. Insulated, ventilation-controlled buildings incorporating *in situ* composting – yet to be clearly established as a viable commercial system (Fig. 10.16).

Growers and finishers

SPECIAL REQUIREMENTS

- None.

DESIRABLE PROVISIONS

- Use of bedding or access to substrate.

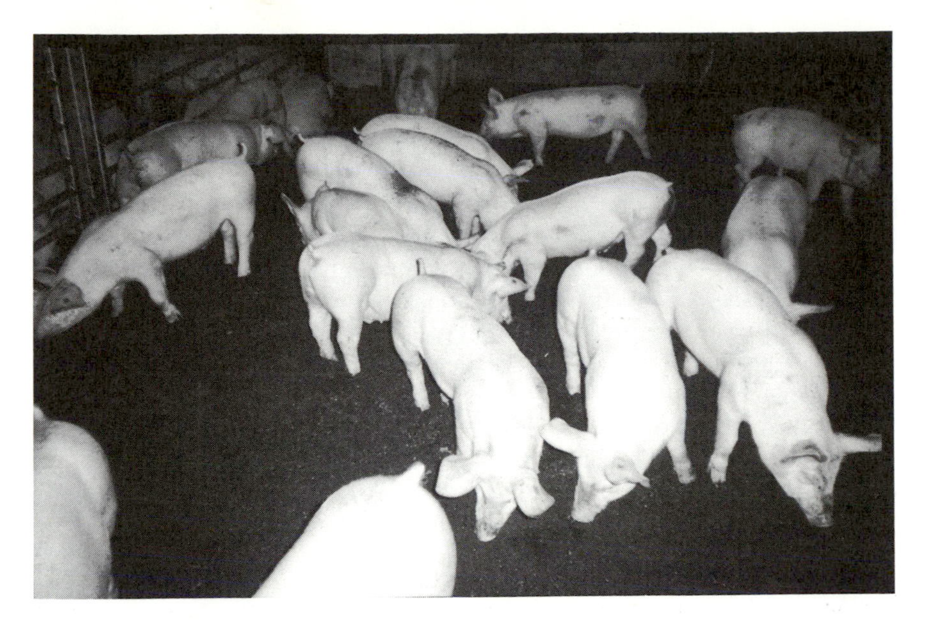

Fig. 10.16. Growing pigs on *in situ* composting bed.

- Utilization of thermal gradients to influence lying and dunging behaviour.

Pressure against fully slatted systems seems likely to increase.

There is a wide range of alternatives in current use many of which have specific merits in particular situations. Those developments which are likely to meet the new demands include:

1. Kennelled accommodation in conjunction with deep straw yards.
2. Insulated temperature-controlled buildings incorporating straw flow and dung fence (Bruce, 1990) (Fig. 10.14).
3. Insulated, ventilation-controlled building incorporating *in situ* composting – yet to be clearly established as a viable commercial system (Fig. 10.16).

Future Housing Systems

For the past 20–30 years production parameters have been the overriding criteria for selection of husbandry systems. Throughout the 1980s a combination of welfare pressure groups and improved knowledge of pig requirements has culminated in consumer and legal pressures for change.

If there is to be a move away from existing systems it must be based on the behavioural and physiological needs of the pig. The development of the

Edinburgh pig park by Stolba and Wood-Gush (1989) marked a turning point in novel housing systems for pigs. The major components in this system are of general utility, especially to those who aspire to develop new systems for the next generation of commercial pig producers. The key features are a sleeping area well away from the feeding area; open-fronted pens; a dunging corridor well away from the lying area; a rooting area; and an activity area.

Wood-Gush (1983) observed among other behaviours, that pigs always built their nests in such a way as to protect them from the prevailing wind and yet with an opening that gave good line of sight. Pigs also always walked a considerable distance from the nest before dunging or urinating. A modified version of the family pens is now under development for commercial application.

A key feature of the family pen system is avoidance of social stress by eliminating mixing and re-grouping. On farms mixing of group-housed sows is inevitable to some extent but can lead to aggression and sometimes injury. Similarly, aggression also occurs whenever growing pigs are re-grouped and mixed. Efficiency of production is then reduced, although the two sexes are not affected equally (Rundgren and Lofquist, 1989).

Comment

Pig production became progressively more intensive between the 1960s and the 1980s. This development followed from increasing knowledge of physiological requirements and the development of environmental control technology. Ethological research in the 1980s has prompted a greater awareness of behavioural needs. The challenge of the next decade is to utilize the recently developed technology and incorporate the emerging knowledge of behaviour needs to meet the aspirations of society.

References

Baldwin, B.A. and Start, I.B. (1985) Illumination preferences of pigs. *Applied Animal Behaviour Science* 14, 233–243.

Barber, J., Brooks, P.H. and Carpenter J.L. (1988) The effect of water delivery rate and drinker number on the water use of growing pigs. *Animal Production* 46, 521.

Baxter, M.R. (1986) The design of the feeding environment for the pig. PhD thesis. University of Aberdeen.

Bruce, J.M. (1990) Straw-flow: A high welfare system for pigs. *Farm Building Progress* 102, 9–13.

Bruce, J.M. and Clarke J.J. (1979) Models of heat production and critical temperature for growing pigs. *Animal Production* 28, 353–369.

Donham, K.J., Zavala, D.C. and Merchant, J. (1984) Acute effects of the work environment on pulmonary functions of swine confinement workers. *American Journal of Industrial Medicine* 5, 367–375.

Edwards, S.A., Armsby, A.W. and Spechter, H.H. (1988) Effects of floor area allowance on performance of growing pigs kept on fully slatted floors. *Animal Production* 46, 453–459.

Ewebank, R. and Bryant, M.J. (1972) Aggressive behaviour amongst groups of domesticated pigs kept at various stocking rates. *Animal Behaviour* 20, 21–28.

Farmer, C. and Christison, G.I. (1982) Selection of perforated floors by new born and weaning pigs. *Canadian Journal of Animal Science* 62, 1229–1236.

Fraser, D. (1985) Selection of bedded and unbedded pens by pigs in relation to environmental temperature and behaviour. *Applied Animal Behaviour Science* 14, 127–135.

Geers, R., Goedseels, V., De Lact, B. and Verstegen, M.W.A. (1986) The group postural behaviour of growing pigs in relation to air velocity, air and floor temperature. *Applied Animal Behaviour Science* 16, 353–362.

Gill, B.P. and Barber, J. (1990) Water delivery systems for growing pigs. *Farm Building Progress* 102, 19–22.

Hemsworth, P.H., Brand, A. and Williams, P. (1981) The behavioural response of sows to the presence of human beings and in its relation to productivity. *Livestock Production Science* 8, 67–74.

Hepherd, R.Q., Hanley, M., Armsby, A.W. and Hartley, C. (1983) Measurement of the water consumption of two herds of bacon pigs. Div. Note DN 1176. National Institute of Agricultural Engineering.

Hunt, K.A. (1987) The effect of stocking density on the performance and welfare of early weaned pigs. University of Aberdeen, Thesis.

Kornegay, E.T. and Lindemann, M.D. (1984). Floor surfaces and flooring material for pigs. *Pig News and Information* 5(4), 351–357.

Kornegay, E.T. and Notter, R.R. (1984) Effects of floor space and number of pigs per pen on performance. *Pig News and Information* 5, 23.

Lawrence, A.B., Appleby, M.C. and MacLeod, H.A. (1988) Measuring hunger in the pig using operant conditioning; the effect of food restriction. *Animal Production* 47, 131–137.

McGlone, J.J. and Curtis, S.E. (1985) Behaviour and performance of weaning pigs in pens equipped with hide areas. *Journal of Animal Science* 60, 20–24.

MAFF (1982) *Pig Environment*. Ministry of Agriculture, Fisheries and Food. Booklet 2410.

MAFF (1983) *Codes of Recommendations for the Welfare of Pigs*. Ministry of Agriculture, Fisheries and Food.

MAFF (1990) *The Welfare of Livestock Regulations*. Ministry of Agriculture, Fisheries and Food.

Marx, D. and Schuster, H. (1982) Behavioural choice experiments with early weaned pigs kept in flat decks. II Types of flooring. *Deutsche Tierargthiche Wochenschrift* 89 (8), 313–318.

Marx, D., Laeffler, M., Buchhaly, B. and Kamanshi, U. (1989) Investigations into the appropriate housing of pigs. *Berl. Munch. Tierarytl Wschr* 102, 218–223.

Mertz, R. (1988) The behaviour of early-weaned pigs in selection experiments with varying use of straw and different flooring. Agricultural dissertation, Hohenheim.

Morrow, A.T.S. and Walker, N. (1991) The effect of the number of single space feeders and the provision of an additional drinker or toy on the performance and feeding behaviour of growing pigs. British Society of Animal Production, Winter Meeting.

NAC (1979–84) Pig Unit Annual Reports, National Agricultural Centre, Stoneleigh.

NRC 89 (1984) Effect of space allowance and antibiotic feeding on performance of nursery pigs. *Journal of Animal Science* 58, 801–804.

NRC 89 (1989) Effect of vitamin C and space allowance on performance of weaning pigs. *Journal of Animal Science* 67, 624–627.

Petchey, A.M. and Hunt, K.A. (1990) The board: size and space requirements. *Farm Building Progress* 99, 17–20.

Petherick, J.C. (1983) A biological basis for the design of space in livestock housing. In: Baxter, S.H., Baxter, M.R. and MacCormack, J.A. Sc. (eds), *Farm Housing and Welfare.*

Robertson, J.B., Laird, R., Hall, J.K.S., Forsyth, R.J., Thompson, J.M. and Walker-Love, J. (1966) A comparison of two indoor farrowing systems for sows. *Animal Production* 8, 171.

Rundgren, M. and Lofquist, I. (1989) Effects on performance and behaviour of mixing 20 kg pigs fed individually. *Animal Production* 49 (2), 311–315.

Schrenk, H.K. (1981) The effect of light and feeding on the diurnal rhythm of piglet activity. Hohenheim: Agricultural dissertation.

Schwarting, G. (1989) Give pigs a warm bed. *Pigs.* Misset International.

Simonsen, H.B. (1990). Behaviour and distribution of fattening pigs in the multi activity pen. *Applied Animal Behaviour Science* 27, 311–324.

Smith, A.T. (1981) Characteristics of pig fattening systems involving partially slatted floors. In: Sybesma, W. (ed.), *The Welfare of Pigs.* Martinus Nijhoff, Dordrecht.

Smith, A.T. (1987) *Current pig production systems.* In: Smith, A.T. and Lawrence, T.L.J. (eds), *Pig Housing and the Environment.* BSAP Occasional Publication No. 11.

Stolba, A. (1981) A family system in enriched pens as a novel method of pig housing. In: *Alternatives to Intensive Husbandry Systems.* Proc. of UFAW Symposium, pp. 52–67.

Stolba, A. and Wood-Gush, D.G.M. (1989) The behaviour of pigs in a semi-natural environment. *Animal Production* 48(2), 419.

Tilbrook, A.J. and Hemsworth, P.H. (1990) Detection of oestrus in gilts housed adjacent or opposite boars or exposed to erogenous boar stimuli. *Applied Animal Behavioural Science* 28, 233–245.

Van Putten, G. (1981) The behaviour of fattening pigs. In: Sybesma, W. (ed.), *The Welfare of Pigs.* Martinus Nijhoff, Anim. Reg Stud 3: 105–118.

Walker, A.J. and Overton, D.C. (1988) Comparison of the performance of finishing pigs fed ad libitum from either conventional or single space feeders. BSAP Occasional meeting. The Voluntary Food Intake of Pigs.

Watson, R.D. and Friend, J.A.R. (1987) Pig housing and human health. In: Smith, A.T. and Lawrence, T.L.J. *Pig Housing and the Environment.* BSAP Occasional Publication.

Wood-Gush, D.G.M. (1983) *The Assessment of Welfare.* Animal Ethology. Chapman & Hall, London.

Dairy Cow Housing

11

R. BLOWEY
Wood Veterinary Group, Gloucester, UK

Introduction

It is not the intention of this chapter to give details of the design and construction of dairy cow housing systems, but rather to express guidelines for the provision of housing which is economic, safe, and promotes positive welfare for both the cow and the stockperson. There is often an association between housing, disease and hence the welfare of the animal. These aspects will be explored, referring specifically to mastitis, lameness, teat injuries and traumatic body damage. All these conditions are influenced by housing construction and by the management of that housing. For example, the same unit, initially designed to hold 60 cows, will probably perform well with 50 cows, adequately with 60 cows, but poorly with 70–80 cows, where both man and cows are under stress in attempting to cope with the system.

The first question to ask must be – why do we house dairy cows? There are probably three main reasons, namely:

1. To protect pastures from the effects of large numbers of cows regularly walking over wet land, an event which would seriously damage the sward and depress grassland production the following year.
2. To protect dairy cows from extremes of environment. Although the moderately low temperatures experienced in the UK are not normally detrimental to dairy cows, a combination of wind and rain, significantly increasing the chill factor, will be deleterious to both productivity and welfare. In hotter climates protection of high-yielding dairy cows against heat stress is essential.
3. To control and thereby maximize nutrient intake and hence production. In areas where land is of high value, economics may dictate that the cows

are permanently 'housed', although the housing may be simply in open sand yards with areas to provide shade from direct sunlight.

Changes in dairy farming systems over the past 20–30 years have seen a dramatic decline in the number of dairy units and, at the same time, an increase in the number of cows kept at each of the remaining units. The progressive squeeze on financial margins and the general problem of attracting suitable labour to farms have together led to increasing numbers of cows being looked after by one man, sometimes without a proportionate improvement in mechanization. In addition, bonus summer milk price incentives in the UK are currently attempting to persuade farmers to start calving earlier in the year (e.g. June or July). Many herds commence housing at the time of calving, to optimize food intakes and hence those herds calving in July may well have the equivalent of a ten-month winter! This can put serious stresses on the design and running of the housing system, since it has to produce a suitable environment for the cows during both the hot summer and cold winter months. As yield per cow increases, so must nutrient intake and consequently heat output. Unfortunately, it is all too common to enter poorly ventilated, hot buildings during the winter months – where attempts are being made to keep the cows warm – only to find cows and fittings coated with condensation, hence exacerbating associated disease risks. Increasing feed intakes must also mean longer time spent eating. Have feeding space allocations been increased accordingly?

Housing systems must be designed to be convenient and user-friendly for both cow and herdsman. If the system itself is difficult to manage, the herdsman will have less time to look after the cows and to carry out the basic, but important, daily tasks which differentiate a good herdsman from a bad one (often points which are difficult for an outsider to appreciate). In addition, if the stockman has spent a frustrating day repairing an outdated piece of equipment which should have been replaced long ago, it is not unnatural that, by milking time, tempers will be frayed and patience in handling cows will be seriously reduced. Housing brings man and cows into a very close association and while this can be beneficial, like any close relationship, it can also have its stormy moments!

Housing Systems

Historically, cows were housed in cowsheds (also known as shippons, byres or stanchion barns) where they were individually tied by the neck and housed, fed and milked in the same standing. The system works well and is still in use today, both in smaller farms and also in very high-yielding herds, where individual attention is required. In some parts of the world, particularly underdeveloped countries, cows are permanently housed in cowsheds. It is interesting to speculate that, while such a system is considered to be perfectly adequate and acceptable for dairy cows, tethering of sows in the UK is to be banned on welfare grounds by 1998. It would appear that what has been carried out historically in low numbers is acceptable, whereas similar housing systems of more recent innovation, which involve larger numbers of animals, are liable to be encompassed under the umbrella of 'factory farming' and deemed by some to be unacceptable!

With the trend towards larger units, milking parlours and a smaller labour force, more efficient housing, milking and management systems were evolved. The two in common use are the cow cubicle, or free-stall housing, and straw yards. Open sand yards are used in hotter climates, with varying systems of protection from heat stress, depending on the ambient temperature. The design and running of these three systems is discussed in the following.

Cowsheds

This is the traditional cow housing and is quite suitable for herds of 30–40 cows, or less (Figs 11.1 and 11.2). Each cow is tied at the neck either by a chain (Fig. 11.2, B) or with a yoke fitted at the front of the standing. Both chain and yoke should be equipped with an emergency rapid-release system, to cater for the occasional cow which becomes recumbent, for

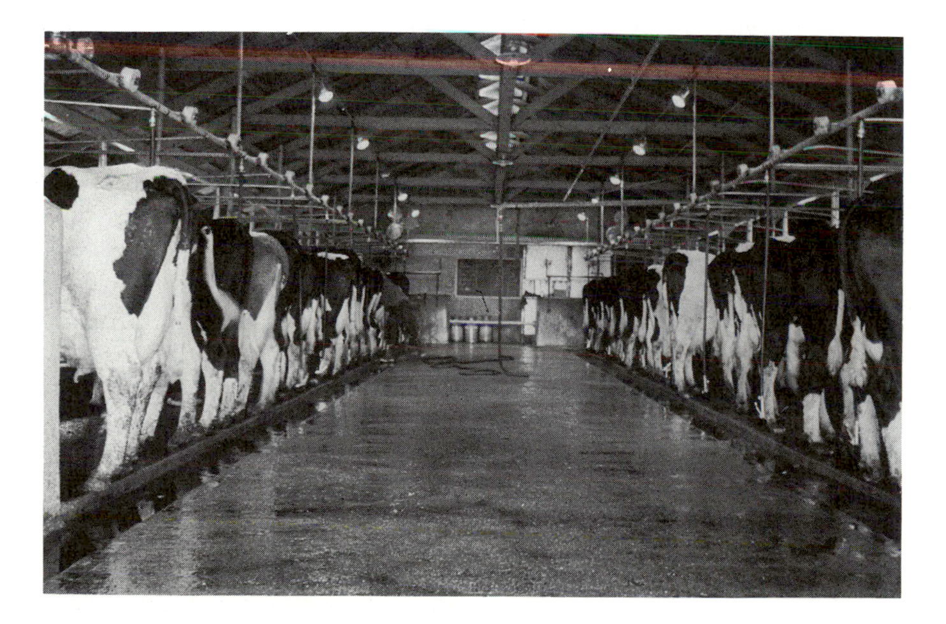

Fig. 11.1. Modern cowshed housing (Stansfield, 1991. Published with permission of Farming Press).

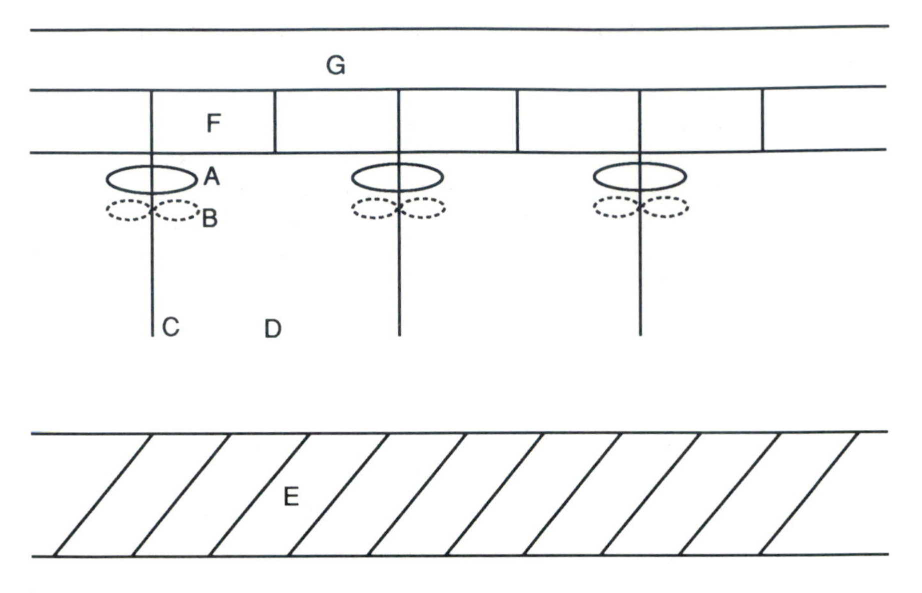

Fig. 11.2. Diagrammatic representation of cowshed.

example as a result of milk fever, or simply by slipping on the floor. In most systems it is impossible to use the normal release mechanism when the cow is pulling against it and high pressure is being applied. Cowsheds traditionally had hay racks at head height or above and mangers (F) at floor level. This tended to produce dust and an increase in respiratory disease. During the early days of eradication of tuberculosis, the overhead racks were removed and all feeding was from a manger. In most systems there is a partition (C) between every second cow, the yoke or chain being attached to the partition. Individual water bowls (A) are provided for each cow, these also being sited on the partition. The cows stand and lie on a wooden or concrete floor (D), raised 150–200 mm above a dunging passage (E). Cows are fed and milked in their standings and may or may not be released into a loafing area once each day for cleaning out and oestrus detection. The major disadvantage with this system is its high labour requirement:

1. Stooping to cow level for milking is uncomfortable and unpopular.
2. Cleaning out is difficult with the cows *in situ*, but individually releasing and retying them every day is very laborious.
3. Traditionally cows were milked into buckets (by hand or machine) and the milk carried to the dairy. Pipeline milking can now be installed, whereby milk is automatically transferred to the dairy. It is difficult to install a system which does not produce vacuum fluctuations over a long pipeline and even with a pipeline, the unit has to be carried from cow to cow.
4. Premilking udder preparation systems are more difficult to operate. The

traditional bucket and cloth was notorious for spreading mastitis. Mobile teat washing units are now available.

5. Feed passages (Fig. 11.2, G) along the front of the cow were rarely wide enough to accommodate a tractor and hence feeding had to be by hand. Concentrates were fed by barrow from the feed passage, but forage was carried across to the stall from the dunging passage (E). The change from hay to silage and the dramatic increase in effort associated with carrying wet and heavy silage to the feed mangers, was a significant factor in stimulating the change away from traditional cowsheds – as I know from personal experience!

6. Because the cows are present in the standing for most of the day, bedding can be a problem. Straw is the bedding of choice, although other materials such as dried bracken and sand can also be used. Over a long period, fouled straw may become compacted, to produce an uneven surface. As they are situated at the front of the standing, leaking water bowls can also produce dirty lying conditions and an increased risk of disease.

The major advantage of the cowshed is the individual attention which can be given to each cow, especially in relation to feed intake. The opportunity exists to feed each cow on a separate ration, frequently throughout the day. Feed refusal can be monitored. Increased milking frequency is easily carried out. There are reports of yields decreasing following a change from a cowshed to group housing systems (Radostits and Blood, 1985). However, moving cows to a specific, easily cleaned and mechanized milking area (i.e. a parlour) must be much more efficient and hygienic.

Loose yarding

Loose yarding and cubicle housing systems both have specific areas for milking (the parlour), feeding and lying. The difference between the two systems is in the lying area. Cubicles consist of individual areas where a cow can lie. Loose yards allow cows to lie where they wish – although they are, of course, encouraged to lie on a clean, bedded area. Apart from hotter climates, where sand is used in open yards, straw is the prime bedding material. A typical straw yard layout is shown in Fig. 11.3 and diagrammatically in Fig. 11.4. Access to the straw-bedded area is from the front, where the cows are able to stand and eat from a feed manger or through the feed fence (Fig. 11.4, C). Often the feed passage (D), which should be wide enough to accommodate a tractor and forage waggon, is itself the manger, the food being delivered up against the feed fence. The standing area (E) should be sufficiently wide to permit the use of a tractor and scraper and also to allow the easy passage and movement of cows when the feed face is fully occupied by other feeding cows. The siting of the water troughs (B) is vital. They should be far enough from the straw-bedded area to avoid

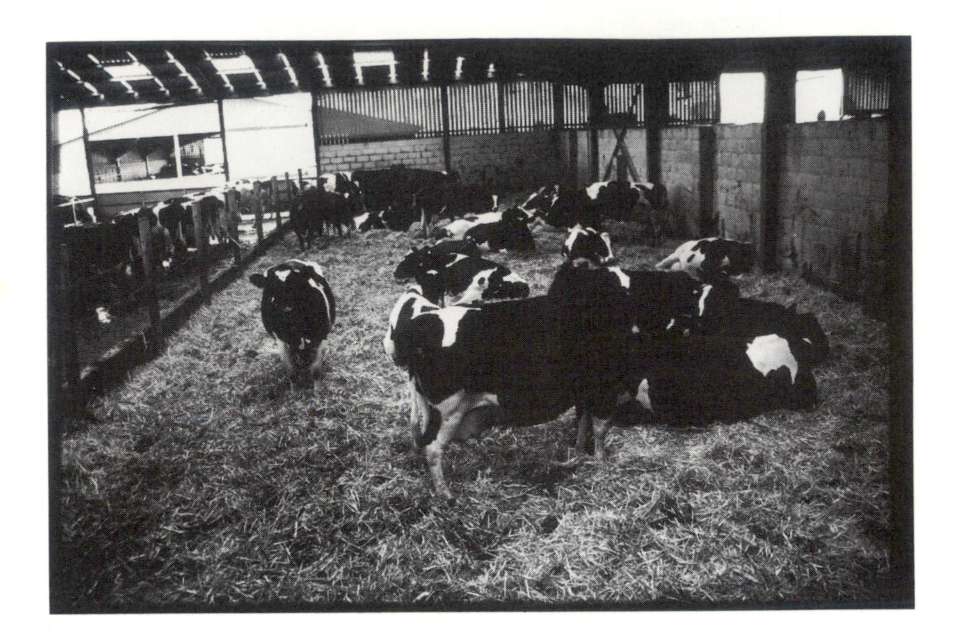

Fig. 11.3. Straw yard.

fouling and yet not sited such that they are liable to become damaged or fouled when scraping out, feeding or rebedding the yards. If placed at B_1, access must be restricted to only those cows in the standing area. If access is permitted from the strawed area (A), serious fouling could occur around the trough and part of the bedded area would then become obliterated. Siting at B_2 is a possibility, but it reduces available feeding space, risks becoming contaminated by food and may get damaged by the feeder waggon. Siting at B_3, is acceptable in layout 2, where there is no division (G) between the bedded and lying area, but in layout 2 it could cause an obstruction to the flow of cows and fouling of the initial bedded area. Opinions vary over the value of the division. Some consider that it reduces straw use, in that less straw is dragged down into the passage on cows' feet. Others consider that it reduces access to the bedded area and in so doing increases both the risk of bullying of heifers and fouling of the bedded area, in that cows are less able and hence less willing to move to the dunging/standing area (E) to urinate and defaecate.

Space allowances per cow have been detailed by Webster (1987a) and are given in Table 11.1. A standard 700 kg Holstein cow requires a minimum 5.8 m^2 of bedded area and, in addition, a further 2.0 m^2 for feeding, standing and loafing. These dimensions are in broad agreement with Stansfield (1991) who quotes a requirement of 6 m^2 per cow and Sumner (1989), who suggests 6.25 m^2 of bedding and 2.25 m^2 for feeding and loafing. Clearly the actual

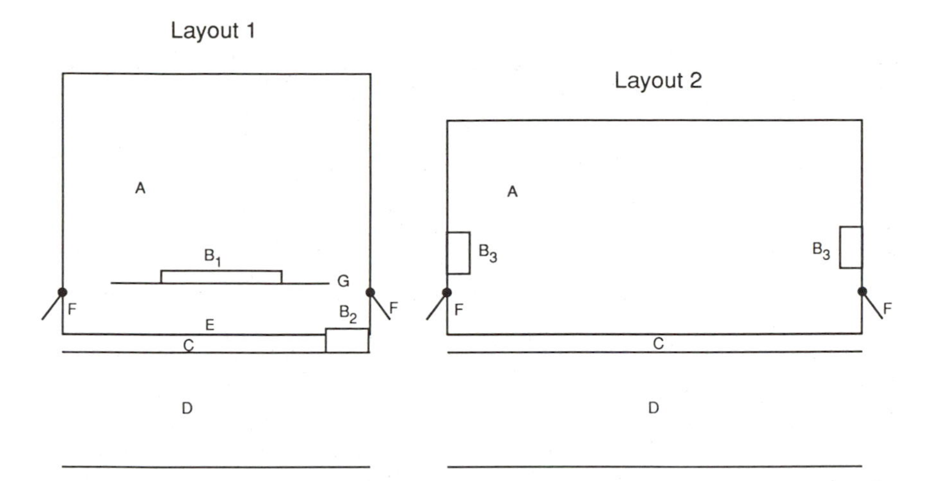

Fig. 11.4. Diagram of two typical straw yard layouts.

space requirement is not a fixed figure, since it depends considerably on the availability and quality of straw bedding, on the yield (and hence faecal and heat output), on the behaviour of the cows and on the time of year. More space is needed during hot summer months and during damp, humid weather than during cool, dry, crisp winter conditions and also for high yielding, early lactation cows and cows in oestrus. The shape of the yard also has an effect (Stansfield, 1991). Deep, long yards, such as that in layout 1, Fig. 11.4 (and in many on-farm situations yards are even deeper than this) are less efficient than the shallow, wide yards shown in layout 2 (Fig. 11.3). Layout 2 gives better access to the bedded area, is easier to clean out and provides a longer feed face. The dimensions of the yard are often at least partly determined by feed face requirements and hence also the siting of the water troughs.

Straw requirements are high. Approximately one and a half tonnes of straw per cow are needed for the winter housing period (Francis, 1989), the actual amount depending on the length of the winter housing period, straw quality and yard stocking density. Yards should be bedded daily and ideally cows allowed to come back into a freshly bedded yard after morning milking. Opinions vary over the ideal frequency of cleaning out and rebedding. Stansfield (1991) states that this should be at least once over the winter period; the author would consider every six weeks to be ideal and Williams (1990, personal communication) suggests that cleaning out every two weeks and only using a thin bed of straw both reduced mastitis and decreased the overall straw requirement. The influence of straw yards on mastitis is discussed in detail in a later section. Straw usage can be decreased by ensuring that the standing/dunging passage is scraped twice daily and that the building is well ventilated. An adult dairy cow evaporates

Table 11.1. Dimensions and space requirements of cows and heifers.

	Cows			Heifers, Friesian
	Jersey	Friesian	Holstein	2-year-olds
Body weight (kg)	350	600	700	450
Height to withers (m)	1.15	1.35	1.50	1.25
Body length (m)*	1.40	1.62	1.72	1.45
Reach of mouth (m)				
at floor level	0.85	0.90	0.92	0.84
300 mm above floor level	1.00	1.05	1.07	1.02
Cubicle dimensions (m)				
length to wall	2.00	2.20	2.40	2.40
length behind trough†	1.40	1.60	1.80	1.60
width between partitions	1.10	1.15	1.20	1.15
height of neck rail	1.00	1.05	1.10	1.05
Feeding face, width (m)	0.55	0.70	0.70	0.65
Loose housing (m^2)				
bedded area/head	3.2	5.0	5.8	4.0
feeding, etc./head	1.3	1.8	2.0	1.5

Source: Webster, 1987a.

*Tailhead to shoulders.
†Where present.

15–20 l of water per day from the respiratory tract and skin (Webster, 1987a), in addition to producing approximately 50 l of urine per day (urine output varying with diet and milk yield). Cattle buildings can be very humid therefore and good ventilation is essential.

It should be remembered that housing exists primarily for protection against rain/snow and wind. Low temperature is relatively unimportant for lactating dairy cows in temperate climates, their lower critical temperature being as low as −25°C (Radostits and Blood, 1985 – see Table 11.2, and Chapter 1). Hence airflow through dairy cow yards should be optimized, to decrease humidity and thereby reduce both bedding usage and risk of disease. Details of ventilation systems are given in Chapters 7 and 12.

The increasingly strict requirements for effluent disposal and reducing odour pollution from livestock buildings, combined with the prohibition of straw burning might well result in an increase in the use of straw yard systems in the future.

Table 11.2. Critical temperatures for cattle.

	Critical temperatures (°C)	
	Lower	Upper
Calf (4 l milk per day)	13	26
Calf (50–200 kg growing)	−5	26
Cow (dry and pregnant)	−14	25
Cow (peak lactation)	−25	25

Source: Radostits and Blood, 1985.

Cubicles (free stalls)

A cubicle system is an extension of a cowshed, but one in which there is a division between each cow and cows have freedom of choice between lying in the cubicle, standing in the dunging passage or loafing area, or eating at the feed face. Figure 11.5 gives a diagrammatic representation of a typical layout, and an example is given in Fig. 11.6. Individual cow lying areas (Fig. 11.5, A) are separated from one another by barriers (B). The front of the cubicle may comprise the outer wall of the building (E_1) or a specially constructed wooden partition (E_2) or two rows of cubicles may face each other (E_3, Fig. 11.5b), when only a few simple rails are needed. The dunging channel (D) and feeding/loafing (F) may be either concrete or slatted. Water troughs (W) are conveniently sited at the ends of cubicle rows. The feed area (G) may consist of a feed passage, as shown in the diagram, or may simply be an outside concrete loafing area with ring feeders and self-feed access to the silage bunker face. Various combinations of systems also exist. With increasing concern over effluent disposal and pollution of watercourses, there has been a trend in recent years to cover as much of the cow standing, loafing and feeding areas as possible. In addition to increasing protection from the elements, it reduces the amount of slurry produced (because rainwater can be channelled direct into the watercourses) and hence it reduces the size of the effluent pumping and disposal operation.

Cubicle beds are raised 150–160 mm above the dunging channel. Too high a step leads to cow discomfort. If it is too low, slurry may contaminate the beds at the end of the tractor's run during scraping. A wide range of materials is available for use as cubicle flooring, but because of its durability, concrete is by far the most common. However, it is not particularly comfortable for the cows and additional bedding is therefore required. Earth floors can be used, but cows tend to erode hollows with continual use. This can allow stones to rise to the surface, producing discomfort, and continued erosion may increase the space under the central cubicle bar (R), allowing cows to get trapped, or even fracture limbs. Floor hollows at the rear of the cubicle can fill with water and act as a mastitis risk. Rammed chalk has also been used. While it is more comfortable than concrete, and may drain well, it can still be eroded to form hollows. Provided that the surface is regularly repaired and maintained, rammed chalk is a useful alternative to concrete. A modification of the earth/chalk floor consists of laying car tyres flat on the cubicle base, so that each tyre touches the adjacent one and the height is level with the kerbstone (K). The space in the centre of the tyres and between them is then filled with compacted earth or chalk. The tyres

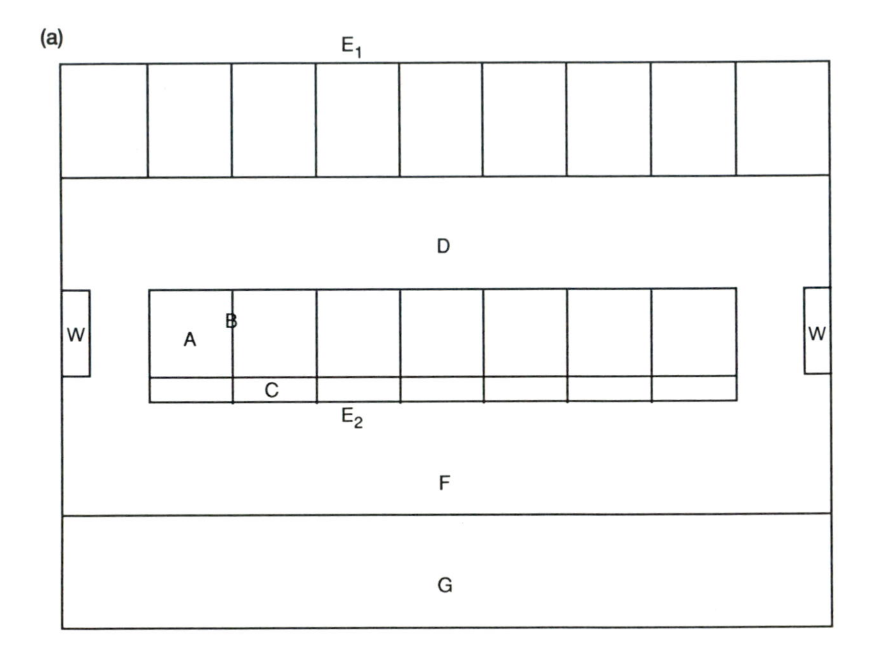

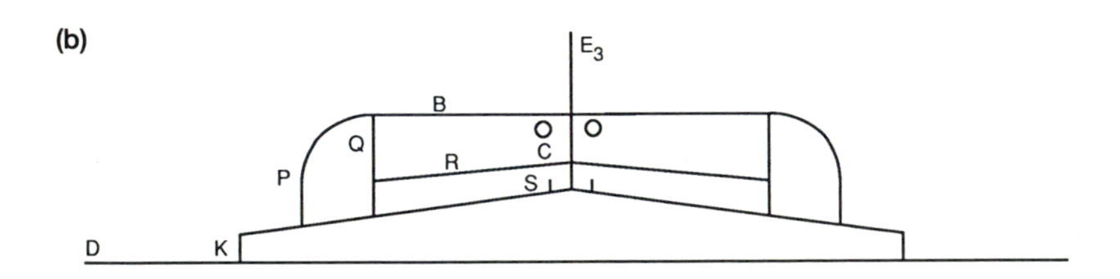

Fig. 11.5. Diagram of cubicle house.

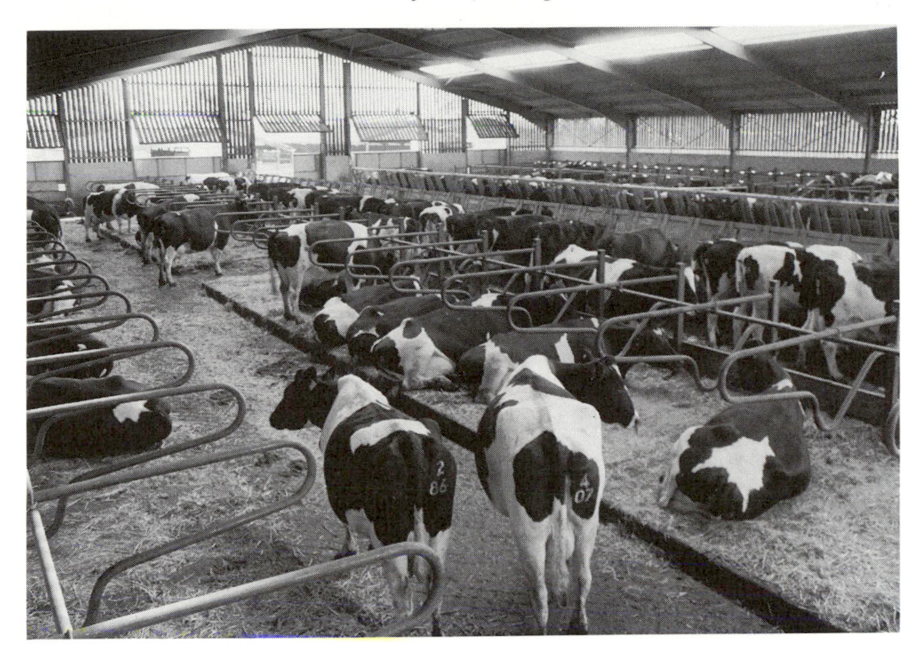

Fig. 11.6. A typical modern cubicle house (Stansfield, 1991. Published with permission of Farming Press).

produce a slightly springy (and hence more comfortable) surface and, in addition, reduce the amount of 'floor hollowing' by the cows.

Whatever the floor surface of the cubicle, bedding is essential to encourage cows to lie down. Cows confined in housing systems attempt to maintain the same activities as if they were outside grazing (Hedlund and Rolls, 1977). For example, during a 24-hour period, 45% of the time is spent lying down.

Housing system	Mean lying time, h
Pasture	11.0
Cubicles or straw yards	11.5
Cowsheds	12.0

The same authors found that during the 15 hours of daylight, cows spent 45% of their time lying down, 26% eating, 22% ruminating, 1% drinking and 2% socializing. Others, for example Cermak (1990) consider that a cubicle housed cow should spend 14 hours per day lying down. More recently, however, Miller and Wood-Gush (1991), comparing the behaviour of a high-yielding Friesian herd, either cubicle housed or outdoor grazing,

Table 11.3. Quantities of bedding (kg) required for cubicle housed cows for a 30-week winter (from summer 1989).

Type of bedding	Quantity (kg)
Long straw	350–450
Chopped straw or rape straw	180–220
Sawdust/shavings/newsprint	250–320
Sand	850–1000

found that the proportion of time spent lying down was much greater indoors (0.57) than outdoors (0.269). They suggested that the increased lying time indoors could be due to a variety of factors including suppression of synchronized group behaviour; easier feed access indoors; the nature of the flooring; the physiological burden of early lactation (cows were in cubicles in early lactation and grazing in mid-late lactation) and perhaps simply that the cows had more spare time when they were housed.

This contrasts with the findings of Hughes (1992) who reported that cows at pasture spent up to 14 hours per day lying down, cudding and regurgitating at two cuds per minute. At the start of each cudding movement, a cow extends her head forwards to her full 2.4m length requirement, presumably to facilitate the uninterrupted passage of cud along the oesophagus. Cows tightly packed in excessively small cubicles must lie with their head flexed to one side. They are unable to extend their necks to ruminate and, in addition, normal rumen motility may be restricted or even totally inhibited by pressure on the stomach by the metal divisions of the cubicle. Under such circumstances the cow may be forced to rise (perhaps by rumen discomfort) to ruminate and may stand half in and half

Table 11.4. In this trial it was found that cows preferred cubicles which were either deeply bedded with chopped straw, or those which had a thick cushioned mat.

Type of cubicle bed	Length of time cows spent resting each day (h)
Bare concrete	7.2
Insulated concrete screed	8.1
Hard rubber mat	9.8
Chopped straw on concrete	14.1
Proprietary cow cushion	14.4

out of the cubicle, which then gives her room to extend her neck to regurgitate her cud. Hughes (1992) reports an increase in yield when cows are moved from cubicles to open yards and speculates that this may be due to an improved efficiency of digestion associated with increased rumination and saliva flow.

The provision of a comfortable and acceptable bedded area is therefore essential, both for the welfare of the cow and in the prevention of disease. Straw is the commonest bedding material used, with a requirement of approximately 350 kg per cow over the winter (Francis, 1989), namely one-quarter of that required for a straw yard. If chopped straw is used (Table 11.3) it compacts into a mat and is less likely to be pulled out of the cubicle than long straw, hence producing fewer problems for slurry handling systems and reducing straw usage. Woodshavings, sand, shredded paper and sawdust have all been used as bedding materials. Large quantities of sand may run into and eventually block slurry handling systems, although sand supports the lowest *Escherichia coli* growth of all materials tested (Francis, 1989). Fresh, soft wood sawdust, on the other hand, may contain *Klebsiella* species which can cause peracute mastitis (Newman and Kowalski, 1973; Francis 1989). Shredded paper is absorbent and supports very limited bacterial growth, but if it is very wet it becomes compacted. Cows with numerous pieces of paper adhering to them may also not be considered acceptable by the owner or herdsman!

Proprietary mats are available and although expensive, they are comfortable and hygienic, but must be kept dry. Wet mats support bacterial growth and become slippery, leading to possible mastitis and leg injuries. Mats are probably no more effective than a well-bedded cubicle (Table 11.4). Cermak (1990) described a low-cost durable mattress for use in cubicle beds.

Other factors influencing cubicle comfort and hygiene include the slope of the floor, cubicle size, the construction of the division, the amount of forward lying space and position of neck rail and cubicle management.

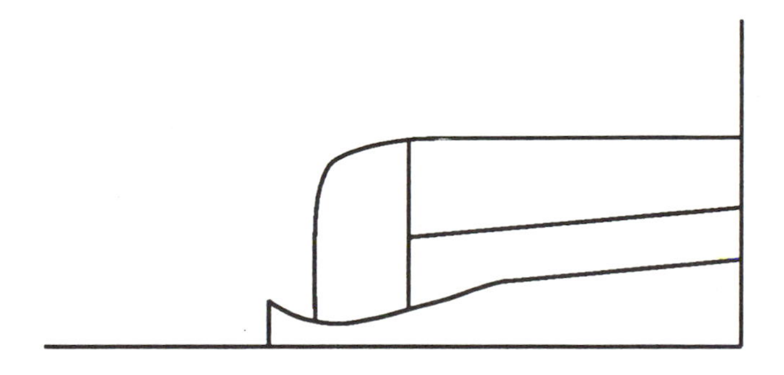

Fig. 11.7. Cubicle design which produced a high incidence of rejection.

Slope of floor

This should be approximately 100 mm from front to rear and should be a straight slope. Cows prefer facing uphill when they lie. One of the worst outbreaks of lameness seen by the author was in a cubicle house where the cubicle sloped from mid-way along the bed (see Fig. 11.7). The presence of a rear lip increases discomfort and, by allowing the pooling of urine, can lead to a soiled wet area which can exacerbate mastitis. However, a lip may be necessary to retain sand bedding (Sumner, 1989).

Cubicle size

Preferred dimensions are given in Table 11.1, where it can be seen that larger cubicles are required with increasing size of cow. Some units are currently installing cubicles as large as 1.2 m wide by 2.33 m long (Sumner, 1989) and Hughes (1990) has proposed that cubicles should be a minimum of 1.2 m × 2.4 m. Length is probably the most important feature and seems to have the greatest influence on cow acceptance. Width requirements are, to a certain extent, modified by cubicle design, since narrow cubicles can be offset by divisions which allow space sharing (Sumner, 1989; Cermak, 1990).

Cubicle division

The division should be of sufficient construction to prevent cows lying transversely across the cubicle, thus occupying two to three spaces and possibly injuring other cows, but at the same time the division should not cause injury to the cow. A wide variety of shapes and materials is available. In some buildings, often referred to as kennels, part of the division acts as a support for the roof. This usually entails a heavy rear upright (a vertical extension of P in Fig. 11.5) which can traumatize the cow's pelvic tuber coxae, leading to welfare problems and obvious discomfort. The best designs are those with minimal materials at the rear, as shown in Figs 11.6 and 11.8. The upright (Q, Fig. 11.5) is a common feature in many designs, but can traumatize the tuber coxae and together with R is best removed. In an evaluation of the four cubicle designs, O'Connell *et al.* (1991) found that cows preferred Dutch Comfort cubicles, rather than Newton Rigg and cantilever types, with Newton Rigg being the least preferred. Preference was assessed by direct observation of total occupancy and frequency of turnover. However, once a cow had chosen a cubicle, continuous lying time was similar, regardless of cubicle type.

The height of the central bar (R)

This is important because too high and the cow can slide beneath it; too low

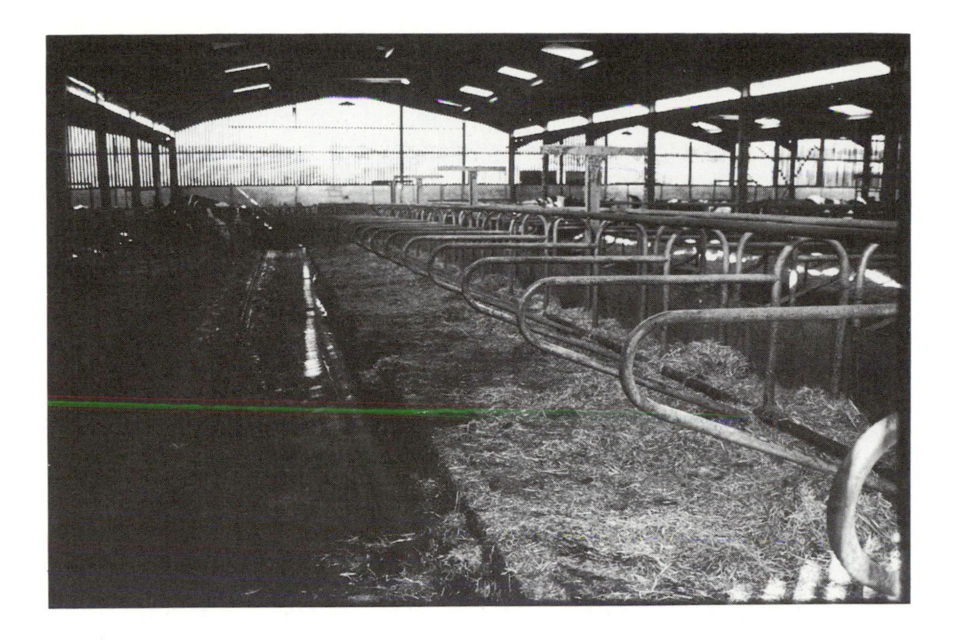

Fig. 11.8. Cubicles with a minimum rear structure. These were installed for particularly large Holsteins.

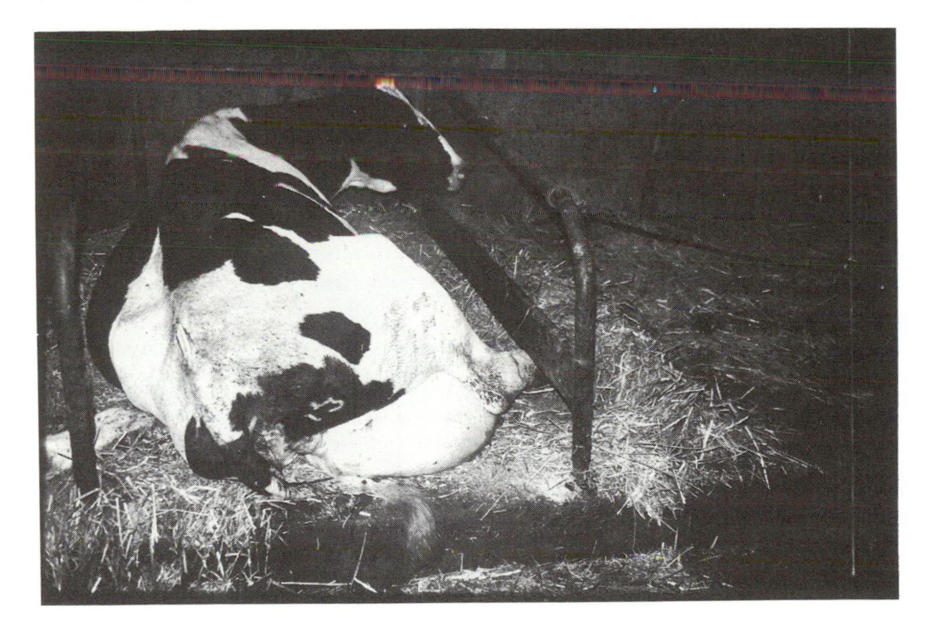

Fig. 11.9. Cubicle beds had been concreted, decreasing the space between the lower rail and the floor. This led to hock bursitis.

and she may trap or even fracture her leg. The cubicle beds in Fig. 11.9 had recently been concreted, thus reducing the available space. This led to a series of cows with severe hock bursitis. The normal accepted height is approximately 400mm for the lower bar and 1050mm for the top rail (ADAS, 1988). In many systems the horizontal bar, R, is replaced by a length of nylon rope, maintained under tension. The disadvantage of ropes is that they may break and hence regular maintenance is required. Some of the worst types of cubicle divisions are home made and of such heavy construction that they reduce the available lying space, in addition to traumatizing the cow as she rises and lies down. A typical example is shown in Fig. 11.10. The cubicles were of varying sizes, with some as little as 910mm wide. The head of a bolt, used to attach the lower rail, protrudes into the cubicle space and was smooth and worn from the cows continually knocking against it. The owner admitted that the cows did not like using these cubicles, particularly the narrow ones!

Forward lying space

When getting up from a sitting position, a cow rises on to her front feet first and in so doing lunges forward (Fig. 11.11). The forward movement may be as much as 0.8 to 1.0m (Cermak, 1983). Ideally a cubicle needs to be long

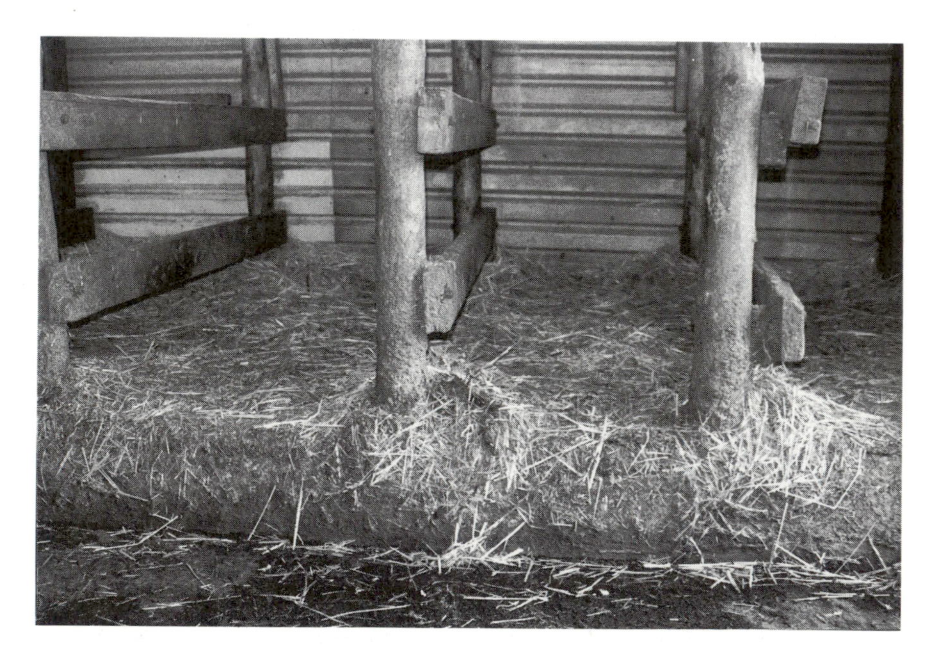

Fig. 11.10. Very narrow cubicles. Note the heavy construction, reducing available space and the protruding bolt.

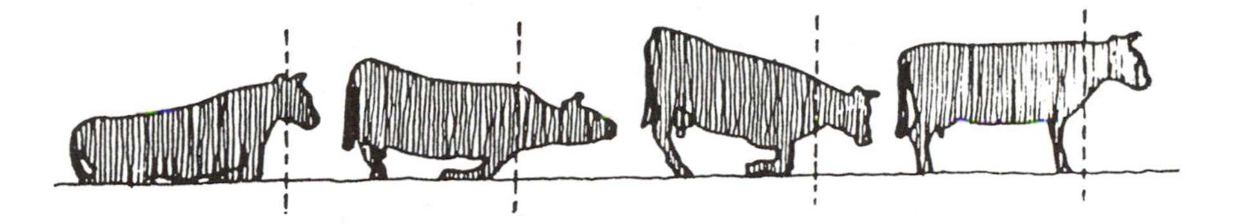

Fig. 11.11. Forward movement of cow on rising.

enough to accommodate this behaviour, but at the same time be short enough to ensure that when standing in the cubicle, her feet are very close to the rear kerb (Fig. 11.5, K), thus ensuring that urine and faeces fall into the dunging channel. This correct positioning can be achieved, either by means of a head rail (C) or a floor-mounted brisket board (S), positioned 1730 mm from the kerb, K, or by having open-fronted cubicles (Fig. 11.5b), which permit front space-sharing, i.e. the cow can put her head through into the opposite cubicle when rising. The position of the head rail can be critical, both in height and distance from the front of the cubicle. Its precise placing depends on the cubicle dimensions and size of the cows.

Cubicle management

Like so many systems, the success of cubicle housing largely depends on its management. Dunging passages should be scraped twice daily, preferably during milking. This has two major advantages, namely:

1. Cows can return to the cubicles along a clean passageway, thus minimizing fouling of the beds by dirty feet, when they lie down.
2. It is one less disturbance of the cows, compared with moving them out of the cubicles specifically for scraping out later in the day.

Dung pats and soiled bedding should be removed from the rear of the cubicles prior to each scraping and the cubicles should be bedded each day (Dodd *et al.*, 1984). Broken central bars (Fig. 11.5, R) should be replaced as soon as possible, to prevent cows becoming trapped. One cubicle (Fig. 11.8) is manufactured as a cantilever system so that it can be lifted to free any cow which gets caught and enables also automatic brushing from the rear of the cubicle.

Cubicle passages

These should be straight to allow easy scraping, have a non-slip surface for cow safety, be wide enough to minimize aggression and fear, especially in younger and less dominant cows, and be sited so that they avoid a wind-tunnel effect. 'Escape routes', i.e. clearways through the cubicles, are needed every 20 cubicles (Sumner, 1989) and these make ideal positions for water troughs.

Calving boxes

Every farm should have a few well-bedded pens where individual sick or parturient cows can be housed. These can be constructed as a row of individual boxes (Fig. 11.12), or even a large yard subdivided by gates. The latter option gives less isolation of cows, but is much easier to construct and to clean out. Calving boxes should have a deep straw bed, be easily cleaned and have a large door at the front, to deal with the unfortunate fatality that will inevitably occur. Boxes should be used for sick and lame cows, so that these animals do not have to compete for food and, of course, for calvings. Handling facilities are essential within the box. These are most easily constructed by installing two gate hinges in the wall of each box, 750 mm from a corner, so that the cow can be penned behind a gate. Calving cows in tightly stocked yards is stressful and counter to welfare, especially for animals which are low in the pecking order. When at pasture, a cow will wander off by herself to select a suitably secluded spot for calving and will stay in that spot to calve, especially when the ruptured placental fluids have imparted the cow's own odour to the area. Cows calving in crowded yards

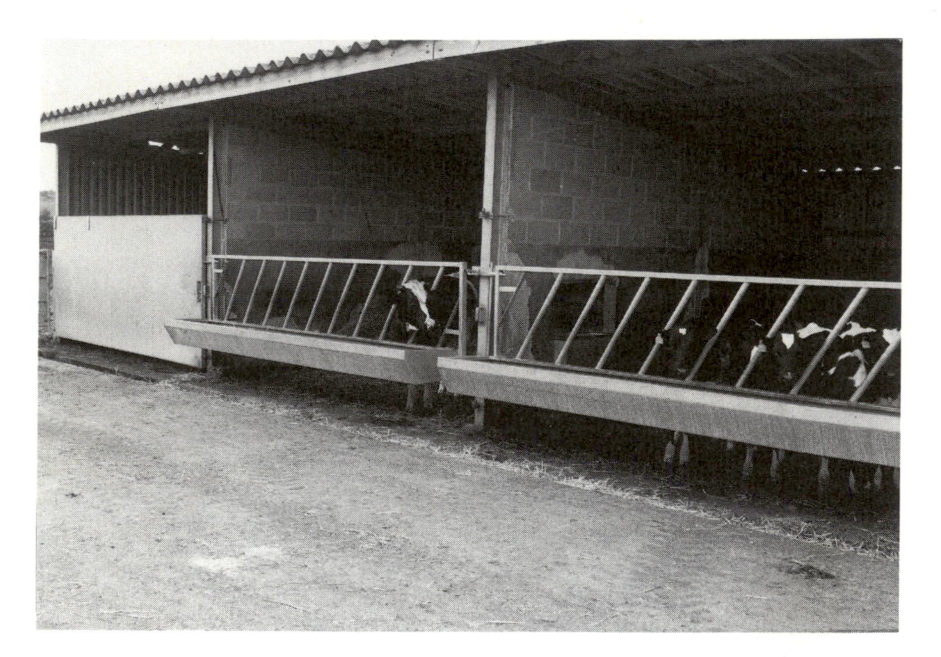

Fig. 11.12. Row of individual calving boxes that can also be used for calf rearing.

Table 11.5. Effect of calving site and degree of supervision on calving performance.

Calving performance	Paddock ($n = 301$)	Yard ($n = 168$)	Pen A ($n = 95$)	Pen B ($n = 54$)
Vulval constriction (%)	2.7	1.8	33.7	57.4
Dystocia (%)	9.0	8.3	43.2	63.0
Stillbirths (%)	13.3	7.7	31.6	22.2

Source: Mee, 1990.

Pen A Observed intermittently
Pen B Observed continuously during stage 2 of calving

(or even in very crowded paddocks) may *try* to select their own area for calving, but if they are low in the pecking order they may continually get moved away to different areas of the yard, thus causing stress and disrupting the calving process. Mee (1990), summarizing the work of Dufty (1981), suggested that the increased incidence of vulval constriction in heifers calving in yards under close confinement and continuous supervision, compared with those left outside in a paddock (Table 11.5), was due to excessive disturbances during parturition stimulating the sympathetic branch of the autonomic nervous system. This leads to contraction of the constrictor vestibuli muscle in the caudal genital tract and hence vaginal constriction. In a large survey involving Friesian heifers, Drew (1987) found that one of the most important determinants of ease of calving was the farm at which the heifers calved, further indicating the importance of management in relation to minimizing stress and improving both ease of calving and animal welfare.

Other Facilities

Feeding system

In this section reference will only be made to those aspects of feeding which affect housing. Feed is the greatest single determinant of milk production and hence every effort should be made to optimize feed intake, both in terms of quality and quantity. These two factors are, of course, related, in that improving feed quality often increases intake. Feed intake may also be increased by presentation, namely providing accessible and adequate feeding space.

Table 11.1 indicates that approximately 700 mm per cow of feeding space is required. At one time it was considered that if cows had 24-hour

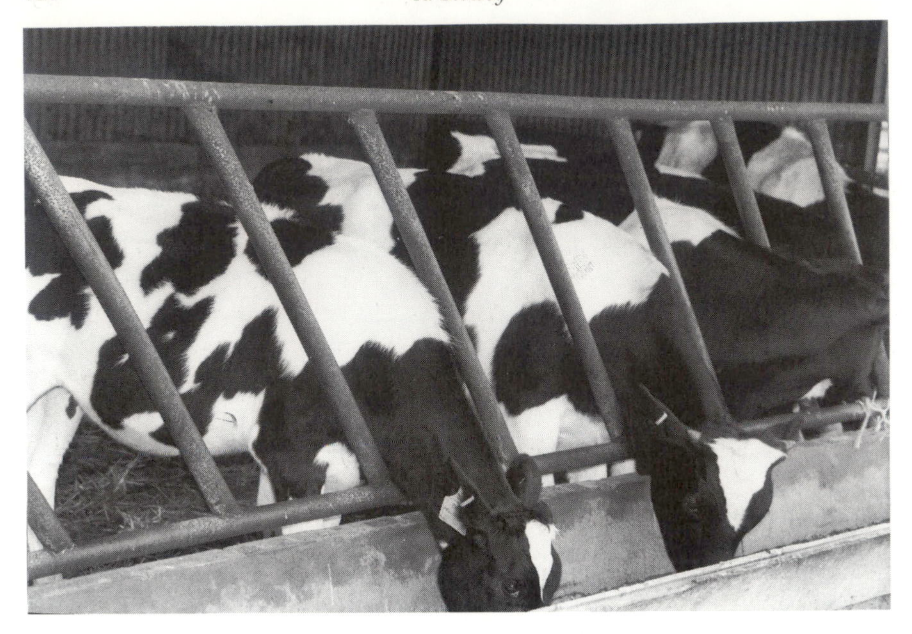

Fig. 11.13. Feed barrier with bars angled diagonally between animals.

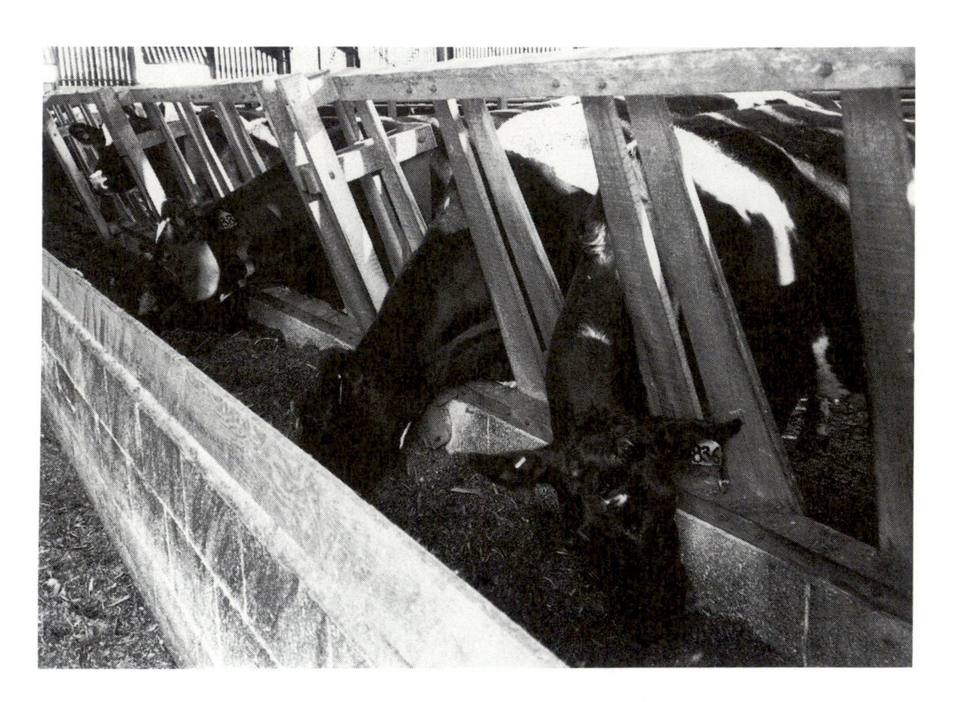

Fig. 11.14. Feed face with barriers tilted forward and diagonal divisions gives the best access (Stansfield, 1991. Published with permission of Farming Press).

access to feed (e.g. silage) then 100 mm per cow was sufficient. However, cows are gregarious creatures and prefer feeding together, with periods of intense feeding, drinking and social activity occurring shortly after morning and afternoon milking and when fresh food is dispensed (Hedlund and Rolls, 1977). Ample feed space needs to be available therefore, especially when concentrates are fed out of parlour. Unless there is sufficient feeding space, shy feeders and heifers will not receive their full allocation. Feed areas should be protected from extremes of weather and should not be excessively far from the lying area. However, heavily stocked, purpose-built buildings, where the manger is immediately behind or beside the cubicles and which do not allow any free loafing area for social activity, can be counterproductive in terms of stress and heat detection. On the other hand, if cows have to stand outside to feed in cold, driving rain, intakes will be reduced.

Although cows normally graze at ground level, access to feed is improved if the manger is slightly raised. Suggested heights vary between 160 mm (Radostits and Blood, 1985) and 300 mm (Webster, 1987a; see Table 11.1). Feed access can also be increased by the design of the feed barrier. Cows prefer to feed from their own feed trough and separated from others (Craig, 1981). Traditionally, vertical bars were used to separate one cow from another, but bars angled diagonally (Fig. 11.13) give better access and also deter cows from changing places when feeding (Stansfield, 1991). The forward movement of a cow is arrested by her shoulders, hence a further improvement is to tilt the feed fence forward at an angle of approximately 10° (Fig. 11.14). Although commonly used, feeding behind an electric fence is not ideal as it decreases voluntary access, especially by some of the shy feeders and heifers; it also fails to provide vertical separation between individual cows when they are feeding and often insufficient feeding space is available to allow cows to express their normal behaviour and all eat together. If an electric fence is to be used, therefore, a much longer feed face needs to be provided (for example, as in strip grazing).

Water

A good source of clean water is an important requirement of dairy cows. As with feeding, cows drink at specific times of the day, namely after morning and afternoon milking (see Fig. 11.15) and hence the provision of large capacity (1600 l) circular tanks, allowing up to 15 cows to drink at any one time, is ideal. These may be difficult to accommodate in some housing systems, but are ideal where there is an outside loafing area and space is not at a premium. The placing of water troughs in straw yard and cubicle systems has already been discussed. Severe restriction of water, by 50% of normal intake, will depress yields, but even a 10% decrease results in behavioural changes (Little *et al.*, 1980).

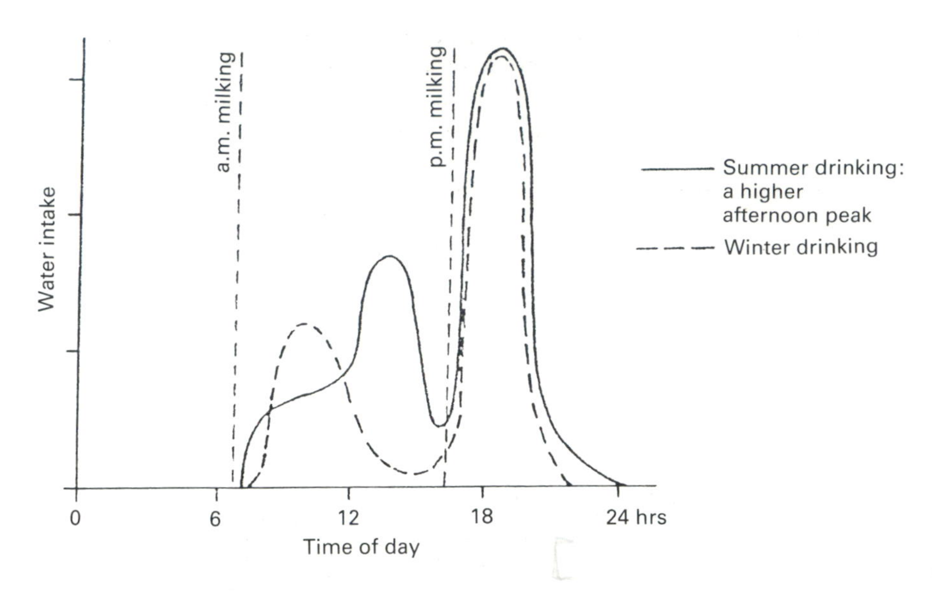

Fig. 11.15. Daily drinking patterns in summer and winter (VBDF, p. 356).

Housing, Disease and Welfare

Because of their close confinement, housed animals are more susceptible to the spread of infectious disease. In addition, the housing environment itself may be a significant factor in the cause of disease, the main syndromes being lameness and mastitis. Disease is probably the single most important determinant of animal welfare (see also this volume, Chapter 2).

Housing and mastitis

The change to loose housing, combined with keeping cows in larger groups, led to a significant increase in mastitis in many herds, especially that caused by the environmental bacteria *Escherichia coli* and *Streptococcus uberis*. In straw yards this can be due to a combination of high stocking density, use of damp straw and inadequate frequency of cleaning out (Blowey, 1989). Under such conditions, the total bacterial count (TBC) of bulk milk may also increase. In one herd, reducing the stocking density from 54 to 45 cows per yard (a decrease of 17%), storing bedding straw under cover and increasing its usage, combined with changes in the milking routine, significantly reduced the incidence of clinical mastitis (Blowey, 1991, unpublished data), with an associated reduction in TBC. With the cost of a single case of mastitis being at least £40 (Blowey, 1986) this represents a considerable saving. In addition, prior to the improvement, the temperature of the straw beds was 40°C,

Table 11.6. The coliform populations supported by different types of bedding, and their effect on the coliform numbers obtained as a teat swab.

Type of bedding	Total coliform count in cubicle bedding	Mean no. of coliforms obtained from a teat swab
Sawdust	52.0×10^6	127
Shavings	6.6×10^6	12
Straw	3.1×10^6	8

Source: Rendos *et al.*, 1975.

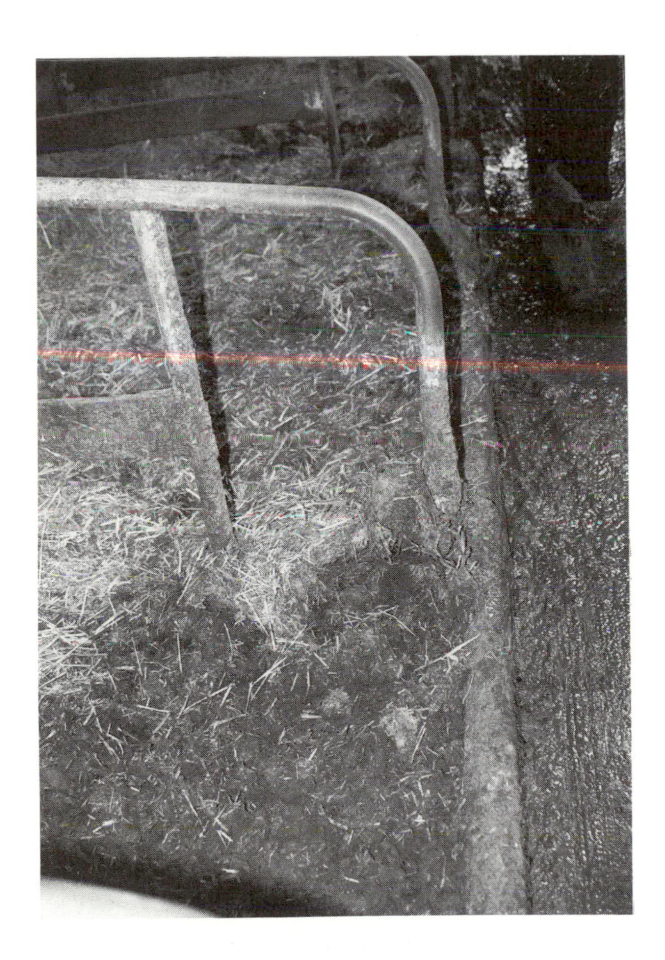

Fig. 11.16. Cubicles with rear tip leading to soiled bedding.

due to fermentation of excreta in the straw. Although such temperatures clearly favour rapid bacterial multiplication, they were not considered excessive. However, Francis (1989) reported that excessively liberal use of bedding materials caused overheating and a bacterial build-up. Mastitic bacteria are usually killed by composting processes in the lower layers of the straw.

Hygiene in cubicle housing is equally important. Soiled bedding should be removed from the rear of the cubicle twice daily, passages scraped twice daily and the lying area rebedded once a day. A combination of milk and urine in the cubicle bed has been shown to support a particularly high (1×10^9) count of *E. coli* (Bramley, personal communication). Levels of coliform bacteria greater than 10^6 per gram of litter predispose to mastitis (Bramley and Neave, 1975). Variations in bedding material also have an effect, with sawdust being able to support the highest bacterial population (Table 11.6). Sand and shredded paper support even lower bacterial populations (Francis, 1989). Cubicles should not be constructed with a lip at the kerb, as this can lead to an accumulation of soiled bedding (Fig. 11.16). The application of a few handfuls of lime twice weekly, prior to rebedding the cubicles, has been suggested (Blowey, 1988) as a method of drying the cubicle bed and reducing the number of bacteria. Cubicle passages should be scraped prior to cows returning after milking. This reduces indirect faecal contamination of beds via the feet and as the teat sphincter does not fully close and seal until 30 min after milking, keeping the cows standing and out of the bedded area (cubicle or straw yard) may be beneficial.

Stress in dairy cows has been proposed as a predisposing cause of mastitis (Bramley, 1989), although its effects are difficult to quantify.

Housing and lameness

Lameness is a major economic and welfare problem in the UK dairy herd, with figures of annual incidence varying between 25% (Whitaker *et al.*, 1983) and 60% (Eddy and Scott, 1980), with 6.5% of dairy cows culled annually because of lameness (Russell *et al.*, 1982). Lameness can have widespread adverse effects on the welfare of cows (Potter and Broom, 1990). Environment has a major impact on the incidence, in that cows which spend excessive periods standing are worst affected. Colam-Ainsworth *et al.* (1989), comparing two identically managed herds, both housed in identical cubicles, showed that by the increased use of straw bedding lying times increased, more first lactation heifers entered the cubicle house and the time between entry and lying was significantly decreased. The higher usage of straw bedding decreased the amount of aberrant behaviour and overall there was a marked decrease in the incidence of lameness (laminitis and sole ulcers) in the first lactation heifers (Fig. 11.17). Many of the cubicle construction and design factors leading to increased cubicle usage and hence decreased

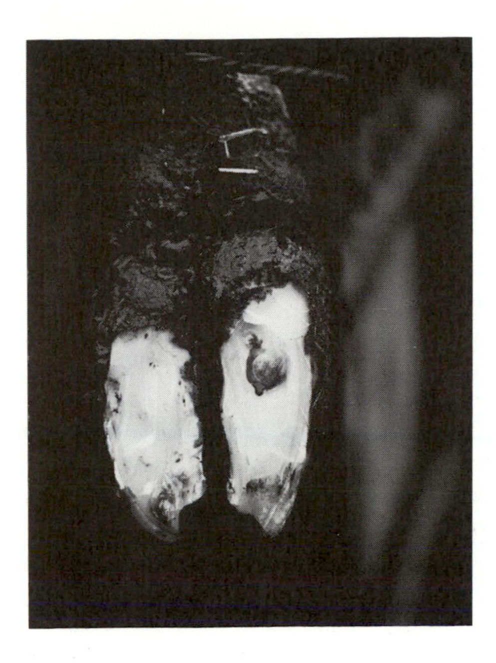

Fig. 11.17. Typical sole ulcer. Note also the extensive soiling of the foot.

incidence of lameness, have been referred to in a previous section.

Cubicle training is also important. Heifers which have been *reared* in cubicles adapt more rapidly when they join the main herd. If separate heifer-rearing cubicles are not available, heifers can be housed for 4–6 weeks during their second summer as a trial period while the cows are at pasture. Heifers introduced into a large dairy herd already have to cope with the stress of parturition, aggression and dramatic changes in feeding. If they are then exposed to a new, foreign and perhaps not particularly comfortable or inviting lying area, they are likely to spend excessive periods standing and hence develop lameness.

A further adaptation, which is being used by a small but increasing number of dairy farmers, is to leave the freshly calved cows and heifers in straw yards for 3–5 weeks after calving, and then transfer them to the cubicles (Blowey, 1993a,b). It is considered that the more 'gentle' environment associated with a well-kept, cleanly bedded low stocking density straw yard significantly increases yields and decreases the incidence of lameness. As the newly calved cows are in a separate group, it is also easy to apply additional management techniques such as premilking teat disinfection and three times daily milking, both of which will reduce the incidence of environmental mastitis. When the move from the straw yard into the cubicle housing occurs, the cows will have recovered more fully from the stress and trauma of calving and cubicle acceptance is, in fact, better than for cows

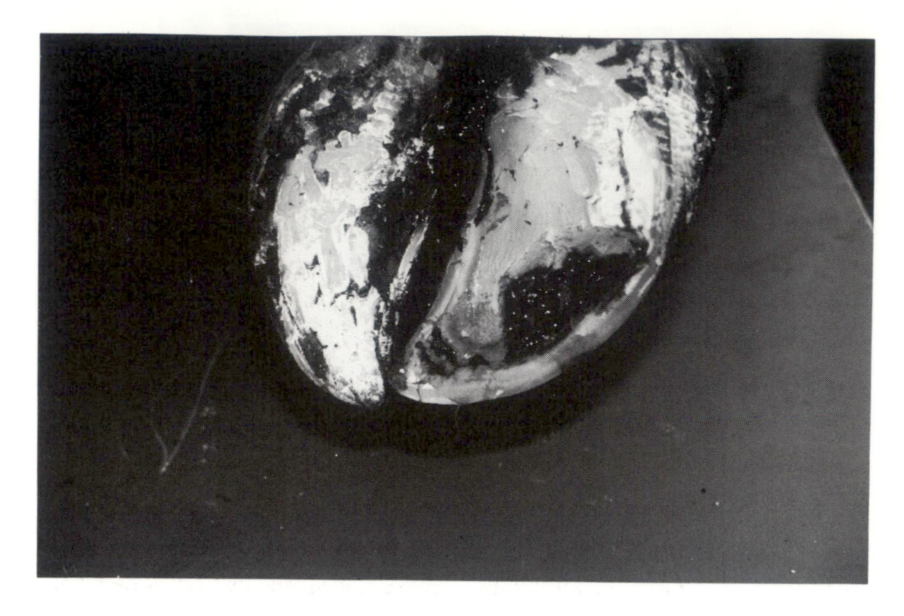

Fig. 11.18. White line abscess, with under-run sole partially removed.

introduced into cubicles immediately post-calving. In their detailed studies of the ultra-structural changes of horn in the white line area, Kempson and Logue (1993) concluded that the physiological and management changes associated with calving have a significant influence on the quality of horn, and this in turn will affect the onset of lameness. Minimizing the extent of these changes therefore, by optimizing the comfort of the environment immediately post-calving, seems a logical step. If it could be proved that the post-calving management regime of 3–5 weeks in straw yards prior to transfer into cubicles also had a significant effect on yield and therefore economic performance, this could be of great benefit to dairy cow welfare.

There is general agreement that there should be sufficient cubicles for all cows to lie at the same time, i.e. equal numbers of cows and cubicles (Sumner, 1989). For low-ranking cows, cubicles act as both a lying area and a 'safety zone', where effective personal distance is increased by the bars of the cubicle (Potter and Broom, 1990). In the study by Miller and Wood-Gush (1991), low ranking cows did not use cubicles as refuges. However, some farmers recommend that late-pregnant heifers should run with the dry cows for a few weeks prior to calving, especially if they are still at pasture. This gives the heifers the opportunity to establish themselves in the pecking order and perhaps start to become accustomed to the postpartum ration before they calve.

Rough, uneven and pitted concrete floors and concrete made with

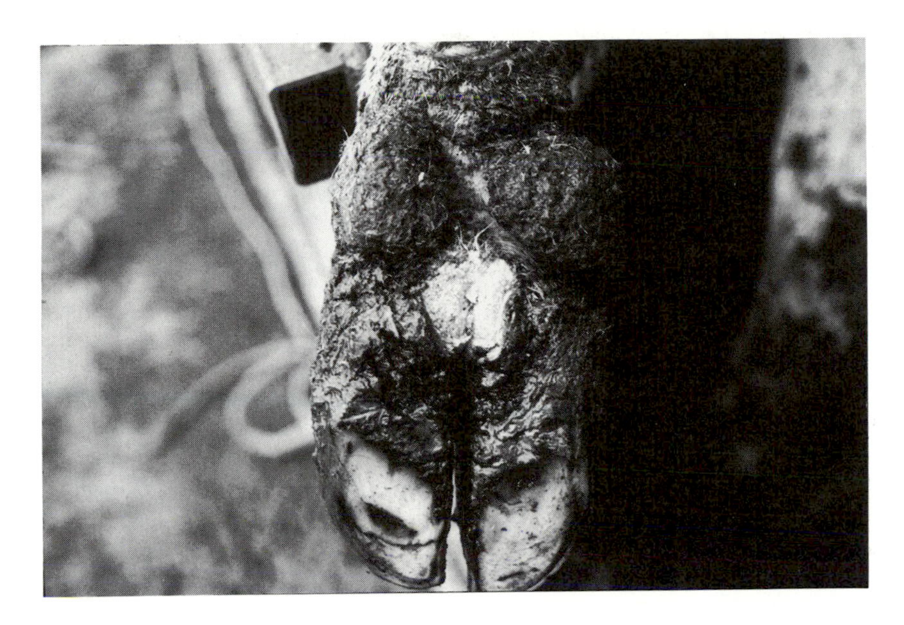

Fig. 11.19. Digital dermatitis and heel erosion.

a sharp aggregate can traumatize solar hooves and predispose to white line infection and abscessation (Fig. 11.18). Sudden turning movements, causing the cow to pivot her weight on a stationary solar horn, leads to tearing and separation of the wall from the sole and further white line abscessation. This is seen when cattle are made to turn through sudden and sharp corners and also when they are forced to make rapid movements, for example the timid heifer escaping from an aggressor, or jostling for priority at an out-of-parlour feeding station, or a feeder where there is inadequate feeding space. Excessive standing and other traumatic events will lead to softening of solar horn and solar haemorrhage. The presence of haemorrhage in horn forms a point of weakness, which might lead to solar penetration, sole ulcers or white line abscessation.

Overcrowding may cause trauma, in that cows do not spend sufficient time walking. This produces poor blood flow in the hoof and as such is similar to the 'trench foot' suffered by soldiers in the First World War.

Unsanitary conditions, for example inadequately scraped yards, especially around feed areas, can predispose to interdigital necrobacillosis ('foul'), heel erosion and digital dermatitis (Blowey and Weaver, 1991). Digital dermatitis (Fig. 11.19) has only recently been reported in the UK (Blowey and Sharp, 1988). Its incidence is associated with winter housing and high stocking densities (Blowey, 1990) and can be controlled by using an antibiotic footbath.

Housing and traumatic injuries

Poor housing, or its poor management can lead to numerous injuries, all of which constitute significant welfare problems. Cows may 'do the splits' or fall on excessively worn and slippery concrete passageways or feed areas, leading to a range of conditions including obturator paralysis, fracture of the pelvis or proximal femur, ischaemic muscle necrosis and rupture of the gastrocnemius tendon. Trauma caused by narrow doors or alleyways, or from protruding water troughs, may lead to haematoma formation, or to fracture and necrosis of the tuber coxae (the 'wing' of the pelvis), especially if cows are rushed and crowded by unsympathetic herdsmen. Cubicles with design faults, inadequate dimensions or protruding parts of divisions and beds may lead to knee or hock bursitis and, if prolonged, stiffness and chronic arthritis (Hughes, 1990). Of particular importance is the lip at the rear of some cubicle beds which can produce hock bursitis, and poorly positioned brisket boards at the front of the cubicles, which may lead to knee bursitis. Both conditions are exacerbated by inadequate littering of cubicle beds.

Teat injuries are a cause for concern to both the cow and herdsman and significantly predispose to mastitis. Traumatic teat damage (Fig. 11.20) is seen in both straw yards and cubicles and may be self-inflicted or caused by

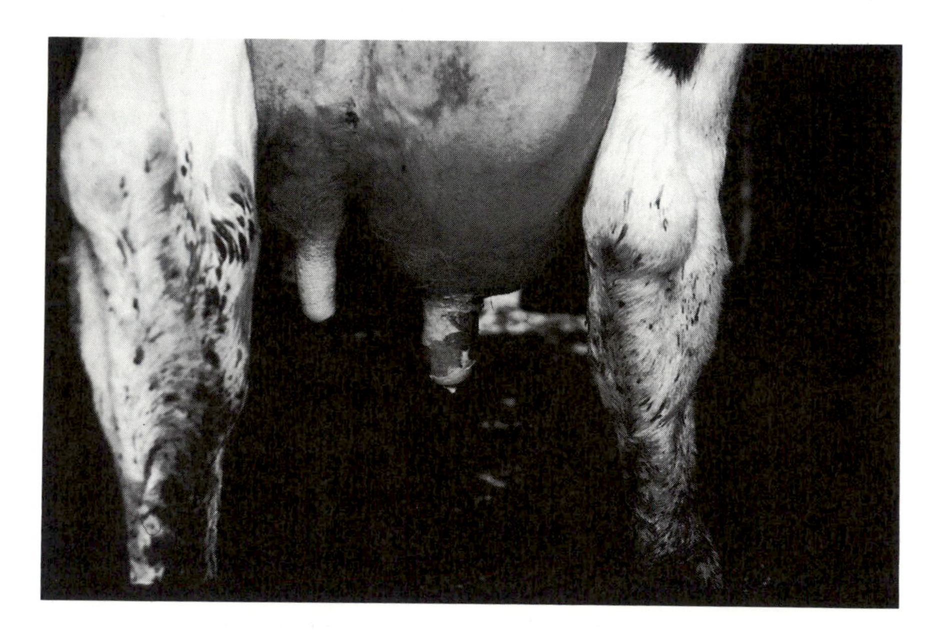

Fig. 11.20. Traumatic teat damage. Superficial skin has been removed and the teat is so swollen that the sphincter is blocked, producing an enlarged quarter full of milk.

other cows. Factors increasing the incidence include poor cubicle design, overcrowding, inadequate cubicle numbers, poor (slippery) floor surfaces and rough handling of the cows, for example rushing them through walkways.

Housing and welfare

Webster (1987b) suggested that welfare can be evaluated in terms of five basic freedoms:

1. Freedom from hunger and malnutrition.
2. Freedom from thermal or physical distress.
3. Freedom to express most normal behaviour.
4. Freedom from disease and injury.
5. Freedom from fear.

Many of these factors have already been dealt with in earlier sections of this chapter, particularly freedom from disease and injury (see also this volume, Chapter 4). Space allowance and design of feed area are important determinants of stress. It has been suggested that cows in loose yards prefer to lie at least 1 m away from other cows (Sumner, 1989) and in tied systems restricted movements lead to stress because the animal is unable to establish its position in the social hierarchy (Bramley, 1989). Cows are social animals, wishing to feed together. If there is a shortage of feeding space, this can have a deleterious effect, for example an increase in movement and chasing behaviour (Metz and Mekking, 1984; Potter and Broom, 1987). If barriers exist between animals when feeding, this produces a more even intake of feed between low and high ranking animals (Broom, 1987). Where no such divisions exist and where there is insufficient feeding space, low ranking animals spend considerable periods walking and waiting. The author (unpublished data) has seen a dramatic increase in cubicle lying times following a simple increase in the availability of feed space for a crowded dairy herd.

Welfare problems certainly exist when animals are being handled, for example for routine tuberculosis testing, or when being loaded on to lorries to be transported. The frustration felt by both man and animals when cows will not walk into a lorry, or into a cattle crush is something which has to be experienced to be understood. It is when large numbers of animals have to be handled in a short period of time that some of the worst excesses can occur and this can only be avoided by careful planning. Figure 11.21 shows two possible handling systems, with for example, dairy cows being held in yard Y prior to being brought into the crush C for testing. In Plan A, gate G will certainly help to deflect cows into the crush, but they will have to be brought forward one at a time, which is highly stressful, and the remainder of the cows will push towards the left corners of the yard each time another cow is selected to be brought forward. This leads to severe stress, often with cows slipping, becoming recumbent and then being trampled by the others. In Plan B, groups of four to six cows can be walked alongside S of the yard and deflected into a smaller holding pen (P) and a race (R) by gate G_1. When the gate is closed (G_2) there might be three cows in the holding pen P, two in the race R and one in the crush C. Such a system is shown in Fig. 11.22. Bars, or one-way gates, placed between cows along the race, prevent further movement and in so doing reduce fear and stress. The extra ease with which cows enter the race and then flow through the crush in Plan B, compared with Plan A, is quite dramatic – and yet it is still surprising and frustrating how many farms do not have similar systems! If routine work is to be carried out on dairy cows, then it is excellent practice to let them run

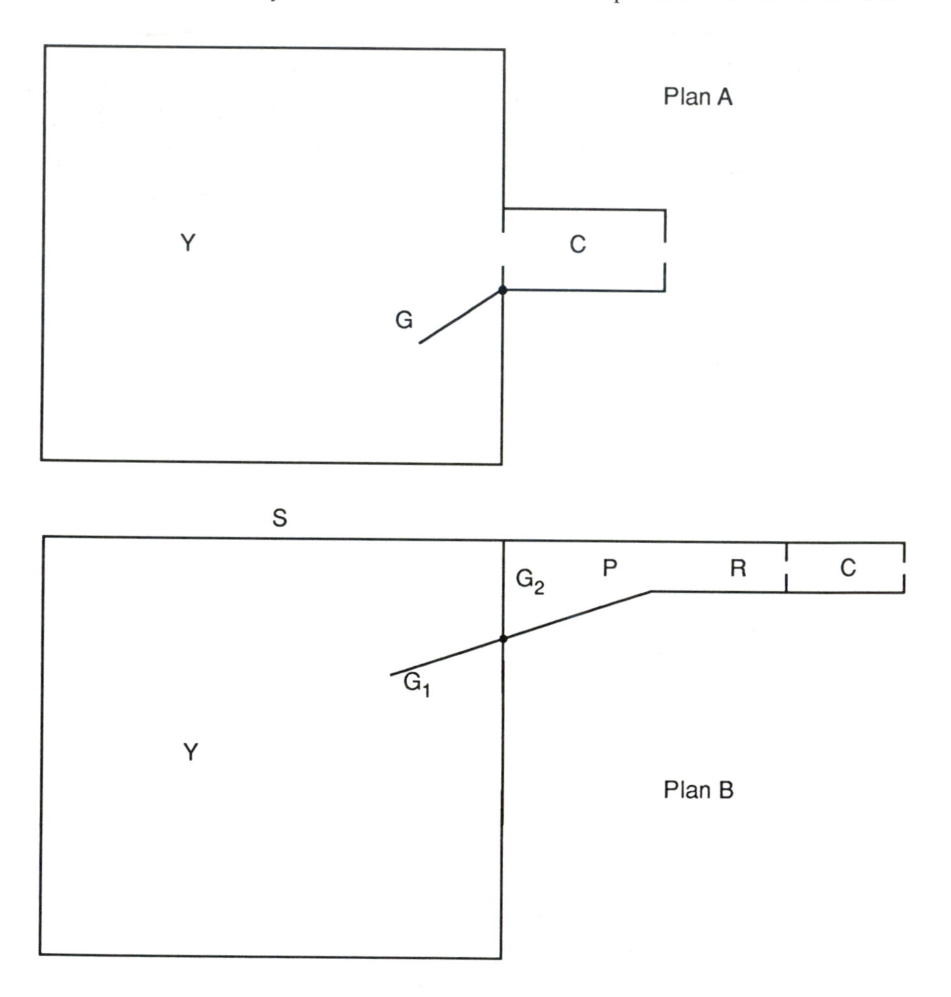

Fig. 11.21. Diagrammatic layout of handling systems.

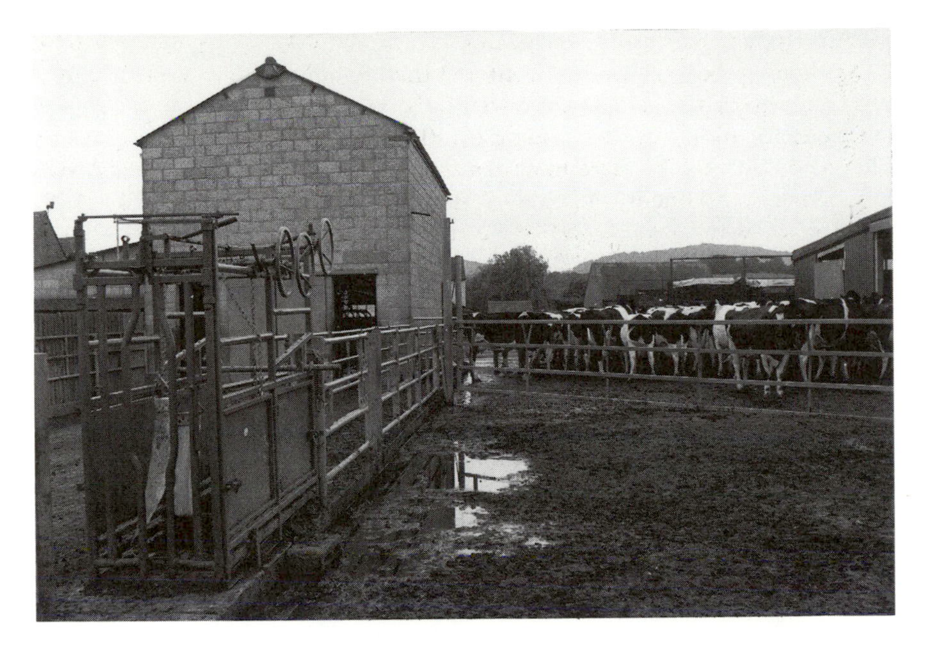

Fig. 11.22. A well-designed handling system.

voluntarily through the handling system, i.e. from the yard, through the race and crush and out (Fig. 11.21, plan B), for a few days prior to catching. Few farmers do this and yet the time it saves and the improvement in animal welfare (less stress and fear, fewer pushings and beatings, etc.) is highly beneficial. Cows generally dislike running down hill and moving from a very bright to a dark environment and vice versa. This should also be considered when constructing a handling system. Similar features apply to loading ramps prior to transport. Ideally, the loading area should be approached along a race and end at a raised platform on to which the lorry tailboard can be dropped, so that cows do not have to walk up an excessively steep ramp on to the lorry. Cows left for AI should have food and water and be restrained in suitable stalls which will not cause injury to cows trying to escape. Selecting an individual animal from the herd and penning it singly is in itself a stressful process.

Acknowledgements

Figures 11.1, 11.6 and 11.14 from Stansfield, M. (1991) *The New Herdsman Book*, The Farming Press, Ipswich.
Figures 11.11 and 11.15 from Blowey, R. (1990) *A Veterinary Book for Dairy Farmers*. The Farming Press, Ipswich.

References

ADAS (1988) Advisory Leaflet 3137 Design & Management of Cubicles. HMSO, London.

Blowey, R.W. (1986) An assessment of the economic benefits of a mastitis control scheme. *Veterinary Record* 119, 551–553.

Blowey, R.W. (1988) *A Veterinary Book for Dairy Farmers.* Farming Press, Ipswich, UK.

Blowey, R.W. (1989) Investigating a herd mastitis problem. In: *Proceedings of the British Mastitis Conference, Stoneleigh,* Ciba Agriculture, Cambridge, pp. 47–59.

Blowey, R.W. (1990) Description and diagnosis of superficial digital lesions in dairy cattle. In: Murray, R. (ed.), *Proceedings of the 6th International Symposium on Diseases of the Ruminant Digit.* BCVA, Liverpool, p. 55.

Blowey, R.W. (1993a) Solar haemorrhage in dairy cattle. *Veterinary Record* 132, 663.

Blowey, R.W. (1993b) *Cattle Lameness and Hoofcare.* Farming Press, Ipswich, p. 75.

Blowey R.W. and Sharp (1988) Digital dermatitis in dairy cattle. *Veterinary Record* 122, 505–508.

Blowey, R.W. and Weaver, A.D. (1991) *A Colour Atlas of Diseases and Disorders of Cattle.* Wolfe Publications, London.

Bramley, A.J. (1989) Why environmental influences on mastitis are important. In: *Proceedings of the British Mastitis Conference,* Stoneleigh, p. 1.

Bramley, A.J. and Neave, F.J. (1975) Studies on the control of coliform mastitis in dairy cows. *British Veterinary Journal* 131, 160–169.

Broom, D.M. (1987) Welfare considerations in cattle practice. *Proceedings of the British Cattle Veterinary Association,* London, p. 153.

Cermak, J. (1983) Cow cubicle design. *Farm Buildings Digest* 18, 7–9.

Cermak, J. (1990) Note on welfare of dairy cows with reference to spatial and comfort aspects of design of cubicles. In: *Proceedings of the 6th International Symposium on Disease of the Ruminant Digit.* p. 85.

Colam-Ainsworth, P., Lunn, G.A., Thomas, R.C. and Eddy, R.G. (1989) Behaviour of cows in cubicles and its possible relationship with laminitis in replacement heifers. *Veterinary Record* 125, 573–575.

Craig, J.V. (1981) *Domestic Animal Behaviour.* Prentice-Hall, New Jersey.

Dodd, F.H., Higgs, T.M. and Bramley, A.J. (1984) Cubicle management and coliform mastitis. *Veterinary Record* 114, 522–523.

Drew, B. (1987) Causes of dystocia in Friesian heifers and its effect on subsequent performance. *Proceedings of the British Cattle Veterinary Association* p. 143.

Dufty, J.H. (1981) The influence of various degrees of confinement and supervision on the incidence of dystocia and stillbirths in Hereford heifers. *New Zealand Veterinary Journal* 29, 44.

Eddy, R.G. and Scott, C.P. (1980) Some observations of the incidence of lameness in dairy cattle in Somerset. *Veterinary Record* 106, 140–144.

Francis, P.G. (1989) Hygiene of litter. In: *Proceedings of the British Mastitis Conference Stoneleigh.* CIBA Agriculture, Cambridge.

Hedlund, L. and Rolls, J. (1977) Behaviour of lactating cows during total confinement. *Journal of Dairy Science* 50, 1807–1812.

Hughes, J. (1990) The cow and her cubicle. In: Murray, R. (ed.), *Proceedings of the 6th International Symposium on Diseases of the Ruminant Digit,* p. 276.

Hughes, J.W. (1992) Practicalities of cow feeding, comfort and behaviour. *Proceedings British Cattle Veterinary Association* July 1992, pp. 43–45.

Kempson, S.M. and Logue, D. (1993) Ultrastructural observations of hoof horn from dairy cows: changes in the white line during first lactation. *Veterinary Record* 132, 524.

Little, W., Collis, K.A. and Gleed, P.T. (1980) Effect of reduced water intake by lactating dairy cows on behaviour, milk yield and blood composition. *Veterinary Record* 106, 547–551.

Mee, J.F. (1990) Dystocia in Friesian heifers. *Veterinary Record* 127, 219.

Metz, J.H.M. and Mekking, P. (1984) Crowding phenomena in dairy cows as related to available idling space in a cubicle housing system. *Applied Animal Behaviour Science* 12, 63–78.

Miller, K. and Wood-Gush, D.G.M. (1991) Some effects of housing on the social behaviour of dairy cows. *Animal Production* 53, 271–278.

Newman, L.E. and Kowalski, J.F. (1973) Fresh sawdust bedding – a possible source of klebsiella organisms. *American Journal of Veterinary Research* 34, 979–980.

O'Connell, J.M., Meaney, M.J. and Giller, P.S. (1991) An evaluation of four cubicle designs using cattle behaviour criteria. *Irish Veterinary Journal* 44, 8–13.

Potter, M.J. and Broom, D.M. (1987) Cattle housing systems, lameness and behaviour. *Current Topics in Veterinary Medicine and Animal Science* 40, 129–147.

Potter, M.J. and Broom, D.M. (1990) Behaviour and welfare aspects of cattle lameness in relation to building design. *Proceedings of the 6th International Symposium on Diseases of the Ruminant Digit*, p. 80.

Radostits, O.M and Blood, D.C. (1985) *Herd Health* W.B. Saunders, Philadelphia pp. 176 and 182.

Rendos, J.J., Eberhart, R.J. and Kesler, E.M. (1975) Microbial populations of teat ends of dairy cows and bedding materials. *Journal of Dairy Science* 58, 1492.

Russell, A.M., Rowlands, G.J. and Shaw, S.R. (1982) A survey of lameness in British dairy cattle. *Veterinary Record* 111, 155–160.

Stansfield, J.M. (1991) *The Herdsman's Book.* The Farming Press, Ipswich, UK.

Sumner, J. (1989) Design and maintenance of housing systems. In: *Proceedings of the British Mastitis Conference Stoneleigh.* Ciba Agriculture, Cambridge, p. 10.

Webster, A.J.F. (1987a) *Understanding the Dairy Cow.* BSP Professional Books, Oxford.

Webster, A.J.F. (1987b) *Proceedings of the British Cattle Veterinary Association* Jan. 1987, London, p. 165.

Whitaker, D.N., Kelly, J.M. and Smith, E.J. (1983) Incidence of lameness in dairy cows. *Veterinary Record* 113, 60–63.

12 Beef Cattle Housing

N.G. LAWRENCE†
ADAS Wolverhampton, UK

The housing needs of the beef animal are generally simpler than those of the dairy cow. The spring calving suckler cow primarily requires confinement during winter to prevent poaching of grassland: ideally, the autumn calver will calve down out of doors for better hygiene. The dairy-bred calf, deprived of its dam and penned for easy management, has more critical requirements. At the other extreme the yearling beast merely needs shelter from wind and rain.

The student of cattle building design would do well to accept the truism that cattle are different from pigs and poultry, especially with regard to their thermoregulatory responses to heat and cold. For example, Webster *et al.* (1970) observed that yearling cattle in Alberta, Canada, can alter both their upper and lower critical temperatures by as much as 20% following adaptation to severe weather. These observations support the predictions of Bruce's (1984) mathematical model of energy exchange, which showed that the benefits of housing for suckler cows in terms of feed saved or reduction of liveweight change over the winter are small. However, Kubisch *et al.* (1991) have recently reported the advantages of partial roofing of feedlot pens for bulls growing in the extreme cold of an Albertan winter. Feed intake was higher and conversion efficiency correspondingly lower in animals denied shelter.

Overall, healthy cattle with a developed and functioning rumen are extremely cold hardy with wide and adaptable zones of thermoneutrality (Webster, 1981, 1988). Thus buildings can rarely be justified on the basis of food saving, liveweight gain or health. The only justification is ease of management. The thermal criteria are different for the neonate or pre-ruminant calf (this volume, Chapter 1).

†Deceased

Calf Housing Specifications

Calf housing should meet the health and behavioural needs of the animals as embodied in the UK Codes of Welfare for Livestock (Chapter 15). The major requirements can be translated into specifications for climate, space allowances, ventilation and pen design.

Floor space allowance

A calf should have space *at least* sufficient to stand up, lie down, turn round, stretch its limbs and groom itself (Brambell, 1965). Mitchell (1976) and others interpret this as a pen width no narrower than the height of a calf's shoulder (or withers). Clearly, the minimum pen width depends on age, sex and breed and Mitchell suggests a minimum width of 750 mm at birth and 900 mm at 12 weeks old. Overall pen lengths of 1.5 m and 1.8 m will suffice for calves up to 4 and 8 weeks old respectively, equivalent to about 60 and 80 kg liveweight. This assumes that feed and water buckets/troughs are on the outside of the pen, each occupying approximately 300 mm, giving an overall length per 80 kg calf of 2.1 m. Passageways should be at least 1.5 m clear width (Fig. 12.1).

Ventilation

Air volume

Mitchell (1976) and Webster (1984) recommend an air volume allowance of 6 m^3 per calf up to 6 weeks and Webster suggests 10 m^3 per calf from 6 to 10

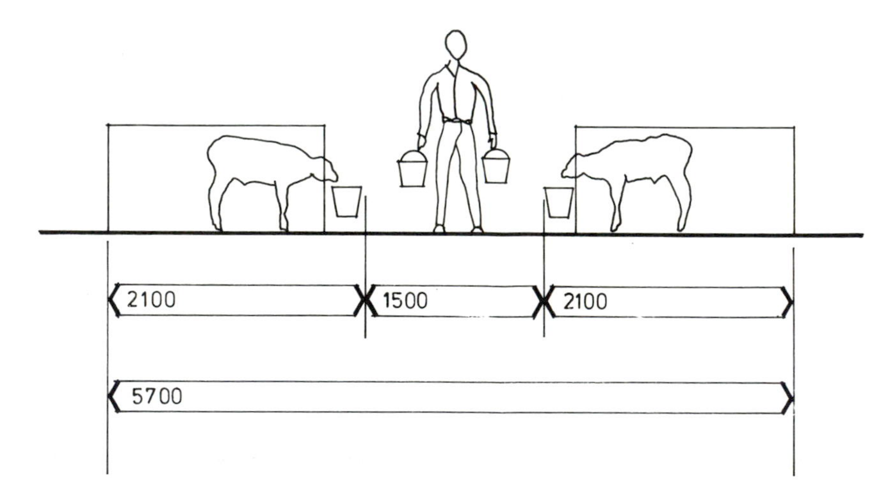

Fig. 12.1. Pen length and passageway width in a two-row calf house.

weeks of age while MAFF (1984) suggests $7\,m^3$ per calf as an absolute minimum. There is not necessarily a conflict in these differing recommendations – it is more likely an acceptance of what actually happens in the UK calf units. On a dairy farm rearing its own calves to 3 or 4 weeks old before sale, $6\,m^3$ of air volume per calf is sufficient. However, the calf rearer often buys-in 3–4-week-old calves that weigh up to 60 or 65 kg but subconsciously ages them as the traditional 10-day-old calf. If he then keeps them in a calf house for another 6 weeks, then Webster's recommendations of up to $10\,m^3$ of air space would be more appropriate.

If the 'ideal' calf house is modelled on a 5.7 m wide building and a halfway compromise of air volume requirement is taken at $8\,m^3$ per calf, then the building should have a mean height of 2.67 m. A roof pitch of 20° is needed to produce an acceptable 'fall' on a ridge building and sufficient height difference between air inlets and outlets. Thus, the overall dimensions become a height of 2.3 m to the eaves and 3.4 m to the apex and a width of 5.7 m (Fig. 12.2). (Increasing the overall height by 0.7 m, would increase the air volume per calf to $10\,m^3$.) If a 'standard' building module of 4.6 m bays is used, then two bays would hold a total of 18 calves in individual pens measuring 1.0 m × 1.8 m.

Air inlets and outlets

A general guide for the outlet area of a ridged roof building is $0.04\,m^2$ per calf. In the building shown in Fig. 12.2 this would equal a gap of 80 mm per metre run. The opening could be an incomplete ridge, a ridge protected by upstand, or a fully protected ventilated ridge (Figs 12.3 and 12.4).

An air inlet area of $0.08\,m^2$ per calf should allow sufficient fresh air

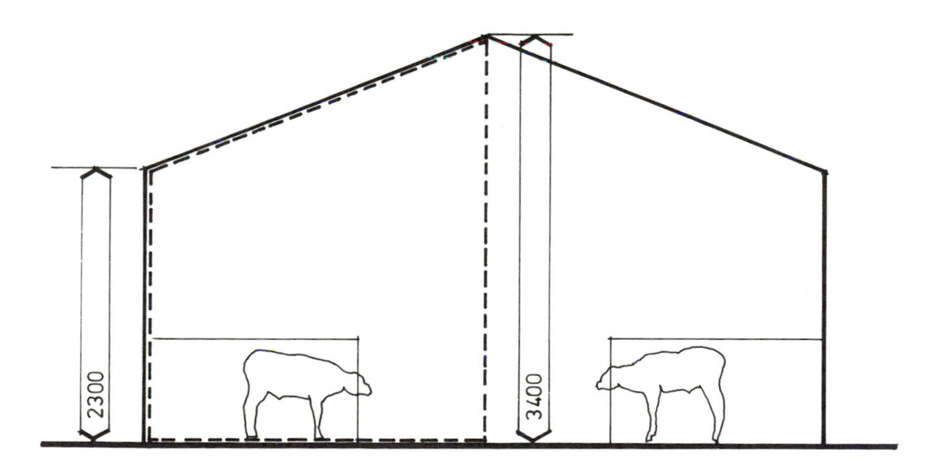

Fig. 12.2. The air space in this calf house is $8\,m^3$ per calf at a building width of 5.7 m.

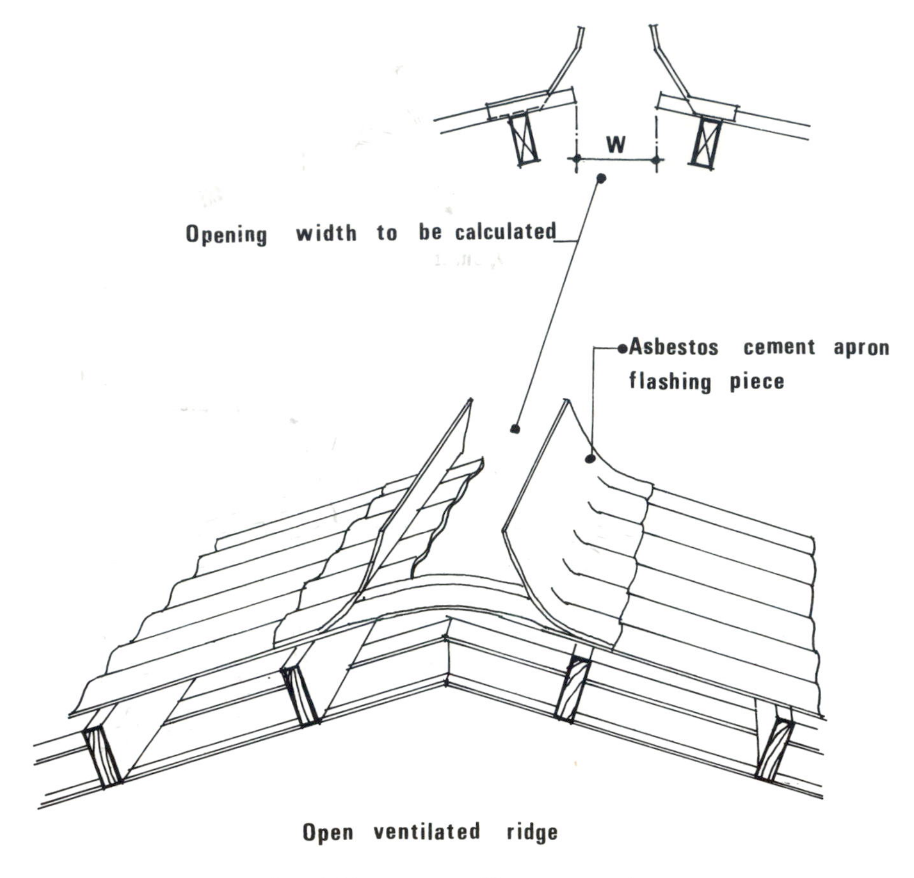

Fig. 12.3. An open ventilated ridge protected by an upstand.

distributed uniformly throughout the building without creating draughts. This can best be achieved by inlets above calf height located along both sides of the building (Fig. 12.5). A continuous inlet is ideal but it should be protected against high windspeeds. In the example the inlet could be provided by space boarding 500 mm high, comprising 125 mm wide boards with a 25 mm gap installed 1.65 m above ground level.

An alternative to the ridged building is the monopitch, which has similar specifications for air volume and floor area. However, the open front functions both as an air inlet at the bottom and outlet at the top. A sheeted gate approximately 1.5 m above ground level eliminates air movement at calf height while space boarding or plastic netting above forms a windbreak. This should have sufficient void in it to allow 0.25 m^2 of opening per calf housed. Buildings less than about 6 m deep do not require ventilation openings in the rear wall. Thickett *et al.* (1986) recommend that a top skirt

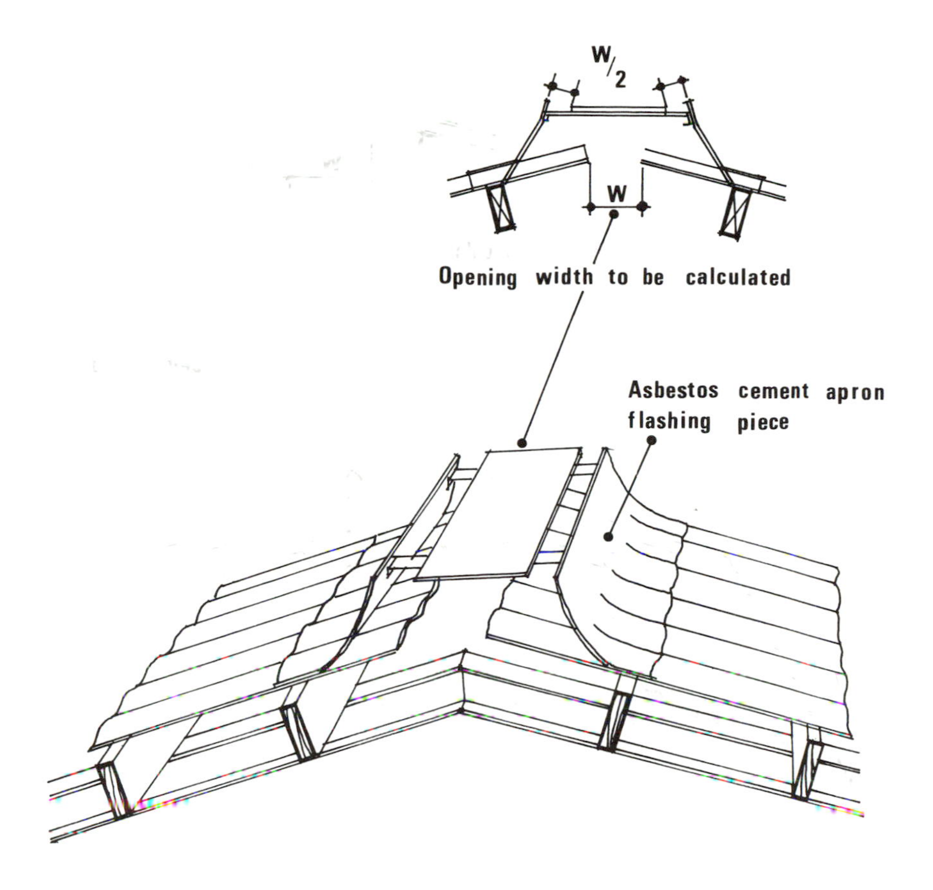

Fig. 12.4. A fully protected ventilated ridge.

along the front of the building prevents down-draughts and entrance of driving rain.

The monopitch calf house has two main advantages over the ridged building; firstly, access by tractor equipped with a foreloader is possible; and secondly, the building can be used as a nursery and follow-on house by permitting the calves to run free after weaning. In the northern hemisphere, the building's front should face south to take advantage of the sun and entry of the prevailing winds. Alternatively, two rows of monopitch houses can face each other in which case they should be constructed on a North–South axis.

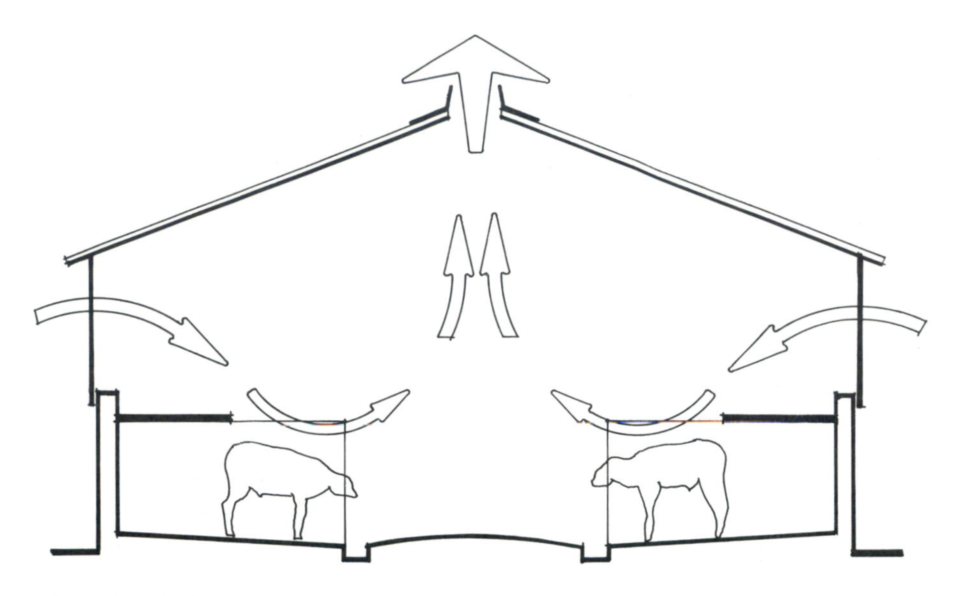

Fig. 12.5. Airflow patterns and floor drainage in a ridged building.

Fan ventilation

Most naturally-ventilated calf houses can achieve the minimum ventilation rate of six air changes per hour, recommended as a minimum by Webster (1984). Converted buildings sometimes pose structural or siting problems and mechanical ventilation may have to be employed. Webster (1984) and Mitchell (1976) suggest design criteria of between 6 and 18 air changes per hour, equivalent to 35–105 m^3h^{-1} at 6 m^3 per calf. Mitchell adds that the fan must always maintain the minimum rate of ventilation while the building is occupied. Details of suitable systems are given in Chapter 7.

Draughts

Whether calves are individually or group penned, they should be in a draught-free environment. A draught is defined as air movement (either vertical or horizontal) greater than 0.25 $m s^{-1}$ in winter (Mitchell, 1976; BS 5502, 1990a) or greater than 0.5 $m s^{-1}$ in summer (Webster, 1984). In individual calf pens, every third pen division should be solid on the basis that an obstruction to air movement (a 900 mm high pen division) is effective in reducing air speed for 3–4 times its height. Downward movement of incoming cool air can be prevented by covering the rear half of the pen with plywood sheets (Fig. 12.5). The cheaper device of stretching wire netting over the rear half of the pen and then covering it with straw is not recommended because of its high fire risk.

Artificial heat

In temperate zones there is rarely need for artificial heat sources. The only exceptions are for the newly born or the sick. If an infrared lamp is used care should be taken to keep it out of the calves' reach. A novel alternative is the quartz heater that can be focused and used to provide a heated area within a group pen. Sick calves may search out the heated zone unlike healthy calves.

Relative humidity

The direct effects of high relative humidity (RH) are twofold. At high ambient temperatures, high RH restricts the loss of body heat by evaporative cooling. At low ambient air temperatures, high relative humidity increases heat loss from the body since humid air is a poor insulator compared to dry air. The indirect effects of high RH have important implications for calf health. At high RH, low ambient temperatures result in condensation on cold surfaces. This has a deleterious effect on building structures and results in damp bedding and unhygienic conditions under which the incidence and severity of respiratory and other diseases may increase.

The exact optimum relative humidity and temperature for calf rearing have not been defined. Jones and Webster (1984), working with veal calves kept at a constant 16°C, found that the concentration of airborne bacteria was at a minimum at a relative humidity of 65–75%. The implication of their results is that the likely risk of airborne transmission of bacterial pathogens will be lowest at these relative humidities. In the UK, control of relative humidity is not normally cost effective other than by ventilation and drainage.

Bedding and floors

In other chapters, the need to prevent relative humidity rising above ambient has been described as has the need to keep a calf's coat dry so as to maintain its insulating properties. The lower critical temperature of a two-week-old calf lying on dry concrete is about 18°C (Webster, 1984). However, if a calf is given a dry straw bed in which to nest then its lower critical temperature will drop by about 10°C. Much of the thermal benefit of a straw bed is negated if it is wet. Furthermore, underfloor insulation is unnecessary since most of the conductive heat loss from the individual animal is transmitted laterally (Webster, 1984).

For calves bedded on straw over concrete, a floor slope of 1 in 20 from the back of the pen to the front will facilitate the drainage of urine from the bedding and keep the calf dry (Mitchell, 1976; BS 5502, 1990a). In front of

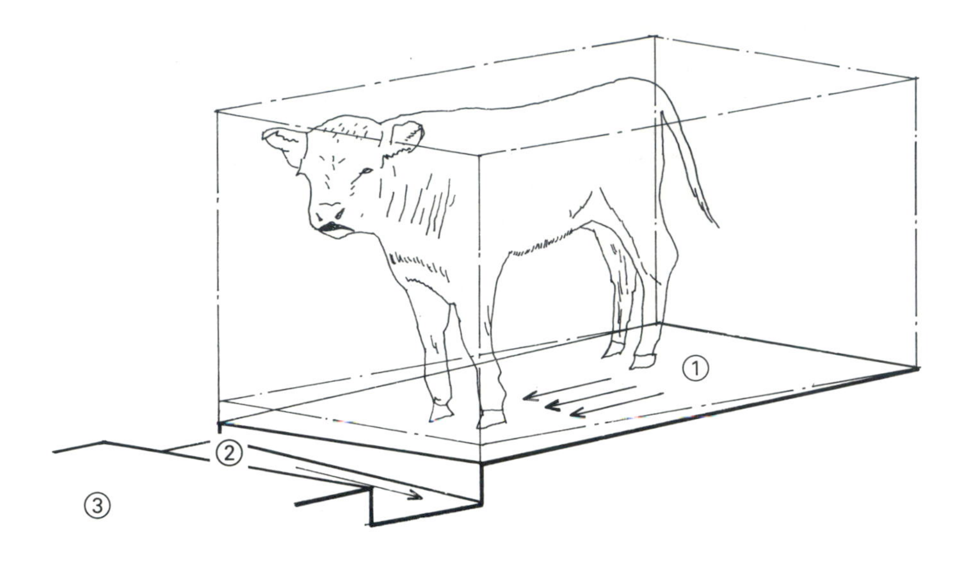

Fig. 12.6. Floor drainage in calf pens: (1) 1 : 20 slope to front of pens; (2) 1 : 40 channel sloped to outside; (3) domed passage with non-slip finish.

the pen, but outside it, preferably just under the feed buckets, a drainage channel should be provided with a fall of 1 in 40. This channel must be kept functional and free of straw and faeces. In some older calf houses drainage channels are positioned incorrectly at the rear of the pen. They quickly become non-functional and the straw bedding becomes wet (Fig. 12.6). Feed passages should have a drain channel on either side. They will be drier if made with a dome (see Fig. 12.5).

Pen design

Over recent years there has been much debate as to the benefits and disadvantages of individual versus group pens. In individual, solid-sided pens the threat of disease spread is theoretically reduced; one calf cannot soil its neighbour's pen and cannot exhale directly into its air space. The calf is fed individually and the calf keeper can readily monitor its health. However, many thousands of calves reared in pens with 'rail' divisions have been observed and in most situations the direct spread of disease from one calf to its immediate neighbours has not been evident (Chapter 6). Instead, the pattern of spread is more random in space. Furthermore, the calf is not so isolated as in pens with solid divisions and can maintain contact with other calves. [The UK Codes of Welfare require that a calf should be able to see another at all times (MAFF, 1990).]

Group penning of six to eight calves is usually associated with automatic and *ad libitum* feeding systems and has proved satisfactory in commercial practice. Group pens have a lower initial cost than individual pens and allow the calves to satisfy their needs for herd membership. However, if calves are fed automatically or *ad libitum*, it is more difficult for the farmer to monitor individuals or identify the onset of disease. Theoretically, disease spread is likely to be faster than in individual pens. In practice, in well-managed units this has not proved to be the case as far as respiratory and enteric diseases are concerned. (Restricted feeding can be practised in group pens using proprietary systems.)

Drinking arrangements and feed preparation

Clean water should be available to stock at all times. Consumption varies from approximately 10 l day^{-1} for a young calf to over 50 l day^{-1} for a lactating suckler cow and will generally increase with the animal's weight, dry matter content of the feed and environmental temperature. Recommended surface areas of water troughs are 0.34 m^2 for 20 cows or 0.3 m^2 for 20 finishing cattle, or one water bowl to 10 beasts. Drinking points should be positioned away from the feed troughs (to avoid feed contamination) and positioned to avoid spillage on to the lying areas. In straw yards troughs should be adjustable in height to allow them to be fixed at a minimum of 800 mm above bed level. A rail should be fixed around them to protect the water trough/bowl, and to protect animals from physical damage. In cold weather, attention should be paid to frost protection by pipe siting, insulation or heating. Where possible, pipes should be kept out of the reach of cattle. The provision of water storage of up to three days of maximum usage should be considered to offset irregularities in and failure of supply.

Since hot water gives off water vapour and thus increases relative humidity, it is recommended that all feed preparation and utensil washing is done in a separate air space to that of the calves.

Calf Hutches

Calf hutches (Fig. 12.7) have been successfully used in the dry cold winters of central US and Canada. Swannack's (personal communication) experiences at Bridgets Experimental Husbandry Farm (Southern England) have also been satisfactory. However, routine handling of calves within the confines of a small hutch only 1.5 m high can be back-breaking while surrounding pasture can quickly become a sea of mud with high rainfall and poorly-drained soils. One solution is to place the hutches on concrete pads but the costs are correspondingly higher. They do, however, make excellent isolation facilities for sick or injured calves.

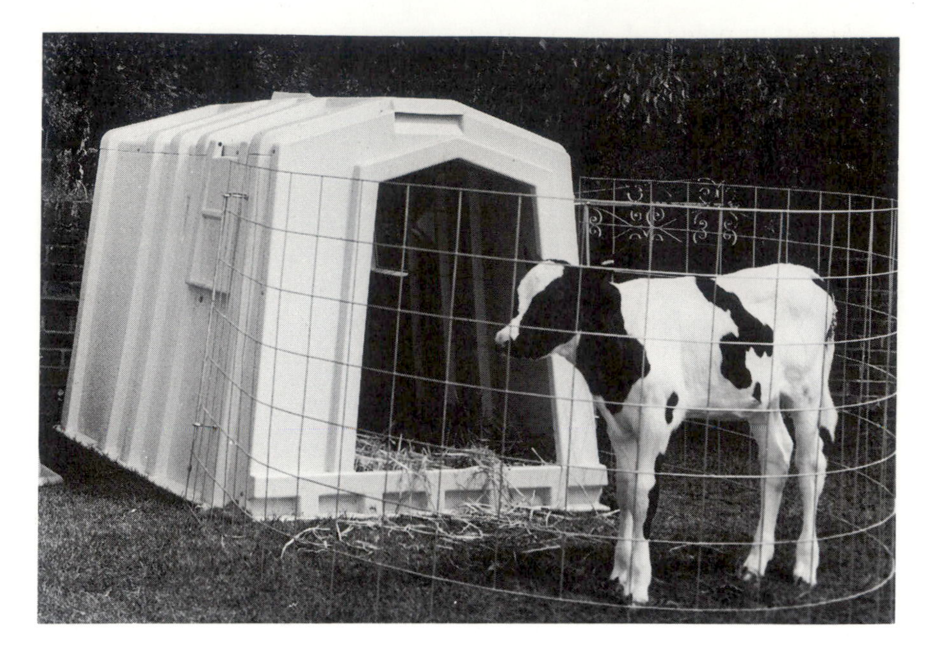

Fig. 12.7. Calf hutches are only suitable on well-drained soils in dry winter climates.

The 'Follow-on' House

Calves are usually weaned at 6–8 weeks old and their needs for housing differ from those of the pre-ruminant calf or yearling beast. The calf's immune status will be low because passive immunity from its dam is waning prior to full immune development. Stresses can also arise from the transition to solid food and mixing with other calves. Taken together these stresses may make a calf more susceptible to infection.

Mitchell (1976) and Webster (1984) recommend that calves should be reared in the rear part of a monopitch bay and then gradually allowed the run of the whole bay or even a pen outside. A good follow-on house also makes an excellent nursery because of the generous cubic capacity and ventilation and the establishment of a stable group of like animals. Experience suggests that a floor area requirement of $3.5\,m^2$, an air volume allowance of $12–13\,m^3$ and a ventilation rate of approximately $1.5\,m^3h^{-1}kg^{-1}$ liveweight will suffice. These figures approximate well with interpolations and extrapolations of data in BS 5502 (1990a) and MAFF (1985) except that the $3.5\,m^2$ of floor area is slightly greater than the $3\,m^2$ recommended in the former for 200 kg calves.

Many farms and calf rearing units have satisfactory accommodation for calves up to 6–8 weeks of age but need extra accommodation for older calves from 8 to 20 weeks. The monopitch built on the above lines is ideal. A bay width of 4.6 m will provide sufficient trough space (at 350 mm per calf) across the front for 13 calves. At 3.5 m^2 floor area per calf this number of calves would need a pen approximately 10 m deep with an average height of between 3.4 and 3.7 m to give a cubic capacity of 12–13 m^3 per calf. Space boarding at the front allowing a void area of 0.25 m^2 above sheeted gates per calf, together with 500 mm high space boarding with a 20% void at the rear, would provide sufficient ventilation.

Growing and Finishing Cattle

The size and layout of beef cattle pens (and hence buildings) depend on the number of cattle, their size and weight, the feeding system (restricted or *ad libitum*), ventilation requirements and type of floor. The latter is in turn dependent upon the availability and cost of bedding materials.

Group size

There are few published experiments on optimum group sizes for housed beef cattle. In general, cattle in bedded yards should be kept in small groups of no more than 20, and those on sloped floors should be housed in groups of between 10 and 20. Hardy and Meadowcroft (1986) recommend similar sizes for beef cattle. The reasons for small groups are twofold. Firstly, stockmen can easily recognize individual animals. Secondly, beef cattle live naturally in herds with an organized social structure and dominance hierarchy that is established quickly within small groups. In groups of housed cattle larger than about 40, individuals may need to establish repeatedly their hierarchical ranking. Thus large groups tend to be less settled with frequent agonistic behaviour, especially with pubertal and mature bulls.

Feeding arrangements

British Standard 5502 (1990a) recommends widths of feeding face per animal if animals are able to feed simultaneously (Table 12.1).

These widths may be reduced by 75% in *ad libitum* systems. Sainsbury and Sainsbury (1979) define manger needs by age rather than weight and suggest somewhat greater allowances earlier in life (Table 12.2).

Table 12.1. Feed faces for beef cattle.

Weight (kg)	Width of feeding face (mm per animal)
200	400
300	500
400	550
500	600
600	650
700	700
800	700

Source: British Standard 5502, 1990a.

Table 12.2. Area allowances for beef cattle.

Type of animal	Manger width (mm)	Pen depth back from manger (including manger) (m)
6 month old	600	6
1 year old	680	8
2 year old	680	10
Bullocks* – dehorned	760	12
Bullocks* – horned	850	14

Source: Sainsbury and Sainsbury, 1979.
*The term 'bullocks' is not defined either in terms of weight or age.

Floor types

Straw yards

In those parts of the country where straw is plentiful then it should be used for bedding (see Table 12.3). Cattle are kept cleaner, spend more of their time lying down, and since little slurry is produced, there is less water pollution. A 50% reduction in use can be made if a scrapeway 2.5–3.0 m wide is constructed immediately behind the feed troughs. This forms a loafing/feeding area on which cattle tend to defaecate and urinate. The disadvantage of a scrapeway is the slurry that is produced.

Table 12.3. Area allowances for beef cattle in straw yards.

Weight (kg)	Bedded area* (excluding troughs) (m^2)	Loafing/feeding area (excluding troughs) (m^2)	Total area per head* (m^2)
200	2.0	1.0	3.0
300	2.4	1.0	3.4
400	2.6	1.2	3.8
500	3.0	1.2	4.2
600	3.4	1.2	4.6
700	3.6	1.4	5.0

Source: British Standard 5502, 1990a.
*For wholly straw bedded yards the total figure should be used.

Hardy and Meadowcroft (1986) note that these area allowances are calculated on the basis of the animal's projected liveweight at the end of a particular stage of housing. Sainsbury and Sainsbury (1979) included the feed trough area in the total floor area and suggested somewhat greater area allowances. Even if the feed trough area is discounted, their suggested figures for the two-year-old (600 kg) animal are approximately 50% greater than those quoted by BS 5502 (1990a), MAFF (1985) and Hardy and Meadowcroft (1986).

If the BS 5502 figures are accepted for feed trough and floor area requirements, then a group of 20 × 500 kg finishing beasts will need a feed trough of 13 m and a pen depth of 6.5 m. Even allowing for 1 m wide manger, this is somewhat less than the 7–9 m depth back from the manger of Sainsbury and Sainsbury. Observations suggest that a reasonable depth behind the feed barrier for 500–550 kg cattle is approximately 8 m.

Orkney sloped floors

Where bedding materials are scarce or prohibitively expensive, then a sloping concrete floor as reviewed by Robinson (1984) has been used successfully. In principle, the Orkney sloped floor comprises pens in which the floor slopes from the feed trough to the pen rear with a steep fall of 1 in 16 (Fig. 12.8c). Cattle activity around the feed barrier treads faeces towards the pen rear. Thus the higher part of the pen remains relatively dry and clean, and the lower part can be mucked out daily with a tractor and scraper. Robinson suggests that the cleanliness of animals kept on an Orkney sloped floor depends on diet. Cattle fed diets that are high in dry

(a)

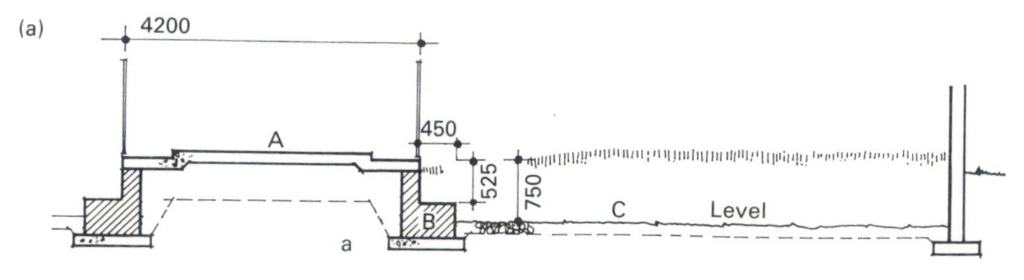

A 150 mm thick concrete
B Solid concrete blockwork
C 225 mm min. thick hardcore

(b)

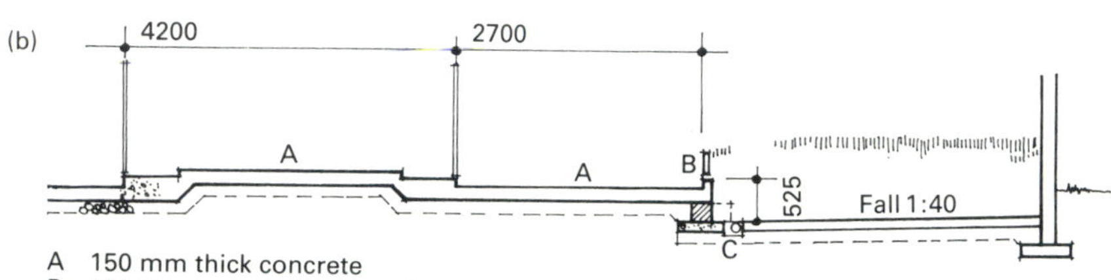

A 150 mm thick concrete
B 150 mm kerb and timber sleeper
C Concrete slot pipe

(c)

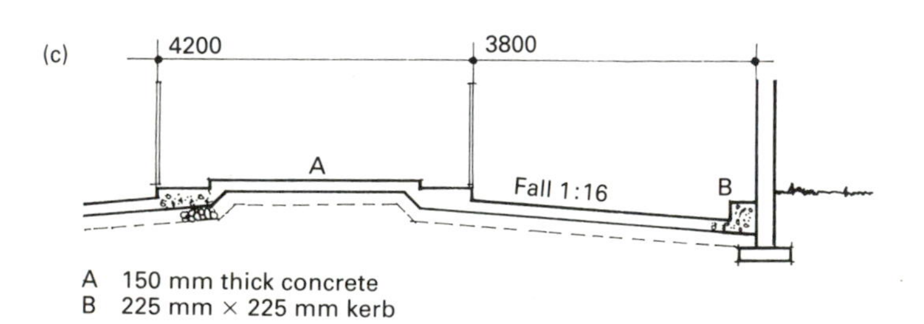

A 150 mm thick concrete
B 225 mm × 225 mm kerb

Fig. 12.8. Typical floor profiles: (a) wholly bedded; (b) part bedded/part scraped; and (c) Orkney sloped floor.

matter and low in protein content produce relatively dry, firm faeces. On the other hand, silage diets coupled with high cereal intakes lead to loose faeces and large quantities of urine, which produce slurry, wet floors and dirty cattle. The ideal pen depth for this system is 3.8 m for cattle weighing 300 kg or 3.6 m with cattle weighing less than 300 kg. Stocking rates generally found in practice are shown in Table 12.4.

Table 12.4. Area allowances for cattle on Orkney sloped floors.

	Weight (kg)	Area (m^2)
Weaned calves	200–250	1.75–1.90
Cattle	300–350	2.00–2.15
Cattle	400–500	2.35–2.50
Cows (excluding calf)		2.80–3.25

Source: Robinson, 1984.

Floor profiles

Typical floor profiles for wholly bedded, part bedded/part scraped, and Orkney sloped floors are shown in Fig. 12.8.

Slatted floors

Another alternative to straw bedded yards is the slatted floor, which gained popularity in the north of England in the 1960s and 1970s, mainly because of the high cost of straw bedding. High stocking rates are essential for successful maintenance of pen cleanliness. Slats are not suitable for animals below 250 kg (Hardy and Meadowcroft, 1986). BS 5502 (1990a) suggests the stocking rates shown in Table 12.5 for fully slatted floors.

Accurate specification of the dimensions of slatted, perforated and mesh floors for beef cattle is vital if the floors are to perform their function (Table 12.6).

Table 12.5. Stocking rates for beef cattle kept on fully slatted, perforated or mesh floors.

Liveweight (kg)	Stocking rate (m^2 per beast excluding troughs)
300	1.5
400	1.8
500	2.1
600	2.3
700	2.5

Source: British Standard 5502, 1990a.

Table 12.6. Recommended dimensions for slatted floors for cattle.

Liveweight and type of animal	Preferred width (mm)	Spacing, diameter of sphere that should: Pass (mm)	Not pass (mm)	Void ratio (%)	Radii of arrises (mm)
Calves and young stock up to 200 kg	80	20	30	18–25	3–5
Beef animals and young stock 200–550 kg	100	25	35	18–25	3–5
Adult cows and stock over 550 kg	125	30	40	18–25	3–5

Source: British Standard 5502, 1990b.

The dimensions given in Table 12.6 satisfy the essential design criteria for slatted floors:

1. The slats should be sufficiently narrow to prevent the build-up of faeces, but wide enough to avoid foot damage.
2. The slat surface should be sufficiently coarse to provide purchase and abrasion, but should not be so coarsely textured as to damage the animal.
3. The slat edges should be slightly rounded to avoid hoof damage.
4. The gap between slats should allow easy passage of faeces.

Kirchner and Boxberger (1987) recommend maximum gap widths of 25–30 mm for dairy cows and 20–25 mm for finishing bulls to avoid hoof damage. These recommendations are based on the need to support at least 70% of the surface area of the hoof with a maximum ground pressure of 2.5 bars. Slat widths of 80 mm will ensure that slats remain clean. Later work by Kirchner (1989) suggested a minimum gap width for bulls up to 250 kg liveweight of 20 mm, increasing to 28 mm for bulls of 650 kg liveweight, and a slat width of 80 mm maximum. The same work suggests floor area allowances of 1.8 m^2 for animals of 270 kg liveweight, 2.3 m^2 for 380 kg liveweight, and 2.6 m^2 for 580 kg liveweight with a minimum pen depth of between 3 and 3.5 m.

The Codes of Recommendations for the Welfare of Livestock – Cattle (MAFF, 1990) state that 'cows should not be kept in a totally slatted area. A solid floor area incorporating straw or a suitable bed should be provided to ensure comfort and reduce the risk of injury to the udder, to which dairy cows are particularly vulnerable. In accommodation for cows, it is essential to provide separate solid floored bedded pens for use at calving time, and a solid floored creep area with bedding should also be provided for the calves where cows with calves at foot are grouped together. This sound advice has withstood the test of time.

Cubicles

Cubicles have been used successfully as low cost housing for dairy cattle and suckler cows for many years (see this volume, Chapter 11 and Table 12.7). However, Hardy and Meadowcroft (1986), and my own personal experience suggest that they are now less favoured by beef finishers, especially those rearing bulls or steers. Entire males exhibit aggressive behaviour and hence tend to damage both themselves and the cubicles during bouts of head butting and riding. Male cattle also urinate in the centre of cubicle beds. Overall, stocking rates per unit area of building are low and slurry disposal can become a problem.

Table 12.7. Dimensions of cubicles for beef cattle.

Liveweight (kg)	Length (including kerb) (m)	Clear width between partitions (m)
200	1.35	0.7
300	1.65	0.8
350	2.0	1.0

Source: British Standard 5502, 1990a.

Roofless or topless units

As described earlier, healthy ruminating beef cattle benefit little from complete housing: they merely need protection from the *combined* effects of wind and rain. In the 1960s and 1970s a number of cubicle, straw yard and sloping floor roofless units were established. It soon became apparent that such units were really best suited to areas with a winter rainfall of less than 350 mm. This restriction has become increasingly more important in the UK as the National Rivers Authority has sought to reduce pollution from livestock units. However, from the livestock point of view, health and cleanliness are usually good in such units although the units are inconvenient for stock keepers.

Housing of the Suckler Cow and Calf

The housing needs of the suckler cow and calf are identical to those of the dairy cow, apart from the provision of a creep area for the calf. The suckler cow is usually mated by natural service rather than artificial insemination. Therefore, provision has to be made for the bull(s) to locate and serve cows on heat and to be handled and fed separately if necessary.

The calf creep

The size of the creep depends on the calving date – an autumn born calf weighs approximately 250 kg at turnout, whereas a calf born in mid-summer could be 100 kg heavier. The smaller calf needs a creep area of 2 m^2 and 450 mm of trough space, whereas heavier animals need 2.5 m^2 of floor area and 550 mm of trough space. The creep unit itself should be part of the main cattle building but cows should be denied access by a creep opening 500 mm wide by 1100 mm high. The creep should be bedded even in a fully slatted house.

Bull accommodation

Where a bull runs with the suckler herd, it is prudent to use stronger structures than normal and provide a separate feed area and a neck yoke. If the cows are fed along the feed barrier, sufficient space should be left for the bull to walk behind the cows during feeding so that he may locate and serve any cow on heat. A 4 m wide feed passage is sufficient. Slippery feed passages may deter the bull from mounting and also cause injury. It is worth remembering that if a bull receives a Pavlovian bump on the head every time he serves a cow, he is likely to give up the whole idea as a bad habit – sufficient head room should be given to allow natural service to be carried out in comfort.

References

Brambell, F.W.R. (1965) Report of the Technical Committee to Enquire into the Welfare of Animals kept under Intensive Livestock Husbandry Systems. Cmd 2836, HMSO, London.

British Standard 5502 (1990a) Buildings and structures for agriculture. Part 40: Code of practice for design and construction of cattle buildings. British Standards Institution, London.

British Standard 5502 (1990b) Buildings and structures for agriculture. Part 57: Code of practice for design and construction of slatted, perforated and mesh floors for livestock. British Standards Institution, London.

Bruce, J.M. (1984) Climate and the value of shelter for suckler cows and calves. *Farm Building Progress* 78, 21–25.

Hardy, R. and Meadowcroft, S. (1986) *Indoor Beef Production.* Farming Press, Ipswich.

Jones, C.D.R. and Webster, A.J.F. (1984) Relationships between counts of nasopharyngeal bacteria, temperature, humidity and lung lesions in veal calves. *Research in Veterinary Science* 37, 132–137.

Kirchner, M. (1989) Pens with slatted floors for fattening bulls. *Proceedings of 11th International Congress on Agricultural Engineering,* Dublin, pp. 1089–1094.

Kirchner, M. and Boxberger, J. (1987) Loading of the claws and the consequences for the design of slatted floors. In: Wierenga, H.K. and Peterse, D.J. (eds), *Cattle Housing Systems, Lameness and Behaviour.* Martinus Nijhoff, Dordrecht, pp. 37–44.

Kubisch, H.-M., Makarechian, M. and Arthur, P.F. (1991) A note on the influence of climatic variables and age on the responses of beef calves to different housing types. *Animal Production* 52, 400–403.

MAFF (1984) *Calf Rearing.* Ref. Book 10, HMSO, London.

MAFF (1985) *Beef Cattle Housing.* Booklet 2512, HMSO, London.

MAFF (1990) Codes of Recommendations for the Welfare of Livestock – Cattle. MAFF Publications, London PB 0074.

Mitchell, C.D. (1976) *Calf Housing Handbook.* Scottish Farm Buildings Investigation Unit, Aberdeen.

Robinson, T.W. (1984) The Orkney sloped floor. *Farm Buildings Progress* 78, 11–14.

Sainsbury, D. and Sainsbury, P. (1979) *Livestock Health and Housing,* 2nd edn. Baillière Tindall, London.

Thickett, B., Mitchell, D. and Hallows, B. (1986) *Calf Rearing.* Farming Press, Ipswich.

Webster, A.J.F. (1981) Optimal housing criteria for ruminants. In: Clark, J.A. (ed.), *Environmental Aspects of Housing for Animal Production,* Butterworths, London, pp. 217–232.

Webster, A.J.F. (1984) *Calf Husbandry, Health and Welfare.* Granada, London.

Webster, A.J.F. (1988) Beef cattle and veal calves. In: *Management and Welfare of Farm Animals – UFAW Handbook,* 3rd edn. Baillière Tindall, London, pp. 47–79.

Webster, A.J.F., Chlumecky, J. and Young, B.A. (1970) Effects of cold environments on the energy exchanges of young beef cattle. *Canadian Journal of Animal Science* 50, 89–100.

13

Sheep Housing

C.F.R. SLADE[1] AND L. STUBBINGS[2]
[1]ADAS Wolverhampton, UK; [2]ADAS Kettering, UK

Can Housing be Justified?

Sheep have a thick fleece which both insulates and sheds water. They thrive readily in the high hills or the best of lowland ground. As long as the ground is not covered by snow for prolonged periods and animals have an opportunity to range for food, their performance is not seriously affected by life outdoors. In Northern Europe most breeds are seasonal breeders and do not have young lambs at foot during the winter, which aids survival through the harsher period of the year. The most numerous pure breeds of sheep in the UK are the main hill breeds, Scottish Blackface, Welsh Mountain and Swaledale (MLC, 1988) and from this basic stock has developed the well-established and unique crossbreeding structure of the UK flock. Crossbred ewes with a hill breed dam or grand dam make up 42% (MLC, 1988) of the national flock and can be found throughout the lowlands and better quality uplands.

Housing of any sort is expensive and, as the sheep thrives outdoors, it is doubtful whether housing is justified on a straightforward 'profit and loss' assessment. There are, however, a number of factors to consider, some of them difficult to assess in simple economic terms, before arriving at a decision on the need to house sheep.

Ease of management

One area which is difficult to quantify is the extra management control that can be gained over housed ewes. Animals can be grouped easily according to body condition and lambing date. Shepherding itself is more comfortable and husbandry assistance or veterinary help can be brought to bear more rapidly. Husbandry treatments, such as foot trimming, drenching or vaccination can be applied at the optimum time. Stock can be inspected easily throughout the night and lambing kept under tight control. These factors all become more relevant if a high performance is required.

Grass supplies

One of the clearest benefits from housing sheep in the winter months is the impact on grassland management. The yield of grass in the spring can be increased by grazing with sheep up to the end of December (Slade, 1986). Reducing surplus growth in the late autumn limits the amount of winter kill. However, if grazing continues through January or February then the yield of grass in April can be reduced by 22% in comparison with ungrazed sward (Slade, 1986). In some intensive units, ewes are concentrated on sacrificial paddocks through the main winter months. This practice saves the remaining grazing area but means that the contribution of the sacrificial paddocks to grass yield is negligible until later in the growing season. The use of a house thus ensures that the maximum area is available for grazing in the spring at a time when ewes' milk is at its peak and maximum lamb growth rate can be anticipated. The corollary of the decision to house in the winter is that stocking rate and fertilizer use can be optimized and reseeding costs minimized.

Ewe losses

In well-managed and well-fed flocks that are not housed, ewe losses during winter and up to parturition are typically between 3% and 6% and are exacerbated by severe weather or disease. Housing a flock would not necessarily reduce any losses due to disease but negates adverse effects of bad weather and poached pastures. In the author's experience at ADAS Liscombe Research and Development Centre (RDC) a well-fed flock of halfbred ewes of mixed ages that were held on a sacrificial paddock from mid-January until lambing in early March suffered losses of just over 4%. Conditions were wet and muddy and a small proportion of ewes stopped eating properly despite adequate food supplies. The main cause of loss was twin-lamb disease. A similar group of halfbred ewes was housed for the first time during the same winter. Losses in these ewes were under 1% and there were no losses from twin-lamb disease because of greater control over management and ewe behaviour.

Lamb percentage

The effect of housing on lambing percentage is not easy to determine. The greater supervision and the closer attention at lambing should increase the

Table 13.1. Lambing percentages at Great House RDC.

	1963/4	1964/5	1966/7	1967/8	Mean
Inwintered ewes	152	145	180	168	162
Outwintered ewes	139	134	163	146	146

Source: Bastiman and Williams, 1973.

number of lambs reared. However, all too often, crowded ewes mean mismothering and build-up of disease may exacerbate losses further. Housing ewes at lambing will only increase the number of lambs raised if the husbandry standards are first class. More than one flock manager has adjusted lambing time so that it coincides with the Easter vacation and allows extra help from (devoted) agricultural and veterinary students.

Early work at Great House RDC has shown some of the gains in lamb numbers that can be achieved by good husbandry (Table 13.1; Bastiman and Williams, 1973). There was a clear gain in each of the four years in the number of lambs reared in the housed flock.

Housing of hill flocks

Housing of hill flocks is apparently less justified than of higher performance lowland flocks. However, many sheep houses were built for hill flocks in the 1980s. The main reasons were ease of management and greater flexibility. Older ewes from many hill flocks are sold after three or four lamb crops for further breeding under more benign conditions on lowland farms. When ewe prices are low, draft ewes can be retained for a further lamb crop and housed in the worst of the winter period rather than left to struggle on the open hill.

The developments in recent years of big bale silage and the move to feed blocks and liquid feeds have given the hill farmer some flexibility in feeding through the winter. Older ewes can be reluctant to eat these feeds at first and up to one-third of the flock may refuse these supplementary feeds. If ewe lambs have been housed through their first winter and trained to eat these feeds, then effective use is more likely when they are encountered later on the open hill.

The practice of away wintering of ewe lambs has always been a feature of hill sheep farming. It is not cheap and where lowland farms have adopted single strand electric fencing for cattle, then the fencing is less suitable for sheep. The availability of a winter sheep house gives the hill flock owner more flexibility in the management of ewe lambs.

Alternative uses for the sheep house

Justification of sheep housing is hampered by the low utilization. In a conventional spring lambing flock the house is only likely to be occupied for 10 to 13 weeks, depending on spread of lambing. In an early lambing flock where first ewes and then growing lambs are kept inside, the house is only likely to be in use for four to five months.

Sheep houses have been adopted for alternative livestock uses in the summer and autumn months, such as calf or turkey rearing. The storage of hay and straw through to the time of housing has also been valuable. At present wool is only worth 4% or less of income (Slade, 1990), however since ewes have to be shorn for welfare reasons it makes sense to get the best possible price for what is basically a by-product. Dirty, wet or contaminated wool is penalized heavily. Many sheep houses are modified temporarily in early summer so that ewes can be housed overnight, shorn and the wool bagged cleanly.

A further use of a sheep house is to finish store lambs in the autumn. Once grass growth ceases, lambs from upland or hill areas may well have to be sold in an uncertain store market. If big bale silage or other feeds are available then the store lambs can be finished for slaughter and a more reliable income achieved.

Basic Requirements for Housing

Sheep are essentially a low output enterprise, whose profits do not usually justify a sophisticated housing system. Fortunately the basic needs of a housed sheep are simple. These are shelter from rain, sufficient air changes to prevent high temperature, high humidity and condensation, adequate space for movement, sensible feeding and watering arrangements and reasonable access to the building (Fig. 13.1). One of the main aims of housing is to provide extra protection and supervision at lambing and the logistics of housing a large flock can be complex.

Organization and management of a sheep house is mainly determined by the husbandry system and type of roughage. Grazing is usually sufficient until December. Where the target is early lambing in late December or January and finished lambs sold in April or May (often referred to as the 'Easter trade'), then ewes are usually housed three to four weeks before lambing. Ewes and suckling lambs are run together until weaning at six to eight weeks of age. Following weaning, lambs remain indoors until slaughter at 12 to 16 weeks of age. Ewes (separated from lambs) may remain indoors, or be turned out if circumstances allow. Each phase of the operation has a different requirement for space and feeding.

A conventional 'spring lambing' flock will be housed in late December

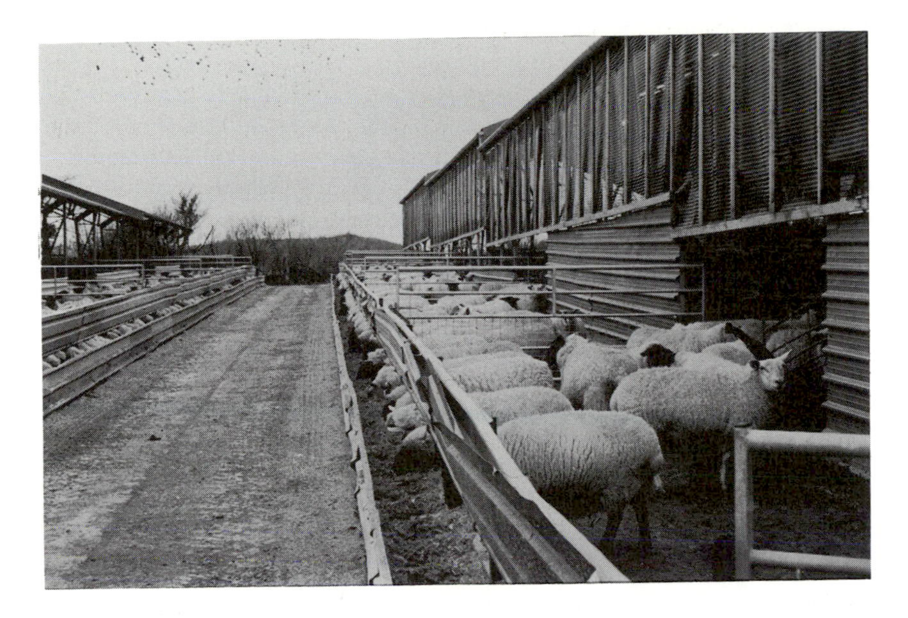

Fig. 13.1. Economical house design, but ewes can get wet during feeding.

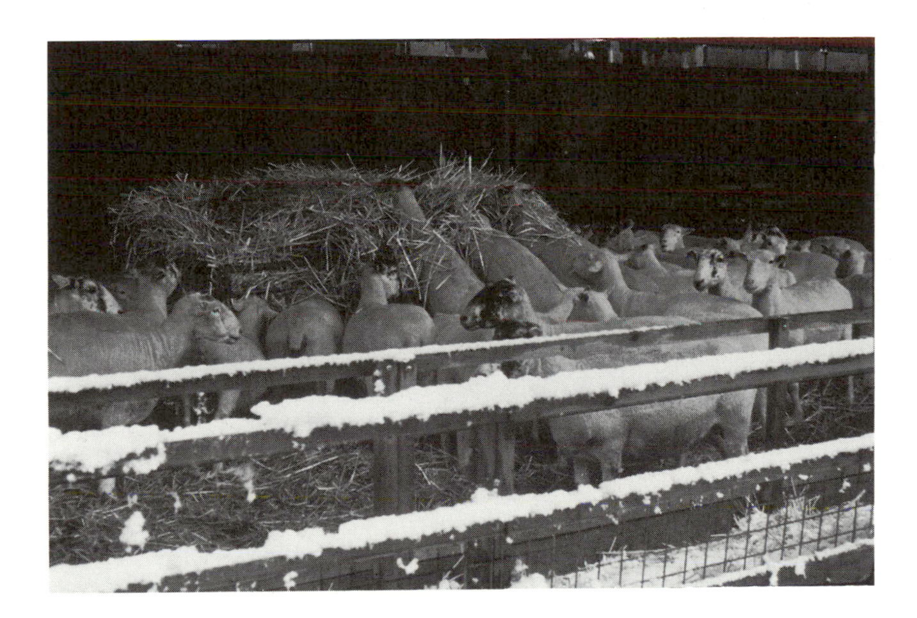

Fig. 13.2. Straw feeding in a monopitch building.

or January, i.e. about six to ten weeks before lambing. Housing requirements are straightforward until lambing and then need individual lambing pens, hospital facilities, fostering pens and pens for bottle-fed lambs.

The feeding system affects the overall internal layout of a sheep house. Hay and straw-based diets offer some flexibility (Fig. 13.2). Interest in straw-bed diets has grown in the UK following the ban on straw burning. However, it is an expensive diet with high concentrate requirements. Hay is a good source of roughage, particularly for ewes in individual pens at lambing, but steady supplies of high quality hay are difficult to guarantee given the vagaries of the British climate. Silage feeding has grown in importance as a sheep feed throughout the last 20 years and its wet bulk imposes constraints on building access and trough design.

Siting a building

Siting a purpose-built sheep building can present a conundrum. Good access is always desirable, particularly if silage has to be carted to the house. Sheep handling pens and feed stores should be sited nearby and access to water and electricity supplies is essential. The shepherd's home should be close at hand to facilitate regular inspection at lambing.

Provision of grazing close to the sheep house will ease the work of moving ewes and young lambs to grass, though if the same fields are grazed year after year the worm burden may build up.

Ventilation

Almost all sheep housing in the UK relies on natural ventilation (see Chapter 7). In sheep houses the air inlet should ideally be positioned above the sheep's back to avoid draughts. Some designs of polythene tunnel have the air inlet at the same height as the sheep. In practice, problems are less than might be expected but draughts may chill newly shorn sheep or young lambs if the location is not sheltered. One important practical aspect is that ewes should be dry when entering a house for the first time and should only be turned out on dry days. Wet fleeces can carry a substantial quantity of water, which makes the house damp. Problems with ventilation can sometimes arise in buildings which have been adapted for sheep from other uses and in certain types of polythene tunnel if stocked very heavily.

Space requirements

Sharples and Dumelow (1990) have developed a set of prediction equations based on body weight to estimate many body dimensions in Mule and Scottish blackface ewes. This knowledge could lead to improved design of houses, feeding equipment and sheep handling pens. In practice, the

Table 13.2. Recommended floor space for sheep.

Type of sheep	Area on slats (m^2)	Area on straw (m^2)
Large ewe 60–90 kg in lamb	0.9–1.1	1.2–1.4
Large ewe 60–90 kg with lambs	1.2–1.7	1.4–1.8
Small ewe 45–60 kg in lamb	0.7–0.9	1.0–1.3
Small ewe 45–60 kg with lambs	1.0–1.4	1.3–1.7
Hoggs 32 kg	0.5–0.7	0.7–0.9
Hoggs 23 kg	0.4–0.5	0.6–0.9
Lamb creep (2 weeks)	–	0.15
Lamb creep (6 weeks)	–	0.4
Ewe + growing lambs	–	2.2
Lambing pen	–	1.5

Source: Loynes, 1983a.

guidelines suggested by Loynes (1983a) from the Farm Buildings Information Centre (Table 13.2) have stood the test of time.

For ewes that have been recently shorn, Loynes suggests that the floor space can be reduced by 10%. ADAS (1987) advice follows Loynes' recommendations, apart from those for lactating ewes with lambs at foot where a 25% (approximately) increase in recommended floor space is suggested.

Dung handling

A mature ewe produces about 2.25 kg of dung and urine per day (Givens, 1992, personal communication). Even on a silage-based diet the dung has a soft, solid form and cannot be described as a slurry. Under slats dung will build up to a depth of 250–350 mm over a 90-day winter period. With a straw-based bedding system, the recommended straw usage (ADAS, 1987) will be about 50 kg per ewe over the same period. Removal of dung either from under slats or in litter systems is not normally necessary during a normal housing period unless there is a specific disease.

Water supply

Sheep consume large quantities of water when housed. Watson (1992) recorded a consumption of about 4.5 l day^{-1} per ewe on a dry hay-based diet and an increase of up to 9 l per day in early lactation. On a silage-based diet, the author has measured a water intake of around 2 l per day in late pregnancy. The water supply must be clean and shallow containers utilized to minimize the risk of drowning by inquisitive lambs. The container should be set high enough to avoid contamination by the build-up of dung. If a cheap and plentiful water supply is available, then a continuous flow through slotted PVC drain pipes offers a practical system that does not normally freeze in cold weather. The alternative is lagged pipes and water bowls or small troughs with ball valves.

Safety and access

Sensible, initial planning to ensure easy access to a sheep building for tractor, man and stock will minimize time spent feeding, cleaning out and in other husbandry routines. Watson (1992) comments that current building legislation requires escape doors at each end for a stock building over 30 m in length. The speed with which fires can spread through agricultural buildings implies that this is a sound provision.

Food and bedding will be supplied every few days, and perhaps even daily in some circumstances. Movement of sheep, e.g. for foot care or at lambing, will be substantially easier if passageways and gate position have been considered during house design. Electricity and hot water are valuable aids at lambing but wiring and power points must be maintained and protected from damp, stock and rodents.

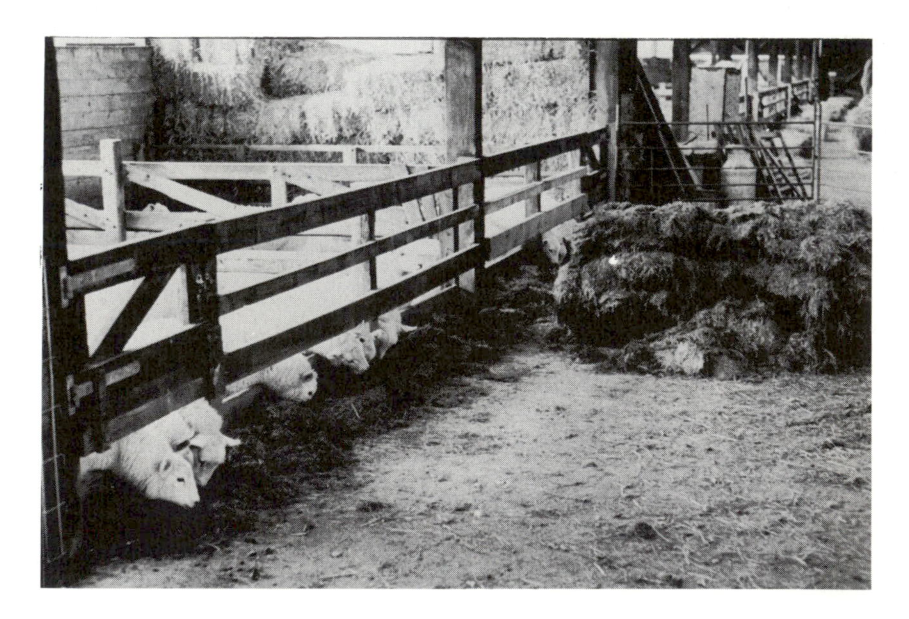

Fig. 13.3. Blocks for silage feeding (Liscombe RDC).

Feeding Arrangements

Feeding is a regular chore when sheep are housed, while lambing is clearly a busy and demanding task. Organization of feed handling and the design of the feeding troughs are key determinants of success. Poor layouts and arrangements can cause unnecessary work. Cartage of feed by tractor requires generous gangways and valuable building space is taken up with passageways that are used infrequently. With some building designs, it is possible to feed silage along the outside wall with protection provided by a cover or overhang.

Part of the building may be needed for hay and straw storage at harvest. Progressive consumption of these stocks can then release valuable extra space at lambing time. Work at Liscombe RDC demonstrated that neatly cut silage blocks did not deteriorate over a ten-day period, and the blocks could be moved weekly into a house and stored in the gangway (Fig. 13.3). Storage of silage or hay in a gangway still requires hand feeding to some degree and access for sheep can be impeded.

Feed quantities

The amount of roughage consumed by a sheep depends on body size and on the quality of the roughage. As the fetus grows rapidly over the last week or two of pregnancy the intake of roughage tends to decrease. Body size in ewes varies from about 35 kg for a Welsh ewe to about 80 kg for a Scotch halfbred. For straw feeding the normal practice is to offer each ewe about 1.5 kg day^{-1}. Ewes will select the most digestible portion leaving the balance for bedding. Silage intake varies from 3.5 to 5 kg day^{-1}, although Brown and Meadowcroft (1989) recorded intakes of 2 kg DM day^{-1} (8 kg of fresh silage) at Rosemaund RDC when feeding very high quality material. Hay intakes are likely to range from 1 to 1.6 kg day^{-1}. Most roughages are offered *ad libitum* although intake of very high quality material should be limited. Uneaten silage is an attractive growth medium for various moulds and the risk of

Table 13.3. Roughage requirements of a 70 kg ewe for a 90 day winter.

	Daily intake (kg)	Winter requirements per ewe (kg)
Silage	4–6	360–540
Hay	1–1.6	100–150
Straw offered	1.5	140
Straw bedding	–	50

listeriosis may increase. Silage that is contaminated with soil or moulds is clearly undesirable. Maize silage in particular can mould rapidly if not eaten quickly. Strict daily cleaning of troughs and removal of uneaten feed will help the control of *Listeria* infection. The total amounts of roughages required for a 90-day winter are shown in Table 13.3.

Trough space

Where roughages are fed *ad libitum* ewes require 150 mm of trough space. In late pregnancy supplementary concentrates will be necessary for the growth of fetal tissue. Although these concentrates are a vital part of the diet, only small amounts are fed. Thus every ewe comes to eat at the same time and the requirement for trough space is increased considerably.

Development work by ADAS (1987) has produced practical guidelines for trough space. These allowances are well tried and tested and are shown in Table 13.4.

Insufficient trough space leads to unnecessary competition for feed. Some ewes may hang back regularly: others will jostle and climb on their pen mates. Some pen designs involve concentrate feeding on three sides. In theory this design is satisfactory, but as the shepherd walks down trough *cum* pen dividers he is often spreading the feed over the ewes' heads and the greedier animals at the front take more than their fair share (Fig. 13.4). Where trough space is insufficient troughs may be placed in the pens. The shepherd must then carry feed into a jostling group of ewes, a time-

Table 13.4. Trough space requirements per sheep (mm).

	Compound	Restricted roughage	*Ad libitum* roughage
Large ewes (70–90 kg)	500	250	150
Small ewes (50–70 kg)	450	200	150
Ewe lambs (not pregnant) and store lambs			
25 kg	300	125	100
45 kg	400	175	100
Lambs under 6 weeks	50*	–	–
Lambs over 6 weeks *ad libitum*	100*	–	–
Lambs over 6 weeks restricted	300*	–	–

Source: ADAS, 1987

*Lambs fed in a creep area.

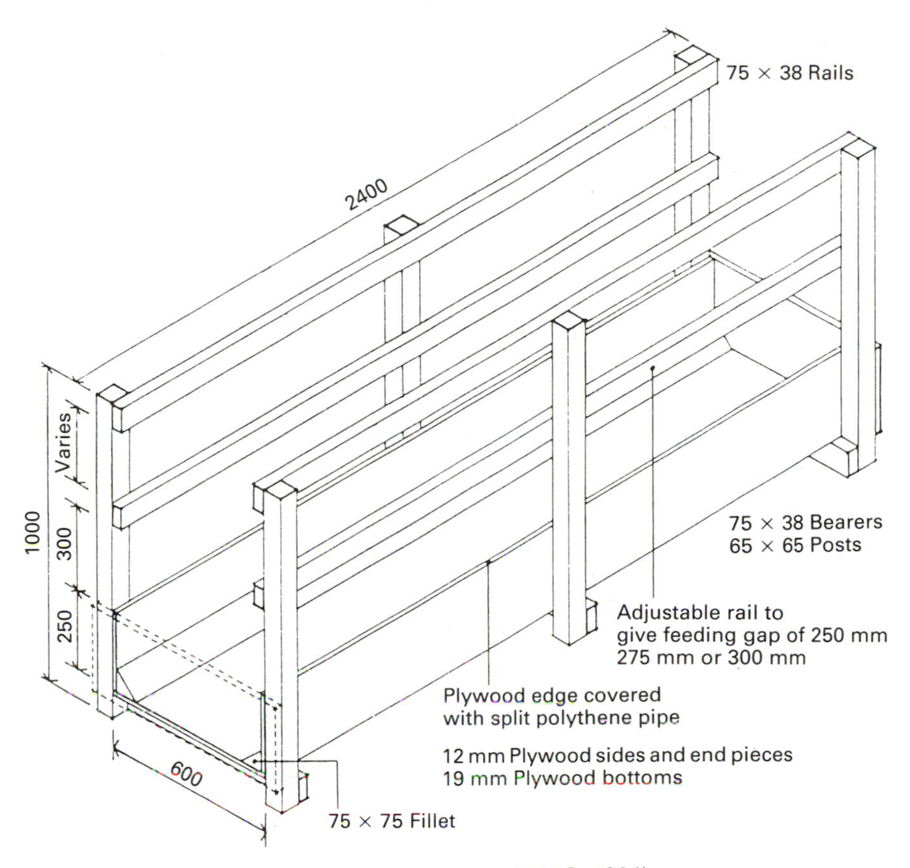

Fig. 13.4. Walk through trough *cum* pen divider (ADAS, 1984).

consuming task. An alternative solution to the problem of matching pen shape with adequate trough space was devised by Brown and Thomas (1990). The concentrate was fed as pellets on the pen floor and ewes then had to root through the straw bedding for their feed. Extra cost was incurred in pelleting but there was no difference in performance from ewes offered the same diet in conventional troughs.

The ideal arrangement of feeding is a long narrow pen with feed supplied along one side (Fig. 13.5). The ideal number of ewes per pen is around 25 to 30. This allows ewes to be grouped according to their anticipated lambing date, body condition and expected lamb numbers. A pen of 30 ewes should be 16 m long and 2.6 m deep. This allows a gateway of 1 m and a feeding trough of 15 m. The space requirement for a 70 kg pregnant ewe of 1.3 m^2 is also satisfied. This specification can be met most readily in long narrow buildings: ewes kept in more conventional buildings will need extra area for feeding troughs or else the building will have more gangway than is absolutely necessary.

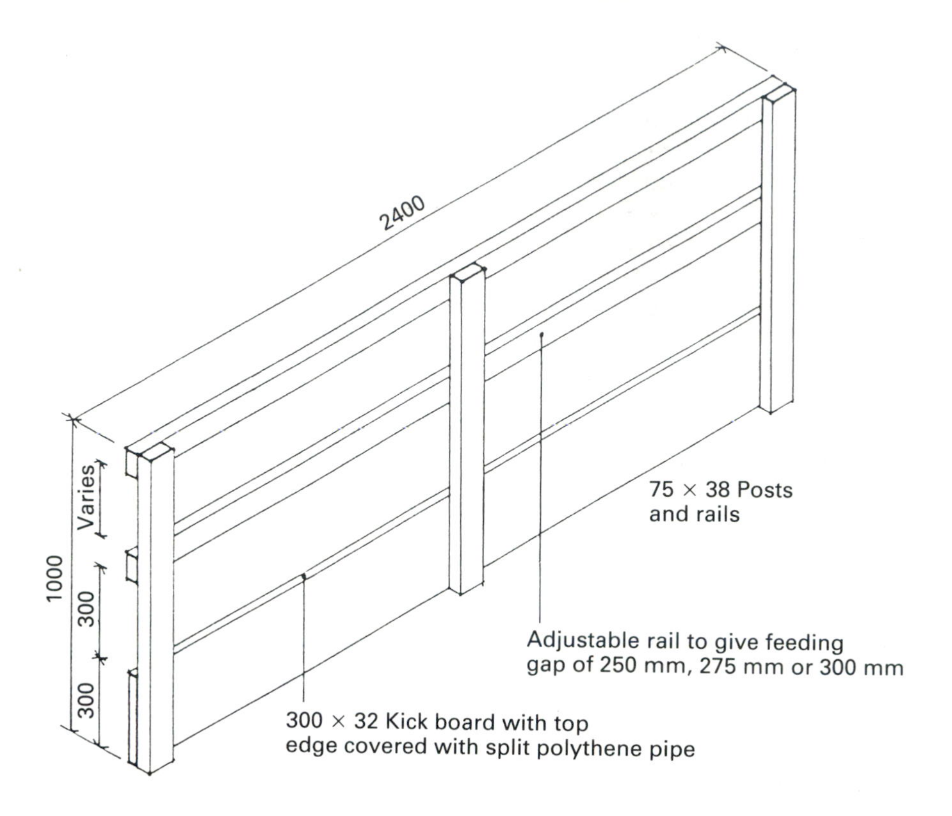

Fig. 13.5. Pen front *cum* barrier feed fence (ADAS, 1984).

The development of big bales has presented difficulties in feeding. If gangways are sufficiently large, big bales can be unrolled along pen fronts. Some front loaders have sufficient reach to drop a large bale into a container within the pen and allow ewes access to the feeder from all sides. The alternative is manual handling of silage into trough *cum* pen dividers.

Gangways

The width of gangway necessary between pens varies considerably according to the feeding method (ADAS, 1987):

Man only	0.6–0.75 m
Man and barrow or trolley	1.25 m
Tractor and trailer or block cutter	2.4–3.0 m
Self-loading trailer or forage box	3.0–4.0 m

Simple pen gateways are also important to ease movement of ewes.

Structures and Floors

Buildings for sheep vary considerably in expense and sophistication (Fig. 13.6). The simplest and cheapest structure is the polythene tunnel. This was originally developed for horticultural use but has since been adapted for a range of other enterprises. More expensive buildings, such as a steel portal frame are often built for general utility on the farm or estate and are difficult to justify for a sheep enterprise by itself (see Table 13.5). British Standard (BS 5502) covers the design and construction of sheep houses.

Open yards and temporary buildings

A few topless in-wintering yards have been built commercially and were evaluated at the National Agricultural Centre, UK in the 1970s. They are a modern development of the open straw yard that can still be seen in the south of England on dry, free-draining soils. Good drainage of topless yards is vital but they have not been adopted commercially, mainly because the wet UK winter makes it very difficult to keep ewes dry.

However, an open-topped yard has been used successfully at Rosemaund RDC for finishing store lambs (Fig. 13.7). The yard comprises an expanded, galvanized steel mesh floor supported by concrete blocks with plywood panels offering shelter against the prevailing wind. The performance of store lambs is comparable with lambs housed in more expensive and conventional roofed structures.

Temporary structures are often erected for extra shelter and accommodation at lambing time. Big straw bales are flexible for this purpose and marquees have also been hired on occasions.

Table 13.5. Comparative costs of sheep housing.

Type	Cost index
Modified existing structure	3–15
Topless yard	7–13
Plastic tunnel	17
Partly covered yard (new mono-pitch)	22
DIY portal frame (second-hand material)	27
DIY portal frame (new material)	40
'Off the shelf' (wooden)	67
'Off the shelf' (portal frame – steel, etc.)	100

Source: Loynes, 1983b.

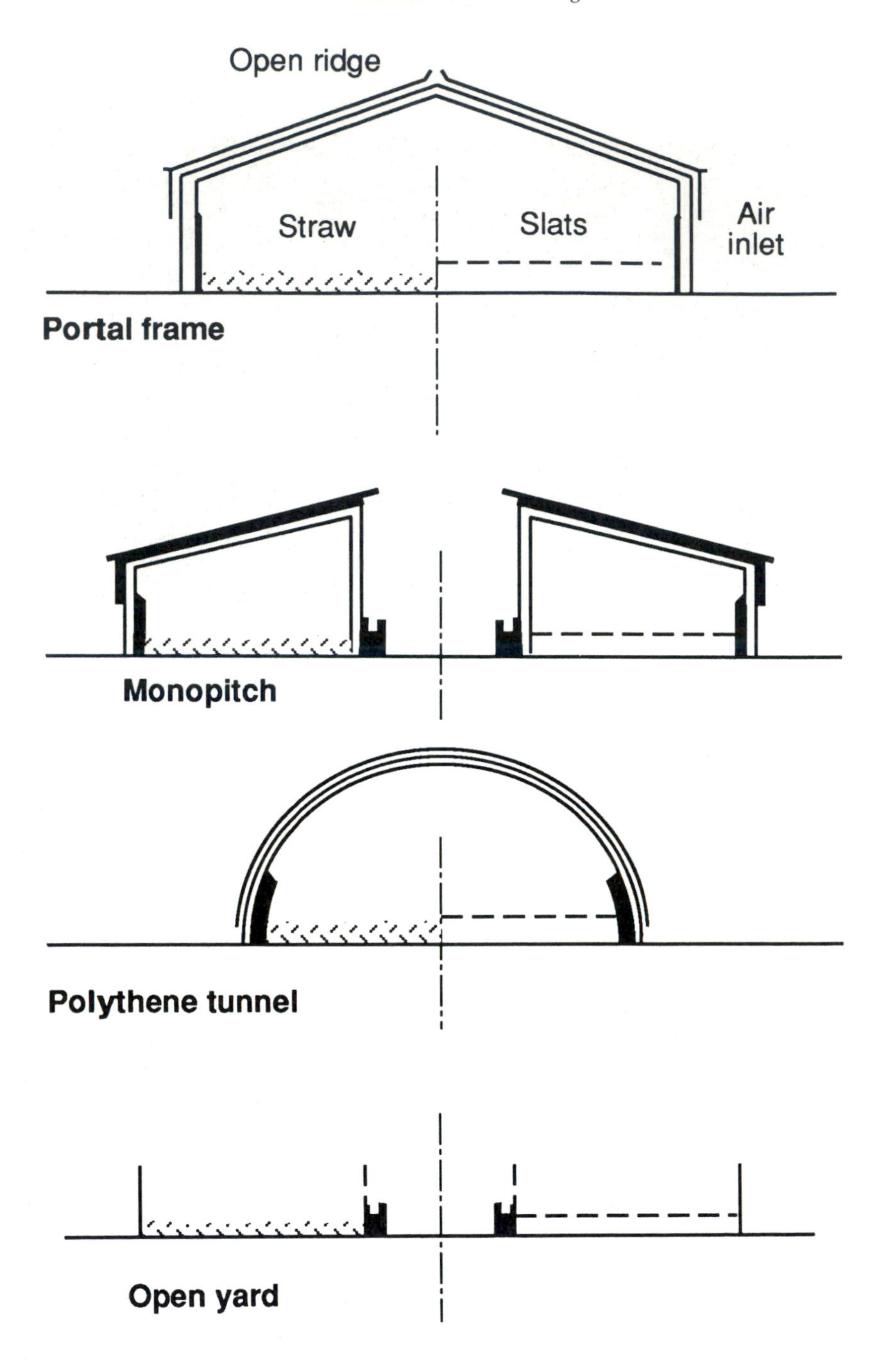

Fig. 13.6. Types of sheep housing (FBIC, 1983).

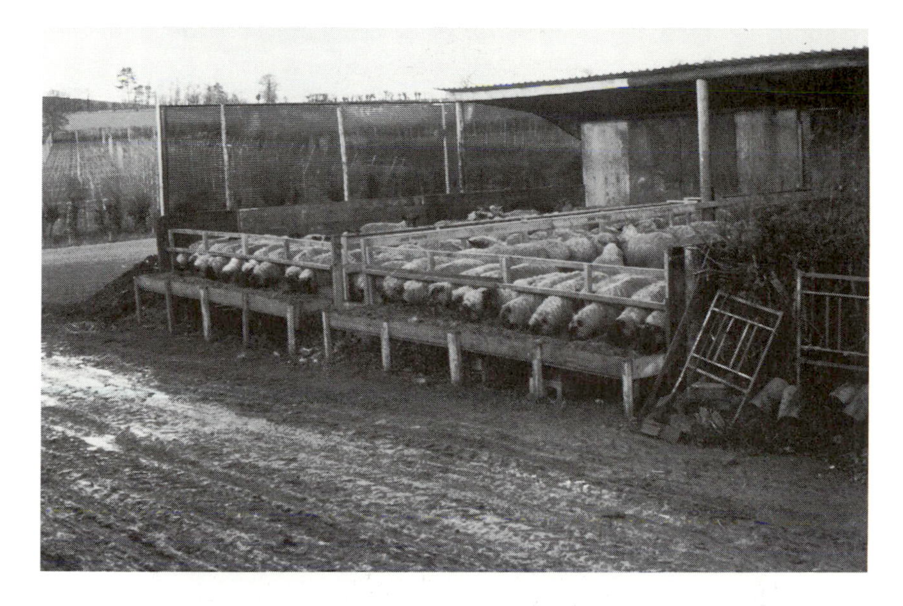

Fig. 13.7. Open topped yard for store lambs (Rosemaund RDC).

Permanent structures

Boe *et al.* (1991) showed clearly that uninsulated buildings are well suited for sheep. In the UK, portal frames are the most sophisticated structure. This type of building can offer the greatest labour saving but is expensive. Stocking rate can be difficult to maximize because of building shape. The ideal sheep pen is long and narrow to provide adequate feeding space and this design is unsuited to a portal frame building.

Timber buildings range from the low cost structure built with local or second-hand materials to those built from sophisticated construction kits with many refinements. Monopitch buildings can provide many of the basic requirements for ewes as well as being ideal for silage transport and feeding. However, they are not readily adapted to other enterprises.

The polythene tunnel has also been used in many situations and has withstood the British climate remarkably well. The long, narrow shape caters well for the basic needs of the pregnant ewe. The major drawback is that the air inlet is at animal height with the risk of draughts for the shorn or recently lambed ewe. An interesting solution to this problem was described by Charles and Stubbings (1992). A trough is set alongside the outside of the tunnel and provides both a windbreak and air inlet which directs airflow upwards and away from the sheep (Fig. 13.8). This design gave an excellent atmosphere in the building and removed the need for a

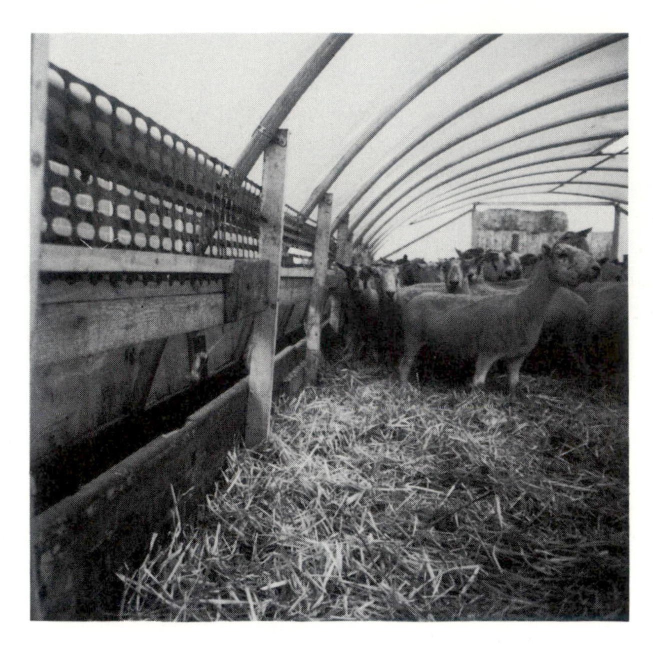

Fig. 13.8. Polythene tunnel with modified exterior feeder.

central feed passage. Ewe numbers in the house were thus maximized. If written off over eight years, the amortized charge per annum was £5/ewe place which was about 30% less than the cost of a tunnel with central feeding.

Floor types

The great majority of UK sheep houses use straw bedding over an earth or rammed hardcore base. This technique works well. The ban on straw burning has increased the availability of straw. Slats are more common in Europe but interest in the UK is largely confined to Scotland where the cost of straw transport is high and the capital cost of slats is easier to justify.

Slats are not well favoured by the Farm Animal Welfare Council (MAFF, 1990) and there is a requirement to cover slats and provide bedding at lambing. Watson (1992) noted that hardwood slats are slippery when wet and difficult to nail. If slats break there is a real risk of injury. The recommended slat width is 60 mm with a 15 mm gap. A range of wooden and concrete slats has been evaluated at the National Agricultural Centre (Court, 1983). Welded mesh, galvanized woven wire mesh, expanded flattened galvanized steel mesh and perforated metal pig slats were all examined. Only the perforated metal pig slats proved unsatisfactory and became clogged with muck.

Lambing

Lambing is the critical time in the sheep year and sheep housing can play an important role in its success. Ideally, extra space should be created at lambing for individual lambing pens. Temporary stores for straw or hay may be taken over gradually for this purpose. Individual pens can be erected in the passageway but this increases manual handling of forage feedstuffs. Ewe and lambing pens should be located together since this will aid movement of ewes and newborn lambs. A few individual pens should be placed in the main lambing area for immediate use. Disentangling three or four sets of twins that have become separated from their mothers can be most frustrating. Individual pens also deter the prepartum ewe from mismothering another's lamb.

Ideally, every postpartum ewe and her lambs should have an individual pen measuring approximately 1.8 × 1.2 m for 24 hours. Sufficient spare pens should be available to cover periods of bad weather. If pressure on space becomes critical and ewes with very young lambs have to be turned out in poor weather then the provision of individual, plastic lamb macs can offer short-term protection. Extra shelter in the form of straw bales or short lengths of plastic netting should also be given.

Two-thirds of ewes in a well-managed flock may be expected to hold to first service and will therefore lamb close together. At this intensity of lambing one individual lambing pen per ten ewes is the recommended guide (ADAS, 1990). Hygiene is paramount during this period but it is often neglected. Afterbirths should be removed regularly, lambing pens disinfected and straw changed between ewes.

Lambing is easier and more successful if hospital or isolation pens are nearby and fostering crates are provided. A well-stocked shepherd's cupboard with medicines, equipment and markers is also invaluable. A lamb warmer box will aid the weak lamb while warm water is needed to thaw frozen colostrum. A microwave oven is unsuitable as colostrum is broken down during heating. Adequate feeding and watering in the individual pen is important as the ewe establishes lactation.

Winter Shearing for Housed Ewes

On warm winter days housed ewes with a full fleece tended to pant and show signs of mild discomfort. A higher respiration rate of unshorn ewes compared with shorn ewes was recorded by Morgan and Broadbent (1980) (Table 13.6).

The lower critical temperature of ewes varies considerably according to climate and fleece length (see review by Charles and Stubbings, 1992).

Table 13.6. Ewe respiration rates one month pre-lambing.

House temperature (°C)	Respiration rate min^{-1}	
	Shorn	Unshorn
+7.5	36	172
+3.5	29	73
−0.5	33	65

Source: Morgan and Broadbent, 1980.

Equally the upper critical temperature of a housed and fully fleeced ewe can be below 10°C. Animals are most efficient thermally in the thermoneutral zone, outwith which there is an extra energy cost and most performance traits, such as growth rate are depressed (Table 13.7).

A series of experiments on the effects of winter shearing were carried out at the ADAS RDCs (see review by Brown and Meadowcroft, 1989). The ewes were housed and half of them shorn in January, eight to ten weeks before parturition. The benefits of winter shearing were an increase in lamb birthweight of around 0.5 kg for all types of lamb, i.e. singles, twins and triplets. This had a carry-over effect on lamb survival and subsequent weights at one month of age. A major commercial benefit was that stocking density in the house could be increased by 20%. It was also claimed that trough space could be reduced by 50–100 mm per ewe. There were other practical benefits: ewe body condition could be observed easily and consequent adjustments to feed levels made. Pregnant ewes were shorn carefully at a slack time of year and newly born lambs were able to find their way to the ewe's udder more easily.

Inevitably there were also some disadvantages. The consumption of roughage increased by 12–16% at an estimated cost of £2 per ewe. At one

Table 13.7. Effect of climate and shearing on lower critical temperature.

	LCT (°C)
Unshorn, dry, calm	−18
Unshorn, windy, wet	2
Shorn, dry, draughty	10
Shorn, wet, windy	15

Source: Charles and Stubbings, 1992.

site the heavier birthweight of single lambs created lambing difficulties. The fleece value was reduced in the first year of winter shearing. Thereafter fleece quality was quite acceptable although the increased risk of straw contamination could cause small financial loss. Shorn ewes proved more difficult to catch at lambing and the treatment of vaginal prolapse proved harder with no wool on which to tie the restraining tapes.

Shorn ewes turned out in March risk cold stress in poor weather as emphasized in the Code of Recommendations for the Welfare of Sheep (MAFF, 1990). Fleece needs at least eight weeks to regrow and ewes should preferably be turned out in mild weather into well-sheltered fields if the risk of lowered milk yield and mastitis infection is to be minimized. Cold stress can also occur before turnout if ewes are shorn in cold weather and little bedding is given. This may cause the ewes to cast their fleece, a condition known as wool-slip (Henderson, 1990). Wool-slip can also take place occasionally in outwintered sheep. The effect is more usually masked by the old fleece which clings to the body until new wool has regrown.

Disease Risks and Potential Problems

Henderson (1990) notes that where ewes are managed or housed intensively then there is an increased risk from some infectious diseases, e.g. enzootic abortion and toxoplasmosis. Sheep should only be housed with dry fleeces if substantial water loads are to be avoided. High humidities favour pneumonias and mycotic dermatitis. The majority of UK sheep houses use straw for bedding and soft conditions underfoot can lead to rapid horn growth and the spread of footrot. Removing the ewes regularly from the house, walking them on a hard surface and regular foot treatment in a footbath are suitable control measures.

Other diseases are associated with poor hygiene at lambing, e.g. *E. coli* infections, particularly the condition of watery mouth which can cause high mortality among lambs. Plentiful use of straw is a sound practice as is regular cleaning of food utensils. Coccidiosis may also occur, particularly where many ewes use the same lambing facilities over a prolonged period.

References

ADAS (1984) Land and Water Services Technical Note TFS 2301 Sheep housing. Ministry of Agriculture, Fisheries and Food, London.

ADAS (1987) Pamphlet P3128. Housing sheep. Ministry of Agriculture, Fisheries and Food, London.

ADAS (1990) Pamphlet P848. Reducing lamb mortality. Ministry of Agriculture, Fisheries and Food, London.

Bastiman, B. and Williams, D.O. (1973) Inwintering of ewes. Part 1 The effect of housing. *Experimental Husbandry* 24, 1–6.

Bøe, K., Nedkvitne, J.J. and Austbø, D. (1991) Effect of different housing systems and feeding regimes on the performance and rectal temperature of sheep. *Animal Production* 53, 331–338.

Brown, D.C. and Meadowcroft, S. (1989) *The Modern Shepherd.* Farming Press, Ipswich.

Brown, D.C. and Thomas, E.M. (1990) On-floor feeding of housed ewes. In: Slade, C.F.R. and Lawrence, T.L.J. (eds), *New Developments in Sheep Production.* Occasional Publication No. 14 British Society of Animal Production, Penicuik.

Charles, D. and Stubbings, L. (1992) Housing and shelter. *Sheep Farmer* 12, 21–24.

Court, K. (1983) Slatted floor trials at NAC sheep unit. In: *Housing Sheep.* Farm Buildings Information Centre, Stoneleigh.

FBIC (1983) *Housing Sheep.* Farm Buildings Information Centre, Stoneleigh, Warwickshire.

Henderson, D. (1990) *The Veterinary Book for Sheep Farmers.* Farming Press, Ipswich.

Loynes, I.J. (1983a) Sheep house design. In: *Housing Sheep.* Farm Buildings Information Centre, Stoneleigh.

Loynes, I.J. (1983b) Putting the right roof over your sheep. In: *Housing Sheep.* Farm Buildings Information Centre, Stoneleigh.

MAFF (1990) Codes of recommendations for the welfare of livestock – sheep. Ministry of Agriculture, Fisheries and Food, London.

MLC (1988) *Sheep in Britain.* Meat and Livestock Commission, Milton Keynes.

Morgan, H. and Broadbent, J.S. (1980) Study of the effects of shearing pregnant ewes at lambing. *Animal Production* 30, 476.

Sharples, T.J. and Dumelow, J. (1990) Prediction of body dimensions of Mule and Scottish blackface ewes from measurement of body weight. *Animal Production* 50, 491–496.

Slade, C.F.R. (1986) The performance of store lambs at grass. In: Pollott, G.E. (ed.), *Efficient Sheep Production from Grass.* Occasional Symposium No. 21, British Grassland Society, Reading.

Slade, C.F.R. (1990) The UK Sheep Industry: Current position, economics and emerging trends. In: Slade, C.F.R. and Lawrence, T.L.J. (eds), *New Developments in Sheep Production.* Occasional Publication No. 14. British Society of Animal Production, Penicuik.

Watson, L. (1992) Safe housing. *Sheep Farmer* 12, 26–27.

Stables 14

A.F. CLARKE
Equine Research Centre, University of Guelph, Canada

Introduction

The horse evolved as a herding, free-ranging grazing animal. Domestication has resulted in some conflicts with this evolutionary pathway. The horse may spend as much as 22½ hours each day in a relatively dark stable with little visual or tactile contact with other horses. The demands of competition and training are often associated with high energy intakes supplied by low fibre, high energy feeds. These feeds can be eaten relatively quickly, leaving the horse with little to do for the rest of the day. These limitations may have adverse behavioural and health consequences for the horse.

Non-empirical recommendations extrapolated from intensively-housed livestock have been used as the basis for many accepted practices for equine stables. However, the housing requirements and performance demands of horses are different from those of food-producing farm animals (Clarke, 1987). One clear example relates to respiratory disease. Minor degrees of respiratory disease can impair a horse's performance, while other farm animals are capable of maintaining high levels of output (e.g. conversion of grain to meat) in spite of frank respiratory disease (Wilson *et al.*, 1986). Meat-producing animals are also slaughtered in early life before many diseases, such as chronically developing respiratory allergies, are manifest. In this chapter the respiratory well-being of horses is emphasized since this body system is most affected by housing. However, it is important that we do not consider the horse as simply a set of lungs to the exclusion of other body systems. Stabled horses have several advantages over other farm animals, e.g. stocking densities are usually more generous (Jones *et al.*, 1987), and higher hygiene standards can be maintained given sound horse and stable management.

Horses travel nationally and internationally to and from competitive events, stud farms and sales. This exchange provides ideal opportunities for the dissemination of agents of infectious diseases ranging from respiratory problems to abortion (Powell, 1985). The incidence of respiratory disease rises with the seasonal influx of new yearlings into racing yards (Burrell *et al.*, 1985). The 'stress' of travel also decreases the phagocytic ability of pulmonary macrophages (Huston *et al.*, 1986), which may lead to diseases such as pleuropneumonia (Sweeney *et al.*, 1985). There are practical methods of decreasing transport stress (Cregier, 1983). Competition and training can also inhibit the phagocytic ability of pulmonary macrophages (Liggit *et al.*, 1985). Rupture of the capillaries in the dorso-caudal area of the diaphragmatic lung lobes causes haemorrhaging and creates an attractive site for secondary bacterial infections (Clarke, 1985). These points highlight the importance of ensuring optimal environmental conditions in stables.

The hygiene and physical environment of a stable can affect the welfare and well-being of horses by:

1. increasing the magnitude of challenges from infectious microorganisms, parasites, noxious gases and allergenic or irritant particles;
2. altering the horse's systemic or local resistance;
3. increasing the risk of physical injury;
4. failing to meet the horse's behavioural needs.

The design and management of a stable follows logically from an assessment of these effects.

Needs of the Stabled Horse

The horse in health and disease – overview of host defence mechanisms

There is a wide range of host defence mechanisms which must be considered in establishing environmental criteria and management practices for stables. The horse's immune status is the major limiting factor governing the occurrence of infectious and parasitic diseases (Hannant, 1990). For infectious agents which act at their site of deposition or ingestion, it is the local mucosal immune system which is of significance. For agents which require a systemic spread to induce disease, levels of circulating antibodies and other systemic immune mechanisms assume a higher importance. Significance of local as distinct from systemic immunity in protecting the horse against infectious respiratory disease has been highlighted by Rouse and Ditchfield (1970) in relation to Equine Influenza virus and Galan and Timoney (1985) and Timoney and Eggers (1985) in relation to *Streptococcus equi* infections. They found no association between levels of bacterial antibody in serum and resistance to reinfection. Immunity also tends to be short-lived when disease results from damage to tissues which the pathogen first encounters and when a short incubation period is involved (Bryans, 1981a). This is in contrast to generally strong and long lasting natural immunity where a systemic spread of the agent is a pre-requisite for disease to occur. Equine herpes virus Type I is a prime example (Allen and Bryans, 1986). The resistance to respiratory disease associated with subtypes 1 and 2 can be as short as 3 or 4 months. However, the length of resistance to abortion associated with subtype 1 is much longer and can be life-long. New vaccines will undoubtedly be beneficial in terms of preventing infectious diseases. However, the ability of viruses to mutate and remain latent in carrier animals make disease eradication by vaccination highly unlikely.

Under certain conditions, the immune system may over-react and induce allergic reactions (Gell and Coombs, 1974). Exposure of sensitized animals to allergens leads to an inflammatory response. The best known example is chronic obstructive pulmonary disease (COPD) which is believed to be an allergic response (or responses) to inhaled mould spores (McPherson *et al.*, 1979; McPherson and Thomson, 1983; Clarke, 1993).

Interactions between different types of pathogens and host responses also occur. For example, COPD has been observed as a common sequel to bacterial and viral infections of the respiratory tract (McPherson and Thomson, 1983). Viral infections of the respiratory tract are known to affect the mucociliary escalator, damage epithelial surfaces and alter the host's immune response (Bryans, 1981a,b; Allen and Bryans, 1986). Tracheal mucociliary clearance can also be inhibited for over a month following a respiratory tract infection (Willoughby *et al.*, 1991, 1992). This inhibition effectively increases the amount of active pathogen present in the lung, i.e. mould spores in the case of COPD. This point is also critical in dealing with viral infections, since good air hygiene is beneficial in terms of minimizing the duration and severity of episodes of infectious respiratory disease (Clarke, 1993). In terms of stable design and management, threshold limiting values for airborne pollutants are effectively decreased when horses have infectious or non-infectious airway disease.

Enteric, locomotion and other diseases

Horses share a very wide range of enteric conditions with other species, including salmonellosis and rota virus infections. *Escherichia coli, Salmonella* and *Pseudomonas* are but a few of the bacteria which may survive for many months in bedding (Curtis, 1983). A review of all of these agents is beyond the scope of this chapter. However, good basic hygiene practices in terms of avoidance of deep litter, clean feed storage facilities and isolation of affected animals are important. Standards of hygiene are critical on stud farms to help prevent rotavirus infection and infectious abortion; the relevant management and stable practices are discussed below.

Gastroenteric parasites are the major cause of deaths from colic in horses. Death is often associated with migration of the larvae, which have also been associated with respiratory disease (Clayton, 1981; Turk and Klei, 1984; Duncan, 1985). Lungworm (*Dictyocaulus arnfieldi*) is often implicated with chronic respiratory disease in horses, especially where horses and donkeys are kept together (Round, 1976). Roundworm (*Parascaris equorum*) has been implicated in cases of hypersensitivity airway disease in horses (Mirbahar and Eyre, 1986). Pasture rotation and management together with the regular use of anthelmintics form the basis of effective control of these parasites. However, the eggs and larval stages of most of these parasites are resistant to desiccation (Curtis, 1983; Duncan, 1985) so that droppings should be removed regularly from stables and deep litter management avoided.

The horse is a 'fright and flight' creature, and injuries can occur as a horse rushes out of a door, slips on a pathway or is kicked by another horse in a narrow passageway. Other locomotion problems that can develop include 'thrush' in a horse's feet, podal dermatitis or an infected foot. Such problems can lead to a horse missing a competitive event or establish chronic problems which may never be resolved. Again, young stock are at particular risk. The risks of foals fracturing their sesamoids or injuries occurring at weaning can be decreased with appropriate management and housing practices (see below).

Respiratory diseases

Manifestations of respiratory disease in horses include life-threatening infections, especially in young foals, subclinical inflammation associated with poor performance in athletes, and debilitating allergic disease in later life. Decreasing the risk of problems in early life leads to longer term benefits as well.

While the severe or overt forms of infectious and allergic diseases are widely appreciated, it is the covert or subclinical problems which warrant special attention since these can be associated with marked loss of performance. Some basic respiratory physiology highlights this point. At rest, an average 550 kg horse has a tidal volume (depth of breath) of approximately 5 litres of air with a respiratory rate of 12 breaths per minute. At the gallop, the tidal volume increases to between 12 and 15 litres per breath with the respiratory rate increasing to over 150 breaths per minute. The respiratory and locomotion cycles are locked in a 1:1 phase during cantering and galloping. Minor degrees of airway inflammation or bronchoconstriction and increased amounts of mucus within the airways can have a marked effect on athletic performance. This problem of covert respiratory disease has been described as lower respiratory tract inflammation (LRTI) (Burrell, 1985) and is diagnosed on the basis of endoscopic examinations of the airways and 'lung washes'. Management and housing practices which help prevent and minimize the severity of episodes of these mild forms of disease in the horse's early life will have longer term benefits in decreasing the incidence of COPD in later life.

Stable dusts

Forage and bedding materials are the main sources of dust in stables and either one or both of these sources are likely to be moulded when high respirable challenges of dust occur (Clarke, 1991; see also this volume, Chapter 6). The highest respirable challenges of dust are associated with the presence of thermotolerant and thermophilic mould species (Gregory and Lacey, 1963). These species produce large numbers of spores with aerodynamic diameters less than 5 μm which can penetrate the deepest areas of the lung when inhaled. There are over 70 species of fungi and actinomycetes to which horses can be exposed (Clarke and Madelin, 1987).

The association between both overt and covert respiratory disease has been discussed earlier. Fungi can also cause a range of systemic and local infections in horses including guttural pouch infections (Hawkins, 1992), abortions (Hyland and Jeffcott, 1987), eye infections (Kern *et al.*, 1983), and kidney and chest infections (Domsch *et al.*, 1980). The ingestion of mouldy feedstuffs may also be associated with systemic mycotoxic disease (Asquith, 1983).

The critical limits or threshold limiting values (TLV) for exposure to fungi and actinomycetes are unknown for the horse (Clarke, 1993). Indeed the horse's response to challenges from these pathogens is likely to be graded and vary between individuals. The presence of concurrent disease, such as viral infections, also increases the horse's susceptibility to stable dusts. Due to the horse's relative longevity compared with other species, the TLV for mould spores must be considered in terms of both acute high level and chronic low level exposures. Years of low level exposure may be as significant as acute high level exposures in terms of sensitizing horses to stable dust. Once sensitization has occurred then tolerance also decreases. It is salient to note that while the current recommended TLV for exposure to dust for humans working an eight-hour five-day week is $10\,mg\,m^{-3}$, handlers of grain continuously exposed to levels of $5\,mg\,m^{-3}$ of dust suffered serious loss of respiratory function (Anon. 1972; Enarson *et al.*, 1985).

Dilution by ventilation is the primary clearance mechanism for airborne dust in stables. The spores of thermophilic and thermotolerant mould sediment from the air at a very slow rate. For example, an actinomycete

Table 14.1. Aerobiology of forage materials for horses.

	Rye (clean)	Rye (dirty)	Lucerne (clean)	Lucerne (dirty)	Horsehage‡	Silage‡
Particles per mg*	980+	65,190	840+	39,270	44	19
Proportion of particles (%)†						
Fungal and actinomycete particles	30	99	55	99	5	5
Plant material	70	ng	45	ng	95	95
Other	ng	1	ng	1	ng	ng

Source: Clarke, 1987.

* Assessed using aerodynamic particle sizer.
† Assessed using a May impactor.
‡ Sealed bags.
ng = negligible.

spore may take up to 30 h to fall 1 m in still air conditions. Furthermore, while the death of an airborne spore negates its ability to induce infection, the risk of an allergic reaction remains. While ventilation is the primary mechanism to remove mould spores from stable air, the best approach is to avoid mould spores at source (Woods *et al.*, 1993). This means avoiding contaminated feeds and beddings or management practices which lead to moulding of materials in stables. Hay and straw can be assessed objectively (Clarke and Madelin, 1987). Alternative forages to hay include barn-dried hay, heat-dried hay, bagged haylage products and cobbed products (Table 14.1; Clarke, 1989). Thorough soaking of hay is another alternative. The best approach involves a half-day soak, i.e. put the evening's hay into soak when the morning's hay is fed out. Dust generated from hay storage areas can still be a problem, especially if the storage area shares an air space with the horses. Hay cleaners and dust extraction machines are also available. Wood shavings, diced newspaper, peat moss and synthetic products are alternatives to straw (Table 14.2). There has also been interest in methods of cleaning and treating straw. It should be highlighted that alternatives to straw, such as wood shavings and paper bedding, can be a significant source of mould spores even though they are relatively clean when first put down in the stable. Heavily insulated, poorly ventilated stables and deep litter management practices are examples of situations where moulding of these source materials can occur (Clarke *et al.*, 1987; Clarke, 1989).

Bacteria, viruses and other infectious agents

A comprehensive review of infectious agents capable of causing respiratory tract infections in the horse is beyond the scope of this chapter (see Clayton, 1981; Mumford, 1992). Horses are the primary source of infectious respiratory pathogens in stables as many of these pathogens are short-lived away from their host. An important exception is *Rhodococcus equi*, an actinomycete associated with peracute pneumonia in foals, which may originate from bedding (Hillidge, 1986; Clarke, 1989). The majority of respiratory pathogens are transmitted via aerosols, though they need not be airborne to enter the host and cause disease. Respiratory disease can be induced by swabbing a horse's pharynx with swabs covered in herpesvirus (Allen and Bryans, 1986). *R. equi* pneumonia in foals is typically associated with an aerosol challenge, but also may follow ingestion and systemic spread of the actinomycete (Smith, 1982).

The likelihood of a horse contracting disease from an aerosol generated by another coughing or sneezing horse will depend on (i) the airborne survival of the pathogen; (ii) the pathogenicity of the microorganism; and (iii) the susceptibility of the horse. Aerosolized bacteria and viruses often only survive a matter of seconds. The latter are particularly sensitive to humidity (Donaldson, 1978). However, not all viruses respond in a similar

Table 14.2. Aerobiology of fresh bedding materials.

	Equibed‡	Diced§ newspaper	Shavings (range)		Straw (range)		Tissue¶
Particle per mg*	19	78	148	873	1,490	28,100	53
Proportion of particles (%)†							
Fungal and actinomycete particles	ng	ng	5	96	90	100	ng
Plant material	ng	ng	95	4	8	trace	ng
Other	100	100	ng	ng	2	trace	100

Source: Clarke, 1987.

* Assessed using aerodynamic particle sizer.
† Assessed using May impactor.
‡ Equibed – Melcourt Industries, Tetbury, Glos. (absorbent synthetic bedding).
§ Diced newspaper – Shredabed, Exeter.
¶ Tissue bedding – F.H. Lee, Greater Manchester.
ng = negligible.

manner. Equine herpesvirus I and equine arteritis virus survive best at low relative humidities while equine rhinovirus survives best at high relative humidities. Bacteria, e.g. haemolytic streptococci, usually suffer increased death rates with increasing temperature.

There are several limitations in practice to minimizing the spread of infectious respiratory disease by altering environmental parameters. Temperature and relative humidity in a well ventilated stable are primarily dependent on outside ambient conditions and can be extremely variable. Furthermore, an environment which decreases the airborne survival of one agent may enhance the survival of another. Infectious diseases can also be spread by means other than aerosols. These include: (i) short-range direct transmission in droplet form following coughing or sneezing; (ii) direct contact between horses, e.g. nose to nose; and (iii) indirect contact between horses, i.e. via harness, staff or by the horse nuzzling contaminated surfaces.

Environmental control of the spread of infectious respiratory disease is likely to be more effective against less pathogenic organisms (i.e. where large challenges are necessary to induce disease) than against more pathogenic organisms. Environmental control is also likely to be effective against pathogens which proliferate and survive for long periods of time away from the host, e.g. *R. equi*.

Isolation and quarantine are practices which lower the incidence of a wide range of infectious diseases, especially with studs or closed herds (Bryans, 1981a, b). In situations where isolation and quarantine are not feasible, management practices should: (i) minimize stress, which may lower an individual's susceptibility to disease; and (ii) minimize the duration and severity of disease through the provision of fresh air in well-ventilated stables and decreased exposure to irritant and allergenic stable dusts (Clarke, 1987; Clarke *et al.*, 1987).

Noxious gases

Noxious gases to which housed animals are exposed include NH_3, H_2S, CH_4 and CO_2 (Nordstrum and McQuitty, 1976). These may act as irritants (e.g. NH_3) or asphyxiants (CH_4 or CO_2). Horses are exposed to a narrower range and lower levels of noxious gases than other intensively housed animals because stocking densities in stables are lower. NH_3 and to a lesser extent H_2S are the primary noxious gases of concern. NH_3 levels tend to rise where deep litter management is practised and where drainage of urine is poor. The TLV for noxious gases in relation to equine respiratory disease is unknown (see also Chapter 6). Since the response of the horse's respiratory tract to noxious gases is likely to be graded, NH_3 levels should be maintained as low as possible at all times.

Environment

Environmental temperature

A healthy, well-fed adult horse has a wide thermal tolerance and, with acclimatization, can withstand temperatures as low as −10°C (Sainsbury, 1981; McBride *et al.*, 1983). The lower critical temperature of a two-day-old foal is approximately 25°C (Ousey *et al.*, 1991), and healthy well-fed foals can tolerate temperatures down to 5°C without a fall in deep body temperature. Disease and malnutrition increase the lower critical temperature because of a decrease in metabolic rate. Wind or draughts also increase the lower critical temperature, especially of wet animals. Foals are the most susceptible to hypothermia and extra heat sources may be required; quartz–halogen radiant heat lamps are particularly beneficial. Rugging and a deep bedding restrict heat loss (Clarke, 1992). Ventilation and environmental temperature are intertwined and are discussed further in this chapter.

Light

Light affects the cyclicity of equine reproduction, shedding of coats, behavioural needs and the survival of airborne microbes. Photoperiod is the primary factor which governs seasonal oestrus activity in mares (Sharp, 1987). Artificial lighting in stables can be used to bring mares into season early in the year. Standard light bulbs or fluorescent lighting will provide suitable light intensities and wavelengths, the target light intensity being between 100 and 200 lux. Extending daylength to between 14 and 16 hours in late November is effective in stimulating early oestrus. The provision of 2.5 hours of artificial light after sunset but before sunrise or a 1 hour exposure to light 9 to 10 hours after natural sunset are other approaches which stimulate mares to cycle. Photoperiod also affects plasma levels of testosterone (Cox *et al.*, 1988), testicular size, seminal characteristics and sexual behaviour in stallions. Photoperiod is also the primary factor which stimulates changes in coat length (Kooistra and Ginther, 1975). Decreasing daylength stimulates the horse to lose its summer coat while increasing daylength leads to the loss of the winter coat. The association between hormone levels and changing hair coat could provide a physiological explanation for the observation of many racehorse trainers that the appearance of the longer winter coat at the end of the racing season is associated with decreasing racing performance.

Ethological studies have shown that horses prefer bright to poorly lit stables (Houpt and Houpt, 1988). Natural light receives inadequate attention in stables. The ultraviolet fraction of sunlight is a natural killer of airborne microbes. Plastic skylights or ultraviolet-pervious glass are preferable to normal glass since the latter does not allow the penetration of ultraviolet rays; 10% of skylight in the roof is suitable as a general guideline.

Behaviour

Domestication has placed many constraints on the behavioural needs of horses (Sweeting *et al.*, 1985; Kiley-Worthington, 1990). The horse evolved as a free-ranging animal that roamed over relatively large areas and grazed a high fibre food. A digestive system with hind gut fermentation evolved as a means of making best use of this diet. High energy concentrate coupled with unnecessarily low fibre has led to changes in feeding behaviour (Meyer *et al.*, 1975; Willard, 1976) and digestion (Noot *et al.*, 1967; Ott, 1981). Coprophagy and wood chewing can be corrected with changes in diet. This is achieved through the provision of extra forage.

The behavioural needs of stabled horses are not met when they spend the majority of their days in individual living areas, often without visual or physical contact with other horses (Houpt and Houpt, 1988). These constraints, and the dietary factors described above, may lead to the development of abnormal behaviour including stereotypies (see Chapter 4). Stereotypies are often known as 'stable vices' and include box walking, crib biting, weaving and kicking. There is much to learn in relation to the avoidance of stereotypic behaviour. The environment in which a horse displays stereotypic behaviour may not be the environment which initiated the habit. Weaning time is believed to be a critical time for their development. Regular exercise, visual and physical contact (through open bars) with other horses, light (as distinct from dark) stables, allowing the horse to put its head out of an open top stable door, the provision of a stimulating environment around stables and access to forage all benefit the behavioural needs of horses.

Stables in Practice

Description of typical designs

There are three basic types of stables:

1. *Stalls.* Horses remain tethered in stalls though controversy exists regarding their use. Objective information regarding the use of stalls should become available within the next few years. Recommendations for the dimensions of stalls are presented in Table 14.3.
2. *Looseboxes* (Fig. 14.1). Looseboxes are typically constructed in rows. An overhang over the front of the boxes can provide shelter for horses and staff in inclement weather. An open top half of the stable door allows horses to enjoy fresh air and a stimulating environment. Looseboxes can also be constructed around a courtyard design. Recommendations for the sizes of looseboxes are presented in Table 14.3.

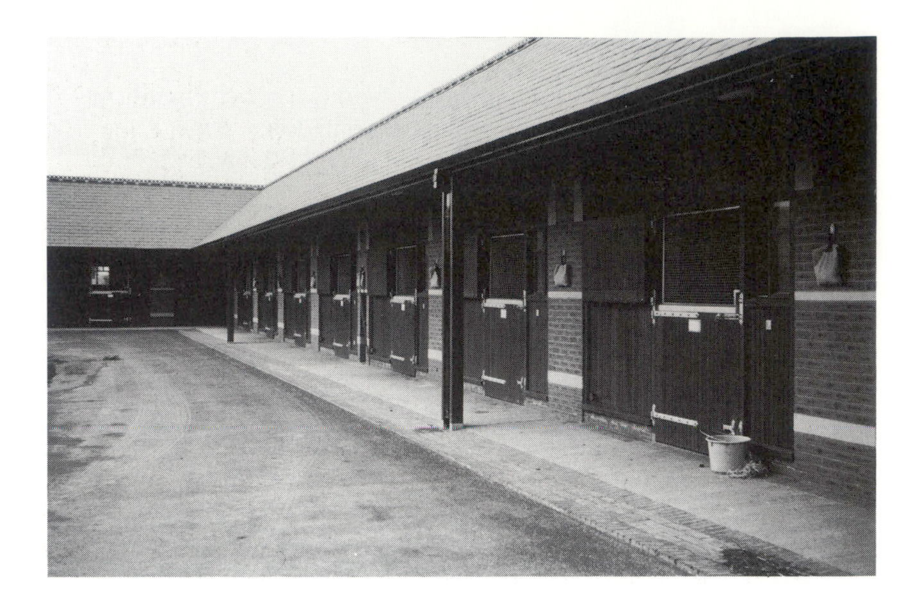

Fig. 14.1. An example of a yard based on individual looseboxes. Note the overhang at the front of the boxes which can be particularly beneficial in inclement weather.

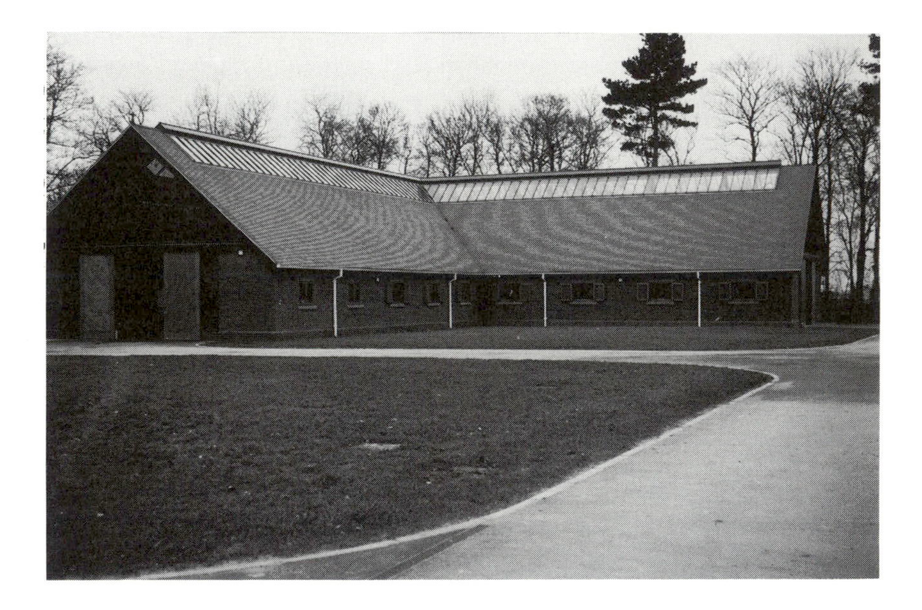

Fig. 14.2. An example of a barn. Note the extensive area of skylight and high level outlets for natural ventilation. Inlets for natural ventilation are at eaves level.

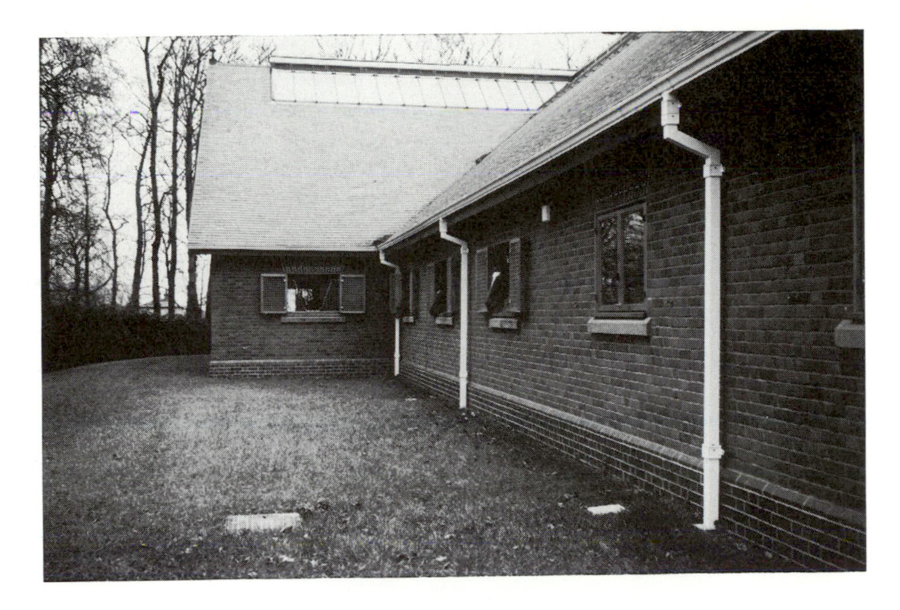

Fig. 14.3. Close up of the barn in Fig. 14.2. Windows can be opened providing fresh air and a more stimulating environment for the horses, helping to avoid potential boredom.

3. *Barns.* Horse barns come in many sizes and shapes ranging from large low barns housing up to 100 horses to mini barns which house a dozen horses (Figs 14.2, 14.3 and 14.4). Barns have many advantages and disadvantages. They are cost effective to build, provide an excellent working environment and use an open concept, i.e. open bars between boxes within the barn, to help meet the behavioural needs of horses. The primary disadvantage is associated with large barns of low height in which proper mixing of air can be difficult to attain (see next section). Mini barns housing between 12 and 20 horses can be used to take full advantage of barn type structures.

There are many variations on the above. For example, one barn type construction comprises effectively parallel rows of looseboxes linked with a roof (Fig 14.5). This type of structure can be particularly useful on stud farms. Greater detail on stable design, structure, layout and fittings is provided by Clarke (1987), Sainsbury (1987) and Smith (1986).

Ventilation

Temperature, water vapour levels and concentrations of noxious gases, dust

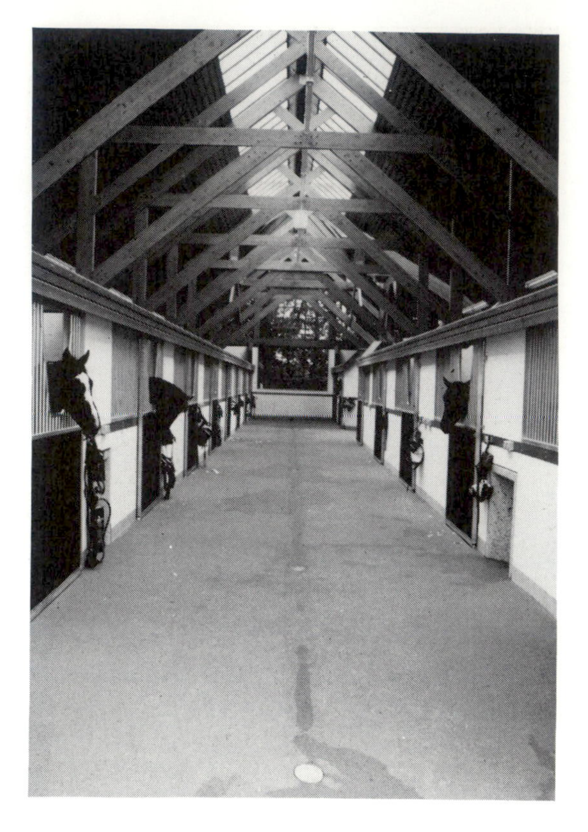

Fig. 14.4. Inside view of the barn in Fig. 14.2. Note natural lighting and open top half of stable door, which again helps provide a more stimulating environment for horses.

and microbes are all affected by ventilation. Ventilation on its own cannot be used to overcome the use of mouldy feeds and beddings (Clarke, 1993; Woods *et al.*, 1993). In addition, ventilation will aid the control of condensation; lower the level of airborne pathogens which cannot be controlled by other means; and aid in the prevention of moulding of bedding materials.

The theoretical principles involved in providing natural ventilation for buildings have been described by Bruce (1978), and are presented in Chapter 7. Natural ventilation is based on the stack effect, i.e. warm air rising from the horse exits the building through high level outlets and draws in fresh air through low level inlets. In designing stables, the minimum rate is four air changes per hour with the top door closed for looseboxes or the main doors shut in a barn. This rate should ensure adequate ventilation all year round. In inclement or windy weather, aspiration and perflation, the other forces of natural ventilation, will increase ventilation above four air changes per hour

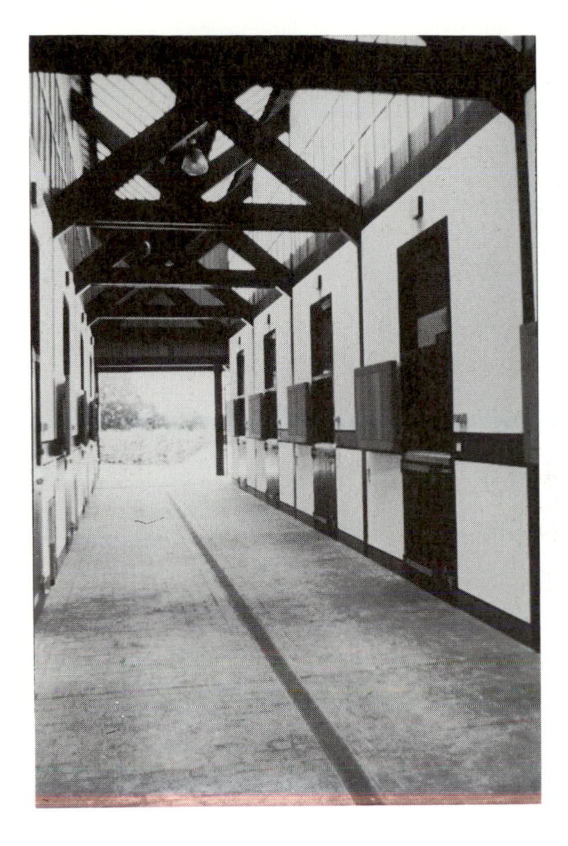

Fig. 14.5. An example of barn design used with studs. Two rows of individual looseboxes are joined with a common walkway.

even when all doors are closed. Examples of a typical loosebox and a barn both with and without insulation are presented in Table 14.4. The figures assume heat loss of 800 W per horse in cool weather. Table 14.4 highlights that a main benefit of insulating stables is to enhance natural ventilation by providing constant air changes with smaller openings than in uninsulated buildings, thereby avoiding draughts.

The distribution of inlet and outlet openings requires special attention, especially in large barns. The guidelines recommended above assume perfect mixing of air within the building. To this end a wide distribution of inlets is required in all stables but especially in large barns. This can be achieved by individual vents or Yorkshire boarding. Capped ridge vents and breathing roofs are also beneficial in large barns. Looseboxes with monopitch roofs should have openings in the front and rear walls in addition to the stable door. Looseboxes with pitched roofs require an opening in the ridge and two inlets at eaves level, in the front wall and rear

Table 14.3. Recommendations for stable dimensions.

Type	Dimension (m)
Loosebox	
ponies (l × w)	3.0 × 3.0
horses	3.6 × 3.6
foaling or isolation box	5.0 × 5.0
Stall	
width, minimum	1.7
length	3.3
rear passageway, minimum	2.0
Door	
height	2.4
width	1.2

Table 14.4. Requirement for natural ventilation of a typical barn and horsebox.

	Box		Barn	
Dimensions (per horse)				
Volume (m^3)	50		85	
Surface area of building (m^2)	41		43	
Height from inlets to outlets (m)	1.0		2.0	
Ventilation rate at 4 ac/h ($m^3\ s^{-1}$)	0.055		0.094	
Ventilation heat loss at 4 ac/h ($W\ °C^{-1}$)	67		114	
	Insulated	Uninsulated	Insulated	Uninsulated
U value of walls and roof ($W\ m^{-2}°C$)	0.4	2.0	0.4	2.0
Building heat loss ($W\ °C^{-2}$)	16	82	17	86
Temperature gradient (°C) at 4 ac/h	8.4	5.2	6.0	4.1
Required				
inlet area/horse (m^2)	0.27	0.34	0.38	0.46
outlet area/horse (m^2)	0.14	0.17	0.19	0.23

Source: Webster *et al.*, 1987.

wall. Inlets may require baffling to prevent the entrance of rain or snow and to decrease the occurrence of draughts.

Mechanical ventilation systems with varying combinations of heating, air conditioning and air filtration are occasionally used in stables. Such systems can be efficient but must undergo regular maintenance. Poorly maintained fans and filters are two main problems. Water-scrubbing filter systems have particular drawbacks especially given the levels of dust and mould contamination in stables. In industrial areas, the filters used in stables may require changing as frequently as every six weeks. Another problem examined by the present author was associated with the close proximity of the inlets and outlets of a mechanical ventilation system. Dust expelled through the outlets was drawn up through the inlet ducts, which led to rapid clogging of the filters. Small filter systems have been developed for domestic dwellings, houses and offices to remove cigarette smoke from the air and have been advocated for stables. These systems often do not have sufficient volumetric capacity to filter effectively the stable air.

Ionizers have been recommended for use in stables as a method of decreasing the burdens of airborne dust and microbes. The author has found no benefit in terms of decreasing dust levels. Similar results were reported by Edwards *et al.* (1985). Philips *et al.* (1964) demonstrated that ionizers enhanced the killing of airborne bacteria. However, this is not likely to be of practical value in a well-ventilated stable. Airborne ions have been shown to enhance mucociliary clearance in some animals and eliminate focal areas of infection in the airways of poultry (Wehner, 1969) but these observations have not been reported in horses. At present, there does not seem to be a sound basis on which ionizers can be recommended for use in stables.

All in all, it can be concluded that suitable air quality of stables can be adequately maintained through the combined use of natural ventilation and appropriate management practices.

Special Needs of Studs

There is a wide range of clinical and research-based information which has practical implications for the equine stud. Many of these factors have been discussed in the earlier sections of this chapter; however, studs are dealt with separately here to highlight some of the unique demands which affect their design, layout and management.

Building design

Stud buildings can be based on traditional individual loosebox design arranged in rows or around a courtyard. Alternatively, large barns may be used. Both have their advantages and disadvantages though a hybrid between the two is the most easily managed in terms of mares and foals (Fig. 14.5). Such a building is effectively two rows of looseboxes facing each other and joined with a covered passageway. The features are that each box has an individual airspace, the mare and foal can be provided with a relatively undisturbed environment from which they can be easily observed, each box can be provided with additional heat as required, and access and working conditions for stud staff and veterinarians provide for the best levels of care.

The importance of providing ventilation without draughts for foals has been emphasized earlier in this chapter. The chilling effects of draughts considerably lower a foal's resistance to cold. Furthermore, foals born in cold, wet environments may need supplementary colostrum to prevent failure of passive transfer of colostral antibodies. Provision should be made to provide additional heat sources. Quartz–halogen heaters provide a particularly effective method of providing supplementary heat in large airy buildings. A dry deep bedding is essential, especially over concrete floors, to avoid excessive conductive heat loss from a foal lying down.

Layout

Several smaller yards are preferable to one main site for the general layout of studs, especially when there is more than one stallion. Approximately 1ha of land is required per mare. A series of smaller yards allows appropriate groups of mares to be segregated. Maiden and barren mares can be kept separate from mares with foals at foot. The logistical problems (and safety risks) of walking mares (with or without foals) to and from an extended main stabling area can be minimized. The best use can also be made of pastures. Paddocks in close proximity to the stable can be saved for mares and foals. In terms of parasite control and hygiene practices, it is best if foals born late in the season can graze on fresh pastures on which early foals have not grazed.

Hygiene

There is a wide range of infectious diseases from which stallions, mares and foals at stud are at risk (Rossdale and Ricketts, 1980). The most devastating of these to a stud farm can be abortion and the best known of these is equine herpesvirus abortion. However, other forms of infectious disease must not be forgotten. Infections of the mares' or stallions' reproductive organs lead to decreases in fertility. Facilities for washing down mares and stallions and the maintenance of good hygiene practices in examination and serving areas must not be overlooked. There is also a wide range of infectious diseases which are particularly harmful and life-threatening for young foals (Brewer and Koterba, 1987; Martens and Carter, 1987; Wilson, 1987; Paradis, 1989). These include septicaemia, pneumonia, arthritis and enteritis.

Equine herpesvirus abortion is a cause for special consideration as a large number of foals can be lost on an individual stud farm. The 1989 Horserace Betting Levy Board's *A Common Code of Practice for the Control of Contagious Equine Metritis and Other Equine Reproductive Diseases for the 1990 Covering Season in France, Ireland and the United Kingdom* reported 37 confirmed separate incidences of virus abortion on 17 premises. The majority of cases (30/37) occurred in unvaccinated mares. However, attention must still be given to management and housing of vaccinated mares and foals. Equine herpesvirus can be shed by carriers such as mares, foals or yearlings and is reported to be more likely to arise when mares are mixed in large stud farms (Ellis, 1987). Pregnant mares at stud should be kept isolated from other horses as far as feasibly possible.

Equine herpesviruses can be transmitted via direct contact between animals, via aerosols and indirectly by infective material transported by grooms or vets on protective clothing. The virus is relatively short-lived in the air and so appropriate spacing of buildings should decrease the risk of spread (Donaldson, 1978). However, the virus may survive for up to several weeks if cleaning and disinfection are not adequate (HBLB Recommendations, 1990). The provision of veterinary examination and clean-down areas at each barn, and allocation of separate staff to each site provide practical means of decreasing the risk of this and other infectious diseases at the stud. An added bonus of a layout based on self-contained yards is that if a problem occurs, e.g. a mare aborts or a foal is taken ill, the risk of the problem spreading throughout the stud can be decreased. It may take several days for conclusive laboratory confirmation and precautionary isolation can be maintained while tests are awaited.

The importance of providing fresh pastures for foals has been mentioned above, along with the advantages of siting their stabling in relatively close proximity to the paddocks. Young foals, like the neonates of other species, can be particularly at risk from infections. Some of these may persist in the environment for weeks or even months, e.g. rotavirus which causes diarrhoea in foals (Harbour, 1985), while others may proliferate in the environment, e.g. *Rhodococcus equi* which causes severe pneumonia in foals (Clarke, 1989). It is clearly beneficial to be able to provide fresh pastures for foals born late in the year.

Injuries and orthopaedic conditions

Special attention must be given to foals at stud to ensure that they grow and develop successfully. There is a range of injuries and orthopaedic conditions of young foals which curtails these opportunities. The risk of some of these (e.g. fractures) can be decreased by attention to stable design, stud layout and management practices.

Foals may suffer various fractures as a result of being kicked, running into objects or running to exhaustion chasing excited or frightened mothers. These fractures may occur at the jaw, spine, pelvis and limbs. The risks of fractures will be increased when horses are brought together in large numbers or mares and foals are frightened or excited. A stud layout based on segregated, separated yards is preferable to one main site.

One specific fracture which warrants special consideration is that of the proximal sesamoid bone in foals (Ellis, 1987). This is the most common fracture in Thoroughbred foals up to one month of age and is caused by foals galloping to exhaustion after their dams. Young, weak foals or foals recovering from other problems may be particularly at risk. Smaller nursery paddocks and exercise areas (see section on barn design) are beneficial. Mares with young foals at foot should not be kept in paddocks with mares with older, more precocious foals. Factors such as lorries delivering feed which may excite or frighten mares with foals at foot should be minimized and located as far away as possible from their paddocks.

Accidents may still occur and measures will need to be taken to correct or avoid developmental problems, which can lead to poor conformation. The sooner problems are recognized and treatment or corrective measures instigated the better. Constant supervision, sound veterinary care, and availability of examination and treatment areas are essential in the short term. In the medium to longer term, continual nursing will be needed along with graded exercise programmes.

Staff

Studs are labour intensive and require around-the-clock supervision. Indeed, the success of a stud is dependent largely on its employees and the care they provide.

Mares usually foal at night. One survey found that 86% of foalings occurred between 7 p.m. and 7 a.m. with 40% happening within two hours either side of midnight (Rossdale and Short, 1967). It is critical that experienced hands are present at such times. Mares must be observed carefully in the lead-up to the birth for signs of problems. Once fetal fluids have been discharged, the foal has from one to three hours to live inside the mare unless it is delivered (Dawson, 1987). The progress of the birth must be monitored and assistance provided where necessary. The foal may need its air passages to be cleared. The mare and foal should be examined for signs of injuries or other problems. The foal may need assistance to get to its feet. It is also critical in these first few hours that the foal receives its first milk or colostrum (Jeffcott, 1987). The foal may need an enema when a few hours old to avoid meconium impaction. Bonding of mares and foals is also important and may be a problem with mares with their first foals, thus necessitating extra attention from attendants. Special attention must be given to mares and foals at this stage to ensure that they have not suffered injury or trauma during the birth and to ensure that the afterbirth has been thoroughly cleared.

Careful observation of mares and foals can detect problems early allowing appropriate therapeutic and management regimens to be instigated. Nursing and treatment of such problems do not fit conveniently into an eight-hour day. Special circumstances apart, the necessary daily routines on stud farms of detecting mares in season, taking mares (with or without foals) to pasture, feeding and bedding down require long days, especially at the peak of the season.

The provision of staff residences at each yard on studs allows constant care and supervision of the horses and the maintenance of security. The advantages of individual yards being self-contained in relation to staff requirements and minimizing hazards associated with infectious disease are often overlooked in the planning stages. It is a point which often requires special emphasis when planning permission for stud developments is sought.

References

Allen, G.P. and Bryans, J.T. (1986) Molecular epizootiology, pathogenesis and prophylaxis of Equine Herpes Virus-1 infection. *Progress in Veterinary Microbiology and Immunology* 2, 78–144.

Anon (1972) Threshold limiting values for substance in work room air with intended changes for 1972. American Conference of Government Industrial Hygienists 1.

Asquith, R.L. (1983) Biological effects of aflatoxins; horses. In: Diener, U.L., Asquith, R.L. and Dickens, J.W. (eds), *Aflatoxin and* Aspergillus flavus *in Corn.* Auburn University, Alabama, pp. 62–66.

Brewer, B.D. and Koterba, A.M. (1987) Neonatal septicaemia. In: Robinson, N.E. (ed.), *Current Therapy in Equine Medicine.* W.B. Saunders Co., London, pp. 222–225.

Bruce, J.M. (1978) Natural ventilation through openings and its application to cattle building ventilation. *Journal of Agricultural and Engineering Research* 23, 151–167.

Bryans, J.T. (1981a) Application of management procedures and prophylactic immunisation to control of equine rhinopneumonitis. *Proceedings of the 26th Annual Conference of the American Association of Equine Practice, Anaheim,* pp. 259–272.

Bryans, J.T. (1981b) Control of equine influenza. *Proceedings of the 26th Annual Conference of the American Association of Equine Practice, Anaheim,* pp. 279–287.

Burrell, M.H. (1985) Endoscopic and virological observations on respiratory disease in a group of young Thoroughbred horses in training. *Equine Veterinary Journal* 17, 99–103.

Burrell, M.H., Mackintosh, M.E., Mumford, J.A. and Rossdale, P.D. (1985) A two-year study of respiratory disease in a Newmarket stable: Some preliminary observations. *Proceedings of the Society for Veterinary Epidemiology and Preventive Medicine*, pp. 74–83.

Clarke, A.F. (1985) Review of exercise induced pulmonary haemorrhage and its possible relationship with mechanical stress. *Equine Veterinary Journal* 17, 166–172.

Clarke, A.F. (1987) Stable environment in relation to the control of respiratory disease. In: Hickman, J. (ed.), *Horse Management*. Academic Press, London, pp. 125–174.

Clarke, A.F. (1989) Management and housing practice in relation to *Rhodococcus equi* infection of foals. *Equine Veterinary Education* 1, 30–33.

Clarke, A.F. (1991) Air hygiene and equine respiratory disease. In: Boden, E. (ed.), *Equine Practice*. Baillière Tindall, London.

Clarke, A.F. (1992) Flecta-rug for horses. *Equine Veterinary Education* 4(4), 207–208.

Clarke, A.F. (1993) Stable dust – threshold limiting values, exposures variables and host risk factors. *Equine Veterinary Journal* 25(3), 172–174.

Clarke, A.F. and Madelin, T. (1987) Technique for assessing respiratory health hazards from hay and other source materials. *Equine Veterinary Journal* 19, 442–447.

Clarke, A.F., Madelin, T. and Allpress, R.G. (1987) The relationship of air hygiene in stables to lower airway disease and pharyngeal lymphoid hyperplasia in two groups of Thoroughbred horses. *Equine Veterinary Journal* 19(6), 524–530.

Clayton, H.M. (1981) Clinical aspects of ascarid and lung worm infections in horses. *Proceedings of the 26th Annual Conference of the American Association of Equine Practice, Anaheim*, pp. 29–32.

Cox, J.E., Redhead, P.H. and Jawad, N.M.A. (1988) The effect of artificial photoperiod at the end of the breeding season on plasma testosterone concentrations in stallions. *Australian Veterinary Journal* 65, 239–241.

Cregier, S.E. (1983) *Road Transport of the Horse: An Annotated Bibliography*. Charlottetown, Prince Edward Island.

Curtis, S.E. (1983) *Environmental Management in Animal Agriculture*. Iowa State University Press, Iowa, pp. 323–357.

Dawson, F.L.M. (1987) Equine reproduction. In: Hickman, J. (ed.), *Horse Management*, 2nd edn. Academic Press, London, pp. 1–56.

Domsch, K.H., Gams, W. and Anderson, T.-H. (1980) *Compendium of Soil Fungi*. Academic Press, London.

Donaldson, A.I. (1978) Factors influencing the dispersal, survival and deposition of airborne pathogens of farm animals. *Veterinary Bulletin* 48, 83–94.

Duncan, J.L. (1985) Parasite diseases. In: Hickman, J. (ed.), *Equine Surgery and Medicine*, Vol. 1. Academic Press, London, pp. 360–392.

Edwards, J.H., Trotman, D.M. and Mason, O.F. (1985) Methods of reducing particle concentrations of *Aspergillus fumigatus* conidia and mouldy hay dust. Sabauroudia: *Journal of Medical and Veterinary Mycology* 23, 237–243.

Ellis, D.R. (1987) Care of the mare and foal. In: Hickman, J. (ed.), *Horse Management*, 2nd edn. Academic Press, London, pp. 57–96.

Enarson, D.A., Vedal, S. and Chan-yeung, M. (1985) Rapid decline in FEV, in grain handlers: relation to level of dust exposure. *American Review of Respiratory Diseases* 132, 814–817.

Galan, J.E. and Timoney, J.F. (1985) Mucosal nasopharyngeal responses of horses to protein antigens of *Streptococcus equi. Infection and Immunity* 47, 623–628.

Gell, G.P.H. and Coombs, R.R.A. (1974) *Clinical Aspects of Immunology*, 3rd edn. Blackwell Scientific, Oxford.

Gregory, P.H. and Lacey, M. (1963) Mycological examination of dust from mouldy hay associated with farmer's lung disease. *Journal of General Microbiology* 30, 75–88.

HBLB Recommendation (1990) A Common Code of Practice for the Control of Contagious Equine Metritis and Other Equine Reproductive Diseases for the 1990 covering Season in France, Ireland and the United Kingdom.

Hannant, D. (1990) Immune responses to common respiratory pathogens: problems and perspectives in equine immunology. *Equine Veterinary Journal* (Suppl. 12).

Harbour, D.A. (1985) Infectious diarrhoea in foals. *Equine Veterinary Journal* 17, 262–264.

Hawkins, D.L. (1992) Diseases of the guttural pouches. In: Robinson, N.E. (ed.), *Current Therapy in Equine Medicine*, vol. 3. W.B. Saunders Co., London, pp. 275–280.

Hillidge, C.J. (1986) Review of *Corynebacterium* (*Rhodococcus*) *equi* lung abscesses in foals: pathogenesis, diagnosis and treatment. *Veterinary Record* 119, 261–264.

Houpt, K.A. and Houpt, T.R. (1988) Social and illumination preferences of mares. *Journal of Animal Science* 66, 2159–2164.

Huston, L.J., Bayly, W.M. and Liggitt, H.D. (1986) The effects of strenuous exercise and training on alveolar macrophage function. 2nd International Conference on Equine Exercise Physiology (Abstract).

Hyland, J. and Jeffcott, L.B. (1987) Abortion. In: Robinson, N.E. (ed.), *Current Therapy in Equine Medicine*, 2nd edn. W.B. Saunders Co., London, pp. 520–525.

Jeffcott, L.B. (1987) Passive transfer of immunity to foals. In: Robinson, N.E. (ed.), *Current Therapy in Equine Medicine*. W.B. Saunders Co., London, pp. 210–215.

Jones, R.D., McGreevy, P.D., Robertson, A.M., Clarke, A.F. and Wathes, C.M. (1987) A survey of the designs of racehorse stables in the South West of England. *Equine Veterinary Journal* 19, 454–457.

Kern, T.J., Brooks, D.E. and White, M.M. (1983) Equine keratomycosis: Current concepts of diagnosis and therapy. *Equine Veterinary Journal* 2, 33–38.

Kiley-Worthington, M. (1990) The behaviour of horses in relation to management and training – towards ethologically sound environments. *Equine Veterinary Science* 10, 62–71.

Kooistra, L.H. and Ginther, O.J. (1975) Effect of photoperiod on reproductive activity and hair in mares. *American Journal of Veterinary Research* 36, 1413–1419.

Liggitt, D., Bayly, W. and Bassaraba, R. (1985) Challenges to the equine lung mucosal defense system. Proceedings of the Annual Sports Medicine Conference for the Equine Practitioner, Washington State University, Pullman, pp. 70–86.

McBride, G.E., Christopherson, R.J. and Sauer, W.C. (1983) Metabolic responses of horses to temperature stress. *Journal of Animal Science* 57, 175.

McPherson, E.A. and Thomson, J.R. (1983) Chronic obstructive pulmonary disease in the horse: I. Nature of the disease. *Equine Veterinary Journal* 15, 203–206.

McPherson, E.A., Lawson, G.H.K., Murphy, J.R., Nicholson, J.M., Breeze, R.G. and Pirie, H.M. (1979) Chronic obstructive pulmonary disease (COPD) in horses: aetiological studies: responses to intradermal and inhalation antigenic challenge. *Equine Veterinary Journal* 11, 159–166.

Martens, R.J. and Carter, G. (1987) Septic arthritis and osteomyelitis. In: Robinson, N.E. (ed.) *Current Therapy in Equine Medicine.* W.B. Saunders Co., London, pp. 225–230.

Meyer, H.V., Ahlswede, L. and Reinhardt, H.J. (1975) Duration of feeding, frequency of chewing and physical form of the feed for horses. *Deutsche Tierarztliche Wochenschrift* 82, 54–58.

Mirbahar, K.B. and Eyre, P. (1986) Chronic obstructive pulmonary disease (COPD) in horses. *The Veterinary Annual,* 26th edn. Scientechnica, Bristol, pp. 146–155.

Mumford, J.A. (1992) Respiratory viral disease. In: Robinson, N.E. (ed.), *Current Therapy in Equine Medicine,* 3rd edn. W.B. Saunders Co., London, pp. 316–324.

Noot, G.W.V., Symons, L.D., Lydman, R.K. and Fonnesbeck, P.V. (1967) Rate of passage of various feedstuffs through the digestive tract of horses. *Journal of Animal Science* 26, 1309–1311.

Nordstrum, G.A. and McQuitty, J.B. (1976) Manure grasses in the animal environment. *University of Alberta, Research Bulletin,* 76 (1).

Ott, E.A. (1981) Influence of level of feeding on digestive efficiency of the horse. Proceedings of the Equine Nutrition and Physiology Symposium, pp. 37–43.

Ousey, J.C., McArthur, A.J. and Rossdale, P.D. (1991) Metabolic changes in thoroughbred and pony foals during the first 24 h *post partum. Journal of Reproduction and Fertility* (Suppl.) 44, 561–570.

Paradis, M.R. (1989) Infectious disease of the equine respiratory tract: from gestation to five months. *Veterinary Medicine,* 1174–1177.

Philips, G.B., Harris, G.J. and Jones, M.W. (1964) The effect of air ions on bacterial aerosols. *International Journal of Biometeorology* 8, 27–32.

Powell, D.G. (1985) International movement of horses and its influence on the spread of infectious disease. Proceedings of the Society for Veterinary Epidemiology and Preventive Medicine, pp. 90–95.

Rossdale, P.D. and Ricketts, S.W. (1980) *Equine Stud Medicine.* Baillière Tindall, London, 564 pp.

Rossdale, P.D. and Short, R.V. (1967) *Journal of Reproduction and Fertility* 13, 341–343.

Round, M.C. (1976) Lungworm infection (*Dictyocaulus arnfieldi*) of the horse and donkey. *Veterinary Record* 99, 393–395.

Rouse, B.T. and Ditchfield, W.J.B. (1970) The response of ponies to Myxovirus Influenza A equi-2. III. The protection effect of serum and nasal antibody against experimental challenge. *Canadian Journal of Comparative Medicine* 34, 7–12.

Sainsbury, D.W.B. (1981) Ventilation and environment in relation to equine respiratory disease. *Equine Veterinary Journal* 13, 167–170.

Sainsbury, D.W.B. (1987) Housing the horse. In: Hickman, J. (ed.) *Horse Management.* Academic Press, London, pp. 97–123.

Sharp, Dan C. (1987) Photoperiod and artificial lighting. In: Robinson, N.E. (ed.), *Current Therapy in Equine Medicine,* vol. 2. W.B. Saunders Co., London, pp. 491–492.

Smith, B.P. (1982) Problems of *Corynebacterium equi* pneumonia in foals. *Journal of Reproduction and Fertility* (Suppl.) 32, 465–468.

Smith, P.C. (1986) *The Design & Construction of STABLES and Ancillary Buildings.* J.A. Allen & Co. Ltd., London.

Sweeney, C.R., Divers, T.J. and Benson, Charles E. (1985) Anaerobic bacteria in 21 horses with pleuropneumonia. *Journal of the American Veterinary Medical Association* 7, 721–724.

Sweeting, M.P., Houpt, C.E. and Houpt, K.A. (1985) Social facilitation of feeding and time budgets in stabled ponies. *Journal of Animal Science* 60, 369–374.

Timoney, J.F. and Eggers, D. (1985) Serum bactericidal responses to *Streptococcus equi* of horses following infection or vaccination. *Equine Veterinary Journal* 17, 306–310.

Turk, M.A.M. and Klei, T.R. (1984) Effect of ivermectin treatment on eosinophilic pneumonia and other extra-vascular lesions of late *Strongylus vulgaris* larval migration in foals. *Veterinary Pathology* 21, 87–92.

Webster, A.J.F., Clarke, A.F., Madelin, T.M. and Wathes, C.M. (1987) Air hygiene in stables 1: Effects of stable design, ventilation and management on the concentration of respirable dust. *Equine Veterinary Journal* 19, 448–453.

Wehner, A.P. (1969) Electro-aerosols, air ions and physical medicine. *American Journal of Physical Medicine* 48, 119–148.

Willard, J.G. (1976) Feeding behavior in the equine fed concentrate versus roughage diets. *Diss. Abstr. Int* 36, 4772-B-3-B.

Willoughby, R.A., Ecker, G., McKee, S. and Riddolls, L.J. (1991) Use of scintigraphy for the determination of mucociliary clearance rates in normal, sedated, diseased and exercised horses. *Canadian Journal of Veterinary Research* 55, 315–320.

Willoughby, R.A., Ecker, G., McKee, S., Riddolls, L., Vernaillen, C., Dubovi, E., Lein, D., Mahony, J.B., Chernesky, M., Nagy, E. and Staempfli, H. (1992) The effects of equine rhinovirus, influenza virus and herpesvirus infection on tracheal clearance rate in horses. *Canadian Journal of Veterinary Research* 56, 115–121.

Wilson, J.M. (1987) Gastrointestinal problems in foals. In: Robinson, N.E. (ed.), *Current Therapy in Equine Medicine.* W.B. Saunders Co., London, pp. 232–241.

Wilson, M.R., Takov, R., Friendship, R.M., Martin, S.W., McMillan, I., Hacker, R.R. and Swaminathan, S. (1986) Prevalence of respiratory diseases and their association with growth rate and space in randomly selected swine herds. *Canadian Journal of Veterinary Research* 50, 209–216.

Woods, P.S.A., Robinson, N.E., Swanson, M.C., Reed, C.E., Broadstone, R.V. and Derksen, F.J. (1993) Airborne dust and aeroallergen concentration in a horse stable under two different management systems. *Equine Veterinary Journal* 25(3), 208–213.

Codes and Regulations IV

15

Codes, Regulations and Mandatory Requirements

D.R. MERCER
ADAS Nottingham, UK

Introduction

Housing for livestock is intended to meet the needs of the stock from several points of view and details are given in other chapters. However, in many countries some constraints are imposed on designers and operators by codes of practice, regulations and statutory requirements. This chapter lists some of the main categories, particularly for the UK and other countries in the European Community. Even for these countries the chapter is not intended to be comprehensive, but rather offers some guidance on the types of constraints which exist and their consequences for building design and operation. Users and designers of livestock housing should seek professional advice on detailed local requirements, and should obtain copies of relevant codes and regulations since detailed quotations are not given. Instead, the chapter indicates the flavour and sentiments of the rules.

Animal Welfare

Historical context

In the UK, codes of practice are voluntary and some regulations are mandatory. Codes of practice represent current consensus on good husbandry, and an infringement is viewed unfavourably in investigations of allegations of cruelty or contravention of statutory welfare regulations. Concern about the protection of the welfare of animals began in the 19th century in the UK while simultaneously animal protection societies were also formed in other countries. These societies, assisted by prominent individuals, lobbied governments to develop standards so that acts of gross cruelty became punishable by law. Some of the standards became written codes of practice or guidelines and eventually many governments created legislation to protect animal welfare.

Cruelty has been defined as 'the unnecessary abuse of the animal'. The principal UK early legislation on cruelty to animals was the Protection of Animals Act (1911). The following acts constitute cruelty and are punishable by fines or imprisonment:

- Cruelly to beat, kick, ill-treat, over-ride, over-drive, over-load, torture, infuriate or terrify any animal.
- To cause unnecessary suffering by doing or omitting to do any act.
- To convey or carry any animal in such a manner as to cause it unnecessary suffering.
- To perform any operation without due care and humanity.
- Fighting or baiting of any animal or the use of any premises for such a purpose.
- The administering of any poisonous or injurious drug or substance to any animal.

Subsequent to the 1911 Act there have been many amendments known as the Protection of Animals Acts 1911 to 1964 (Porter, 1987). This group of Acts is intended to prevent cruelty to animals and to alleviate their sufferings. Similar legislation is present in many other countries.

Current public interest in animal welfare continues to be intense. In the Western world, acts of gross cruelty to animals are rare, though public perception of what constitutes cruelty varies greatly. For example, many vegetarians believe that anyone who keeps animals for food is cruel. However, most meat eaters consider that as long as farmers care for their animals respectfully and with regard to animal welfare then the use of animals for food is quite acceptable. Such opinions influence governments, who continue to react to public pressure by setting more demanding codes of practice, guidelines or legislation. Indeed, government officials and various animal protection societies regularly prosecute offenders who are cruel to animals.

Many books have been written about the morals of keeping animals, and the rights of animals (e.g. Dawkins, 1980). Some authors argue on philosophical grounds that animals have neither interests nor moral rights. Cooper (1987) states 'since animals have no legal status, rights and responsibilities with regard to these must be vested in their owners or keepers. Legislation to their benefit, such as welfare or conservation, can only impose requirements on, and enforce law against, human-beings.' Different groups make stands on issues they firmly believe in. Some claim that factory farms cause pain and suffering to animals. However, farmers and others involved in animal production do not share this view, and farm businesses invest heavily in welfare protection measures.

Current UK codes of recommendations for the welfare of livestock

The UK welfare codes aim to improve the welfare of livestock by meeting ten basic needs:

1. Comfort and shelter.
2. Readily accessible fresh water and a diet to maintain animals in health and vigour.
3. Freedom of movement.
4. The company of other animals, particularly of like kind.
5. The opportunity to exercise most normal patterns of behaviour.
6. Light during the hours of daylight, and lighting readily available to enable the animals to be inspected at any time.
7. Flooring which neither harms animals, nor causes undue strain.
8. The prevention, or rapid diagnosis and treatment, of vice, injury, parasitic infection and disease.
9. The avoidance of unnecessary mutilation.
10. Emergency arrangements to cover outbreaks of fire, the breakdown of essential mechanical services and the disruption of supplies.

The following are some examples of the recommendations from the editions of the codes current at the time of writing, illustrating their spirit and intentions. Copies of the full codes should be obtained by all designers and users of livestock housing in the UK. They are available, free of charge, from offices of the Ministry of Agriculture, Fisheries and Food. Codes are available for cattle, sheep, pigs, goats, rabbits, fowls, turkeys, ducks and geese.

Other regulations of principal relevance to animal housing are given below.

The UK Battery Hens Regulations (1987)

For hens housed in cages there is a legal stocking limit provided in the UK Welfare of Battery Hens Regulations (1987), that implements a European Community Directive 86/113/EEC. Thus, from 1 January 1988 all new cages must have a minimum cage area of:

1000 cm^2 where 1 hen is kept in a cage;
750 cm^2 where 2 hens are kept in the cage;
550 cm^2 where 3 hens are kept in the cage;
450 cm^2 where 4 or more hens are kept in a cage (see also Chapter 9).

This legislation will apply to all British cages by 1 January 1995. There are also other requirements in this Act for design, construction and maintenance of cages, the provision of food and water, ventilation, lighting and inspection of birds and machinery. This regulation also specifies the need to have an alarm system to warn the stock keeper of failure of any essential automated ventilated equipment. In addition, alternative ways of feeding and of maintaining a satisfactory environment must be available for use in the event of a breakdown of any automatic or mechanical equipment essential for the health and welfare of the birds.

A European Community Directive was published in 1986 for all new installations of cages, and existing installations must comply by 1 January 1995, making a requirement for at least 10 cm of feed trough length per bird and a minimum floor area of 450 cm^2 per bird. The Regulation also stipulates detailed dimensions, like the internal height of cages, that are allowable and will restrict the use of steeply sloping cage floors. Table 15.1 gives example details of policies on stocking densities and the banning of cages in Europe.

The UK Welfare of Livestock Regulations (1990)

This legislation was designed to reinforce the Welfare Codes for farmed livestock. The major parts of these regulations came into effect on 1 January 1991 and deal comprehensively with factors affecting animal comfort and staff training.

There are further additional requirements covering alarms and back-up ventilation systems, which came into force on 1 January 1992. An alarm must be provided, to warn of failure of the ventilation system or the power supply. It

Table 15.1. Policy on hen battery cages.

Country	Policy on cages	Minimum stocking density (cm^2 per bird)
Switzerland	Banned in 1992	600
Sweden	Banned in 2004*	600*
Denmark	Permitted	600
Norway	Permitted	700
Germany	Permitted	550**
UK	Permitted	450
Spain	Permitted	450
USA	Permitted	310–350
The Netherlands	Permitted	450
EEC	Permitted	450

Source: After Elson, 1993, personal communication.
*Conditional on progress with research on perches and nesting areas in cage designs.
**For hens over 2 kg

must work even if the power has failed, and it must be tested every seven days. There must also be '... additional equipment (whether automatic or not) which, in the event of failure of the ventilation system, will provide adequate ventilation ...'. On large intensive pig and poultry units generators are, quite rightly, usually standard equipment. Like alarms they should be tested every seven days and kept in working order. However, generators can only guard against electrical failure, and that is why failsafe ventilation equipment is advisable for large units. Suitable equipment includes electromagnetic drop out panels, appropriately designed according to the numbers and types of stock in the building, usually linked to an off-limits temperature sensor.

In cases of legal dispute courts are empowered to interpret the application of the regulations. Whatever technical steps are taken to provide 'additional equipment' the onus will be on the owner or stock keeper to show that the equipment and precautions taken are adequate.

The UK Welfare of Pigs Regulations (1991)

These regulations prohibit the installation of new close confinement stalls or tether systems and ban the use of such existing systems from the end of 1998. They prohibit a person from keeping a pig in a pen or stall unless the following requirements are met:

1. the pig must be free to turn round without difficulty at all times;
2. the area of the stall or pen is not less than the square of the length of the pig;
3. none of the sides of the stall or pen has a length which is less than 75% of the pig.

There are limited exceptions from these restrictions for acceptable management purposes, e.g. for farrowing sows. These regulations may be amended by impending European Union directives on minimum standards for pig welfare.

In particular, one proposal is that a minimum unobstructed floor area must be available to each weaner or rearing pig as follows:

0.15 m^2 for an average weight of the pigs of 10 kgs or less.
0.2 m^2 for an average weight of the pigs of between 10 and 20 kgs.
0.3 m^2 for an average weight of the pigs of between 20 and 30 kgs.
0.4 m^2 for an average weight of the pigs of between 30 and 50 kgs.
0.55 m^2 for an average weight of the pigs of between 50 and 85 kgs.
0.65 m^2 for an average weight of the pigs between 85 and 110 kgs.
1 m^2 for an average weight of the pigs of more than 110 kgs.

Protection of animals from fire

More research is necessary to reduce losses in fires within livestock buildings. Fire and smoke detectors are generally unreliable in the hostile environment present in livestock buildings. In the presence of dust, moisture and gases produced from housed livestock there are too many false alarms from fire alarms currently on the market.

The UK MAFF has published several booklets on how to deal with emergencies on livestock farms and fire emergencies are dealt with in the welfare codes. Most of the details of prevention of fires are common sense, i.e. the use of fire resistant materials, prevention of vermin chewing through wires. However, if the worst happens and a fire results then the emergency services must have good access to the farm, and have adequate water supplies to put the fire out. Generally high standards of maintenance and good management will prevent huge losses and limit damages should the worst occur.

Summary of animal welfare considerations

Although each country may have its own standards for farmed livestock welfare protection, usually initially presented as codes of practice, governments are increasingly reacting to public comments by legislation. Whereas certain European countries have even prohibited some systems of production, e.g. Switzerland banned cages for layers in 1987, other countries are conducting research programmes to study whether or not alternative systems are efficient and viable.

In the UK sow stalls and tether systems are to be phased out by the end of 1998, with an immediate ban on the installation of new units. The UK Government suggests that alternative husbandry systems have been developed to the stage where they might replace the stall and tether system. Farm animal welfare standards are beginning to be harmonized throughout the European Union where concern for animal welfare appears to be more of an issue than elsewhere. In the US individual states have recommended standards for farm animal welfare. In addition to this state legislation, retail outlets are imposing their own standards. Generally, these improved standards for welfare protection will increase the costs of production. If the consumer is willing to pay more for the product, and if the retailer is willing to pay more to the producer, then the standards set for the welfare of housed livestock will continue to improve. However, in Britain, where there has been a choice between cage produced or alternative systems of egg production for many years now, still the majority of the population (over 85%) choose the cheaper battery cage-produced egg.

Building Construction

Planning requirements and local by-laws

In the UK local authorities require that planning permission is obtained before buildings are erected, though there are some exemptions under certain conditions. National requirements come under the Town and Country Planning, England and Wales Statutory Instruments. There may be local structure plans in addition to national regulations. These local plans can be modified over time so there may be existing settlements where further development may be inappropriate.

The general presumption is that the best and most versatile agricultural land, e.g. Grades 1 and 2, should normally not be built on unless there is no other site suitable for the particular purpose. When non-agricultural development is necessary on agricultural land it will, wherever possible and appropriate, be located on land of a lower rather than a higher grade.

New developments are also covered by the General Development Order (1988) which specifies a 400 m minimum distance between livestock buildings and residential dwellings. New livestock housing may be allowed within 400 m of a residence but only if pollution control techniques, an odour plume analysis, visual impact assessments and landscaping have been offered in planning applications, so as not to detract from the amenity of the area. Under some circumstances the 400 m rule has been regarded as negotiable at public inquiries.

From 2 January 1992 any development consisting of the erection of a building, or its significant extension, or significant alteration, or the formation or alteration of a private way, is permitted only subject to certain conditions. The following extract from the Town and Country Planning, England and Wales SI (1991), illustrates the types of constraints.

a. The developer shall, before beginning the development, apply to the local planning authority for a determination as to whether the prior approval of the authority will be required as to the siting, design and external appearance of the building or, as the case may be, the siting and means of construction of the private way;
b. The application shall be accompanied by a written description of the proposed development, the materials to be used and the plan indicating the site together with any fee required to be paid;
c. The development shall not begin before the occurrence of one of the following:
    i. The receipt by the applicant from the local planning authority and a written notice of their determination that such prior approval is not required.
    ii. Where the local planning authority gives the applicant notice within 28 days following the date of receiving his application of their

determination that such prior approval is required, the giving of such approval.

iii. The expiry 28 days following the date on which the application was received by the local planning authority without the local planning authority making any determination as to whether such approval is required or notifying the applicant of their determination.

There are various building regulations and standards. The British Standards Institution has published a series of documents pertaining to requirements of standards in agricultural buildings, particularly the series BS 5502. These British Standards have codes of practice for designs of various livestock buildings, milking premises, storage tanks and reception pits, chemical stores, and alarm systems. There are also British Standards for various features of building design such as the rate of spread of flame in structural materials.

Regulations Concerned with Food Hygiene and Disease

Many livestock products are ultimately used as human food and there has been increasing public concern in the UK and in Europe in recent times about improving the standards of food hygiene. In the UK particular emphasis has recently been placed on food safety, and the Food Safety Act (1990) regards farming operations as food production. The Act imposes certain new constraints on the keepers of livestock. Many of these constraints are simply good housekeeping. For example, there are recommendations for keeping surfaces clean and hygienic and for keeping pets and other animals away from livestock.

There are numerous items of legislation aimed at the control of diseases but the detail is beyond the scope of this book. An example illustrates their consequences for livestock housing.

Following certain food poisoning incidents in the UK, the Testing of Poultry Flocks Order (1989) imposed some requirements on egg producers. The order has since been revoked, but some controls are still placed on hatcheries and on breeding flocks. While most of the requirements are not directed at housing as such, the risk of contamination has imposed new standards of hygiene and cleaning requirements upon the design of accommodation for laying hens, breeding stock and replacement pullets. Internal surfaces now need to be smooth and easily washed and cleaned. Surfaces, as well as equipment and ventilation apparatus, need to be as free as possible from unwashable dust traps and inaccessible, difficult to clean nooks and crannies. Complicated equipment should preferably be at heights where it can be cleaned without ladder work.

Pollution

The UK Ministry of Agriculture, Fisheries and Food has published Codes of Good Agricultural Practice for the Protection of Water, Soil and Air. These codes are practical guides to help farmers avoid causing pollution.

The Code of Good Agricultural Practice for the Protection of Water (1991)

The UK National Rivers Authority is responsible for the prevention of water pollution (the Water Act 1989). Controlled waters covered by the Water Act include groundwater and all coastal or inland waters, including lakes, ponds, rivers, streams, canals and ditches. People responsible for allowing pollution to occur can be prosecuted and fined for up to £20,000 in a Magistrates Court or be fined an unlimited fine in a Crown Court. The codes are available free of charge from MAFF offices.

Certain farm wastes from animal housing have a high pollution potential, the unit of measurement is the Biological Oxygen Demand (BOD). Whereas treated domestic sewage has a BOD of about 20–60, the BOD from cattle slurry is 10,000–20,000, silage effluent BOD is 30,000–80,000, and one of the worst is milk which has a BOD of over 140,000.

All storage facilities for waste should be designed and constructed to BS 5502, Part 50, 1989. There may be grant available from MAFF for up to 25% of the cost of these facilities, but only after strict compliance with the relevant British Standards, and after meeting other conditions set by MAFF.

This code also sets out limits to the applications of fertilizers, particularly restricting nitrogen fertilizer applications between 1 September and 1 February each year. The nitrogen limit is set at $250\,kg\,ha^{-1}$ of total nitrogen in organic manure in any 12 months. It is best practice to apply any fertilizer when the crop needs the nutrients, and that is normally to growing crops in the spring.

Nitrate Sensitive Areas Regulations (1990) exist in the UK to protect boreholes and surface waters where nitrate levels of the water used for drinking supplies are now close to, or exceed, the EC limit of $50\,mg\,l^{-1}$. Farmers in these areas are to be advised of specified limits to fertilizer and manure applications. The European Commission agreed the Nitrate Directive in 1991 which directs member states to identify and adopt measures to control pollution in vulnerable zones where nitrate levels are unacceptably high.

The Code of Good Agricultural Practice for the Protection of Air (1992)

There are many British and European laws covering pollution of the air. Air pollution measures to control agricultural activities include controls on dark smoke nuisance, controlling odours from animal slurries and animal housing, and restricting ammonia release from animal housing. Ammonia has been identified as one of the several contributors to acid rain. There are various European Community regulations concerning the control of aerial pollution. In The Netherlands there are controls on the emission of ammonia from livestock buildings. By the end of the century the emission of ammonia must be curtailed by at least 50% of pre-legislation outputs (1986 emission).

Very odorous operations are defined as 'prescribed' processes and come under the remit of Her Majestys' Inspectorate of Pollution (HMIP) which possesses powers to enforce the prevention of air pollution. Prescribed processes include large scale incinerators and the treatment and processing of animal or vegetable matter.

The Clean Air (Emission of Dark Smoke) (Exemption) Regulations 1969, provide for the exemption of the burning of certain matter from Section 1 of the Clean Air Act 1968. This helps farmers to arrange for the safe disposal of dead stock from animal housing. Under certain circumstances the regulations allow the burning of carcasses of animals and containers contaminated by pesticides, provided, amongst other things, there is no other reasonably safe and practicable method of disposing of the matter other than burning.

This code also recommends the minimizing of odours by adopting methods of good agricultural practice. The code explains techniques to reduce odours from animal housing, from better methods of manure storage and handling to the spreading of livestock waste on agricultural land. This code also gives details of various methods of treatment of livestock wastes, methods to reduce smoke pollution, and how to reduce the effects of greenhouse gases from agricultural activity on the environment.

Health and Safety

In Britain there are rules for the protection of owners and operators from certain dangers associated with work. The Control of Substances Hazardous to Health Regulations (COSHH, 1988) give specific standards for particular hazardous materials, including dust, gases, chemical and disease organisms. There are also Regulations concerning the safety of electrical equipment (e.g. 1989). All deaths and severe injuries to people at work must be reported to the Health and Safety Executive under the RIDDOR Regulations (1989). Further regulations on health and safety at work are required under a recent EC directive (UK Statutory Instruments, 1992).

Fire

All agricultural premises, especially those containing housed livestock, are recommended to approach their local Fire Services Department to evaluate the risks of fire and to adopt measures for fire prevention. All the welfare codes pay particular attention to fire risk. There is a British Standard relating to fire precautions, the advice of which should be carefully followed.

Summary

The above list of codes and regulations, which is not claimed to be comprehensive, appears at first sight rather formidable. But most codes and regulations do not differ substantially from the normal practices and opinions of sensible stockmen, so that compliance should be a matter of routine. This is just as well, since the full range of regulations is vast and daunting. Cooper (1987) lists 115 Statutes relevant to animals for Great Britain, though many of these are irrelevant to animal housing. She also lists 110 Statutory Instruments. Specific legislation for other countries is mentioned including 16 laws for the US, 7 Council of Europe Conventions, 4 Directives and 2 Regulations for the EC and 10 items of international legislation. Readers should take professional advice about the details.

References

British Standard 5502. Buildings and Structures for Agriculture. The BSI, Milton Keynes, UK.

Codes of Recommendations for the Welfare of Livestock; Cattle (1990) MAFF Publications, London, PB 0074.

Codes of Recommendations for the Welfare of Livestock; Domestic Fowls (1990) MAFF Publications, London, BL 556.

Codes of Recommendations for the Welfare of Livestock; Ducks (1987) MAFF Publications, London, BL 556.

Codes of Recommendations for the Welfare of Livestock; Pigs (1990) MAFF Publications, London, PB 0075.

Codes of Recommendations for the Welfare of Livestock; Rabbits (1988) MAFF Publications, London, BL 5566.

Codes of Recommendations for the Welfare of Livestock; Sheep (1989) MAFF Publications, London, Leaflet 705.

Codes of Recommendations for the Welfare of Livestock; Turkeys (1990) MAFF Publications, London, PB 0077.

Cooper, M.E. (1987) *An Introduction to Animal Law.* Academic Press, London.

Control of Substances Hazardous to Health Regulations (1988) HMSO, London.

Dawkins, M.S. (1980) *Animal Suffering. The Science of Animal Welfare.* Chapman & Hall, London.

Electricity at Work Regulations (1989) HMSO, London.

Environmental Protection Act (1990) This Common Inheritance. HMSO, London.

Porter, A.R.W. (1987) *Legislation Affecting the Veterinary Profession in the United Kingdom,* 5th edn. The Royal College of Veterinary Surgeons, London.

Reporting of Injuries, Diseases and Dangerous Occurrences (Amendment) Regulations (1989) HMSO, London.

The Control of Pollution (Silage, Slurry and Agricultural Fuel Oil) Regulations (1991) Department of Environment, Welsh Office.

Town and Country Planning, England and Wales. Statutory Instrument No. 2268 (1991) HMSO, London.

UK Statutory Instruments (1987) *Animals. Prevention of Cruelty. The Welfare of Battery Hens Regulations.* HMSO, London.

UK Statutory Instruments (1990) *Animals. Prevention of Cruelty. The Welfare of Livestock Regulations.* HMSO, London.

UK Statutory Instruments (1991) *The Welfare of Pigs Regulations.* HMSO, London.

UK Statutory Instruments (1992) *The Management of Health and Safety at Work Regulations.* HMSO, London.

Index